Medicine, Money, and Morals

Medicine, Money, and Morals

Physicians' Conflicts of Interest

MARC A. RODWIN

OXFORD UNIVERSITY PRESS

New York   Oxford

Oxford University Press

Oxford   New York
Athens   Auckland   Bangkok   Bombay
Calcutta   Cape Town   Dar es Salaam   Delhi
Florence   Hong Kong   Istanbul   Karachi
Kuala Lumpur   Madras   Madrid   Melbourne
Mexico City   Nairobi   Paris   Singapore
Taipei   Tokyo   Toronto

and associated companies in
Berlin   Ibadan

Library of Congress Cataloging-in-Publication Data
Rodwin, Marc A.
Medicine, money, and morals: physicians' conflict of interest.
Marc A. Rodwin.
p. cm.   Includes bibliographical references and index.
ISBN 0-19-508096-3
ISBN 0-19-509647-9 (Pbk.)
1. Medical care—United States—Decision making—Moral and ethical aspects.
2. Physicians—Professional ethics.
3. Medical care—United States—Cost control—Moral and ethical aspects.
4. Conflict of interest.
I. Title.   [DNLM:
1. Conflict of Interest.   2. Economics, Medical.
3. Ethics, Medical.   4. Morals.   5. Physicians.
W 58 R697m] R725.5R63 1992   174'.2'0973—dc20
SNLM/SLX for Library of Congress
92-49488

2 4 6 8 10 9 7 5 3 1

Printed in the United States of America

For
Lloyd
Nadine
Victor
Julie
&
Wendy
Sine Qua Non

Contents

Foreword

Medical care in America has become dangerously expensive. Consuming more than $800 billion in 1992 and growing at a compound rate of about 10% per year, medical costs now thwart efforts to reduce the deficit and threaten the viability of our economy. At the present rate of growth more than 16% of our gross domestic product would be devoted to the health sector by the end of this decade—a circumstance that would be disastrous for competing public and private needs.

The American medical care system has also become heavily commercialized. In addition to the thousands of businesses, large and small, that supply medically related products and services, at least a third of all facilities providing medical care are controlled by investor-owned corporations. Even the so-called "not-for-profit" hospitals have caught the entrepreneurial fever, as they compete for their share of the new health care market. What was formerly a community-based social service has become a vast industry which, like other industries, seeks to maximize its revenues and expand its markets. Over nine million people work in this industry, including about 600,000 physicians who play the key role in directing health expenditures. This industry's revenues are the health care expenses that business, government, and private consumers are forced to bear.

Practicing physicians are at the center of the health care system and they are its controlling element. Although their professional fees and salaries constitute less than 20% of all health care expenditures, their decisions, opinions, and recommendations account for the expenditure of most of the rest. If our health care system now faces a cost-crisis—and there is nearly universal agreement that it does—the proximate cause of that crisis must be sought in the behavior of physicians. The behavior of physicians has many determinants. In practicing their profession, physicians must respond to the clinical problems their patients bring to them, and these problems become increasingly numerous and complicated. In conducting their practices, doctors are expected to make the best use of a constantly expanding array of drugs, tests, equipment, and procedures being provided by advances in medical science and technology. As the population ages, and the medical problems of old age become more pervasive, and as the consequences of drug abuse, violence, smoking, and other unhealthy lifestyles take their increasing toll, doctors are obliged to do more and use more resources in the practice of their profession. Public expectations of medical care are constantly rising and this, too, increases the demand for physicians' services and the medical resources they command. An increasingly litigious environment and the ever-present risk of malpractice suits have also forced physicians to become more active in prescribing tests that might protect them against future litigation. All of these facts certainly contribute to the increasingly expensive style of medical practice.

But beyond all these considerations, medical practice has been influenced by the fact that the climate of health care is far more commercialized and profit-oriented than ever before. The medical care system has become a competitive, revenue-seeking industry in which many physicians have an economic interest that goes beyond their personal services. This development undoubtedly affects many of the decisions doctors make, and it certainly adds to the cost of medical care. Since doctors make the great majority of purchasing decisions on behalf of their patients, medical businesses and revenue-seeking medical institutions of all kinds look to the physician as their primary customer. It is the physician who refers patients to hospitals and other facilities, prescribes the drugs and the tests, and orders the other medical services— all in the name of the patient, who must rely on the physician for advice. The physician is his patients' fiduciary, but he has become the target of all kinds of financial arrangements designed to influence his recommendations in favor of particular purveyors of medical goods and services. These arrangements tend to increase the income of the purveyors as well as the income—or other benefits—of the physician. The effect on patient care is more problematic.

In this book, Marc Rodwin examines in depth the economic conflicts of interest now facing American physicians. He describes the numerous ways in which conflicts arise and how they affect the behavior of physicians and the welfare of patients. He discusses how medical professional organizations have dealt with this problem over the years and he looks at the responses of other professions that have also faced conflicts of interest. He explains why this issue is of such great social importance and he considers the various ways in which it might be resolved through political or legal action.

Altogether, this is a unique contribution to our understanding of a problem that is at the heart of our health care system's ills, but which has received inadequate public attention to date. This book will be an invaluable resource for all those who wish to understand the interplay between professional ethics and economic interests in the determination of medical behavior. In the long run, no solution to the problems of the health care system will be effective unless it deals with the issues so thoughtfully and comprehensively analyzed by the author.

Arnold S. Relman, M.D.
Professor of Medicine and of Social Medicine,
Harvard Medical School
Editor-in-Chief, Emeritus
The New England Journal of Medicine

Introduction

I would probably not have become interested in physicians' conflicts of interest were it not for an incident that occurred while I was practicing law.

In the fall of 1984 I had finished working for the health policy adviser of the Mondale presidential campaign and was looking for more secure employment. To make ends meet during my search, I worked part time for several law firms and Blue Cross/Blue Shield. I also volunteered my services to the Massachusetts Attorney General's Office on asbestos litigation. Massachusetts had many buildings which contained asbestos. The Attorney General's Office was then considering whether there were legal grounds for bringing suit against asbestos manufacturers to get them to pay for its removal.

Shortly thereafter the law firm I worked for asked me to help defend asbestos manufacturers in litigation. This was not the kind of work I wanted to do. Yet if I flatly turned down the firm's assignment, my employer might not have been pleased. Then I recalled that conflict-of-interest law and ethics might preclude me from representing a new client if it would undermine loyalty or confidentiality to a previous one. I thought I was off the hook.

No such luck. Attorneys for my firm and the state conferred among themselves and then representatives from both sides discussed the issue. These discussions revealed that the state was not even a potential party in the suits my firm was representing, so there was no state interest that I might compromise. Also, the firm and its clients had no worry that I might not adequately represent asbestos manufacturers due to my previous work or commitments. Cleared to do the work, I turned it down anyhow, and much to my relief, another lawyer came along who wanted the litigation experience.

What impressed me about the incident was the process of checking and resolving legal conflicts of interest. There were codes, court rules, legal cases, and traditions. What counted were not my own personal impressions but the relevant legal standards. Over time I learned that there is a great deal of conflict-of-interest law for other professionals as well—government employees, financial advisers, business professionals and others. Indeed, the idea of conflict of interest was an example of how simple legal concepts had come to permeate institutions in contemporary American society.

Some years later when I specialized in health law and policy, I worked with doctors and learned more about medical ethics. I was surprised to find how little conflicts of interest—particularly financial conflicts—figured in traditional medical ethics or the new field of bioethics. Codes of medical ethics didn't even use the term. The three-volume Encyclopedia of Bioethics didn't address the issue. Moreover, despite the extensive regulation of medical care and our health care financing and delivery system, there was hardly any conflict-of-interest law or policy. Why should this be so?

The more I explored this puzzle, the less satisfied I was with answers I found. There seemed to be a gap in the law, an absence of accountability, a growing problem—and it was clear that doctors had very different conceptions from lawyers and other professionals of what ethics was about. Moreover, when doctors did address various conflicts, they often treated them as discrete problems unique to medicine. There was little awareness that other professionals had long dealt with such conflicts, that medicine would soon have to, and if not, society might impose standards and rules on physicians as they had for other professionals.

When I began my research for this book in the spring of 1988, there was little interest in physicians' conflicts of interest. When I made inquiries, it took a long time to explain what I was up to and why. Dr. Arnold Relman had discussed the problem cogently and so had a few other doctors, but by and large the topic was neglected. When I raised the issue with doctors and people working in health policy, the most typical reaction was bemusement. Many people simply did not understand why I felt it was important. A few good friends suggested I choose some more fruitful line of research. Some counseled against my trying to write a book on a topic that had hardly appeared in legislation or policy.

Very quickly this changed. Legislation introduced by Representative Pete Stark proposed to restrict physician self-referral—a classic conflict of interest—in the Medicare Program. About the same time, the Department of Health and Human Services began a public process of issuing Medicare regulations that would define the scope of payments considered akin to kickbacks (because they induce referrals) and therefore improper. These two events galvanized the medical care industry and led to widespread media coverage. As a result, the issue became more comprehensible to many people in health policy circles and the general public.

And yet it didn't. Now the assumption was that I was interested mainly in kickbacks, self-referral, and how they increased health care spending. This was true, but only part of the story. I wanted to examine a whole range of related questions. How did such conflicts of interest affect medical practice? What kinds of challenges did they pose for traditional physician commitments to act on behalf of patients? How did the medical profession's response to conflicts change over time? What could be learned from the way society dealt with the conflicts of interest of other professionals? And what steps could the medical profession or society take to cope with physicians' conflicts of interest in the future?

*

This book shows that current practices often provide doctors with financial incentives to promote various goals that may be at odds with the interests of patients. They tie the doctor's personal financial well-being to that of medical care providers such as hospitals, medical suppliers, and pharmaceutical firms; also to insurers and other third-party payers. They predispose doctors to dispense too many or too few services, or to make referrals that may be inappropriate to providers with which doctors have financial links. Although doctors still profess to act in the interest of patients, other parties have much more leverage over their behavior than in the past.

By compromising the judgment and loyalty of doctors, conflicts of interest bias the clinical choices they make and the advice they provide. Patients may receive poorer quality care than they otherwise would, sometimes undergoing painful, dangerous, and unnecessary medical procedures, losing valuable time and money for services they don't need. Other patients do not receive beneficial or necessary medical services. And the relation between patients and doctors in general deteriorates.

In addition, society as a whole also loses by paying for wasteful services, for adverse consequences when patients lack medical care or receive the wrong kind of services, and for social losses not reducible to money. Indeed, physician conflicts of interest are not just an issue of a few patients and doctors. They are part of what is wrong with our health care system today.

As this book goes to press there is a renewed debate about the direction of our health care policy. That debate, crystallized by the election of Bill Clinton, has focused on two pressing issues: the need to provide health insurance coverage to the nearly 37 million people who lack it and the need to rationalize our health care system, particularly to stem the soaring increase in medical care spending.

Both issues are linked to physicians' conflicts of interest. Today the United States has a medical care payment system that provides doctors with skewed incentives to offer more services. The burdensome and costly oversight of doctors' clinical decisions stems from a roundabout effort to cut costs, but it does not address the underlying problem. New reimbursement mechanisms now offer doctors financial incentives to make fewer referrals and use fewer resources in order to control expenditures, but they can lead to underservice and other distortions. Instead of eliminating the existing conflicts, recent practices and policies have created new ones and in the process expanded the range and severity of the problem.

The organized medical profession's response to financial conflicts of interest over the last century is not encouraging. Codes existed early on that addressed a few conflicts, but they were not well enforced. Since the mid-1950s, the strictures of professional ethics have become much weaker. The organized medical profession still does not accept the need for public or enforceable standards or for measures to preclude doctors from entering into situations subject to abuse. It frames the issue as a problem of individual physicians and patients: mere personal ethics.

As yet, there is no effective policy to hold physicians accountable for their financial conflicts of interests even though physicians are regulated in many other ways, some of which address the issue indirectly. As a result, doctors are held to lower standards of conduct than other professionals.

In contrast, society recognized conflicts of interest as a problem in other professions long ago and developed legal and institutional mechanisms to address many of them. While these programs are not without flaws, they have much to teach physicians and all of us. For although there are differences between these conflicts as well as the various contexts in which they arise, the main issues are the same.

The law considers many other professionals—lawyers, federal government officials, certain financial professionals—fiduciaries, that is, individuals obligated to work for the benefit of others and held to the highest legal standard of conduct. Fiduciary law aims to protect the party for which fiduciaries act. It prevents the professional from entering into situations that give rise to conflicts of interest. It reduces the risk that professionals will abuse discretion by subjecting them to oversight. And it establishes sanctions for breach of trust when it occurs despite these other measures.

Today, many writers on medical ethics refer to doctors as fiduciaries and espouse a fiduciary ethic. The main contribution of fiduciary law, however, is to introduce standards and institutional approaches where individuals would otherwise have to rely on trust or the market. The problem for the future is to develop means to hold doctors accountable to their fiduciary ideals.

Marc A. Rodwin, J.D., Ph.D.
Associate Professor
School of Public and Environmental Affairs
Indiana University
Bloomington, Indiana
December 30, 1992

PART I

The Problem and the Profession's Response

■

1

Physicians' Conflicts of Interest

Do not allow thirst for profit, ambition for renown and admiration, to interfere with my profession, for these. . . . can lead astray in the great task of attending to the welfare of Thy creatures (The Prayer of Moses Maimonides)[1] [Markus Herz].

[T]he object of the medical profession today is to secure an income for the private doctor; and to this consideration all concern for science and public health must give way when the two come into conflict. Fortunately, they are not always in conflict[2] (George Bernard Shaw).

The Patient-Physician Relationship

Most physicians strive to heal patients, extend their lives, and relieve their pain. But doctors are made of the same stuff as other people. They have the usual passions, follies, virtues, and vices. Ideals may attract them—yet they must also make a living. Medicine almost inevitably involves a tension between the physicians' commitment to healing others and their economic self-interest.[3] Doctors, like others, can do well by doing good. But the tension often creates problems.

1

The classic general practitioner had a solo practice and was paid by patients for each service rendered. This species is now all but extinct. Norman Rockwell immortalized it in two *Saturday Evening Post* covers from 1929 and 1958 (Figures 1-1 and 1-2).[4] The 1929 cover portrays an portly, elderly male doctor with white hair sitting in a chair, with a young girl standing next to him. Looking worried, she holds her doll out to the doctor. Resting his stethoscope on the doll's chest, the doc listens intently, bemused. In the 1958 cover a young boy, seen from the back, is standing on a chair inspecting the doctor's medical license on the wall while pulling down his trousers to expose his buttocks. Meanwhile, the white-smocked doctor, a middle-aged man, fills a hypodermic needle with a serum to inoculate the lad. The office is modest: two wood chairs, scales, and a cabinet covered with basic medical equipment. The kind of practice these pictures depict is often invoked fondly by patients and doctors alike, embodying the dedicated, virtuous practitioner in a technologically simpler and ethically untainted era. Physicians and patients knew each other, while today they are often strangers who meet in impersonal institutions.[5]

But the solo practitioner in fact faced a classic economic conflict of interest: fee-for-service payment. The more services the doctor provided, the greater was his income. Physicians needing more money had to raise fees, see more patients, or offer more services to existing patients.

Except for George Bernard Shaw, who discussed it at length as early as 1911 in his play *The Doctor's Dilemma,* this conflict of interest was hardly mentioned in professional or popular writing about medicine in the United States until the late 1960s. Shaw argued that the medical profession was no different from others in self-interest, notably economic. All professions, he maintained, were "conspiracies against the laity."[6] It was clear to Shaw that fee-for-service medicine biased the judgment of physicians in providing services and distorted their judgment.

> And what other men dare pretend to be impartial where they have a strong pecuniary interest on one side? Nobody supposes that doctors are less virtuous than judges; but a judge whose salary and reputation depended on whether the verdict was for plaintiff or defendant, prosecutor or prisoner, would be as little trusted as a general in the pay of the enemy. To offer me a doctor as my judge, and then weigh his decision with a bribe of a large sum of money and a virtual guarantee that if he makes a mistake it can never be proved against him is to go wildly beyond the ascertained strain which human nature will bear.[7]

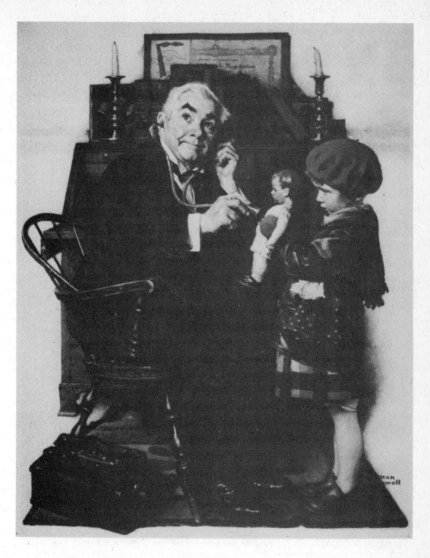

Figure 1-1

3

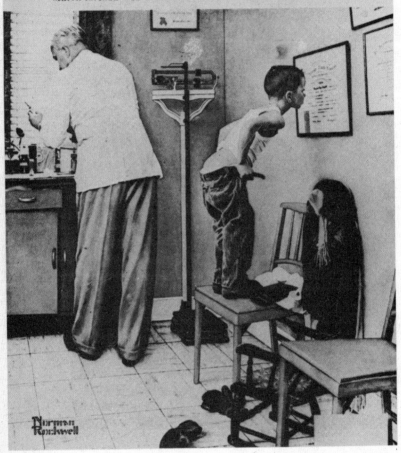

Figure 1-2

According to Shaw, the problem was due to the way society organized the provision of medicine and the payment of physicians. Social institutions created or at least tolerated the problem by allowing private fee-for-service practice, thus offering financial incentives for dispensing medical services whether or not they were needed.

> That any sane nation, having observed that you could provide for the supply of bread by giving bakers a pecuniary interest in baking for you, should go on to give a surgeon a pecuniary interest in cutting off your leg, is enough to make one despair of political humanity.[8]

Shaw believed that poverty—at least its prospect—reinforced the doctor's need to perform services. Most physicians in Shaw's day could not make ends meet; this strained their commitment to patient welfare. Removing the "wolf from the door," thought Shaw, would greatly alleviate the problem. But he also noted that entrepreneurial physicians who earned large sums of money from ties with nursing homes (which were, in effect, small proprietary acute care hospitals) posed a threat to patients. Their interest in the cure they prescribed was even greater. Indeed, many such physicians had developed a high style of living that required a steady flow of income. Shaw's remedy? State sponsorship of physicians. The state could also provide a solution to another contributing cause: the lack of clinical standards and training for physicians.

Shaw's analysis is still relevant. True, today the problem of medical poverty does not exist. In fact, physicians are among the best-compensated professionals in the United States. Physicians' average annual income after expenses and before taxes in 1990 was $155,800—more than seven times the average salary. Their average annual income rose to $164,300 in 1991.[9] Fee-for-service practice still thrives and provides perverse incentives—compounded by doctors now having more frequent and extensive financial ties to medical suppliers and institutional providers, which multiplies the incentive to supply services.

Shaw called attention to a central problem of the patient-physician relationship: the difficulty of ensuring that doctors act in the interests of patients; of devising ways to hold physicians accountable for breaches of trust; and of providing remedies and redress for patients who are harmed by their doctors. Traditionally, this tripartite problem has been left to the medical profession, which has dealt with it through self-regulation and by inculcating in physicians a patient-centered ethos.

An ethos can strongly affect conduct. It has certain advantages over external forms of regulation. And perhaps no regulatory approach can monitor all behavior or foresee the variety of situations that can arise. It is always hard to get people to do something they don't want to do. Far more effective to convince people that they want to act in a certain way: for if they do, then there are fewer problems in ensuring compliance. Very possibly, the medical ethos promotes the conduct of physicians where patients are concerned. Yet we can't measure its effect.

However strong or weak the past fidelity of physicians to patients, patients confront greater risks from conflicts of interest in their doctors today. Medical practice, finance, and organization have been transformed in the last century. These changes have created new problems that, at the very least, complicate fulfillment of the traditional Hippocratic oath.

Norman Rockwell's doctor is long gone. The August 1990 cover of *Health Care Financial Management* reflects the change (Figure 1-3).[10] A male physician, dressed in a blue smock, viewed from the back, stands beside a male hospital administrator wearing a business suit. They smile at each other and each scratches the other's back with a long back-scratcher. No patient is present. Instead, the doctor engages in a financial give-and-take with the hospital that is pleasing to both.

The change from Rockwell's image of the doctor to that portrayed on the cover of *Health Care Financial Management* is significant because patients depend so heavily on doctors. Circumstances can intensify or lessen a patient's dependence. Some patients are very ill, young, scared, uninformed, or incompetent—conditions that render them particularly vulnerable. And patients lack the specialized knowledge of doctors. Physicians understand illness, the range of treatment options, and the pros and cons of alternative interventions. Where they lack knowledge about specific issues, they know how to get it.

Physicians also control patients' access to medical care. They alone can authorize prescriptions. Except in medical emergencies, only physicians can admit patients to hospitals. And within hospitals physicians control surgery, diagnostic tests, nursing care, and diet. They decide when patients should be discharged or transferred to another facility. They channel access to medical specialists, diagnostic and laboratory tests, nursing homes, and home health care services.

Even in routine encounters, patients are vulnerable. They expose their bodies and reveal their most intimate histories, physical and otherwise. They assume a sick role, which increases their psychological dependence.[11] When patients participate in medical decision making, they still turn to physicians for advice. Whether relying on physicians to make decisions or carry out their choices, patients must allow physi-

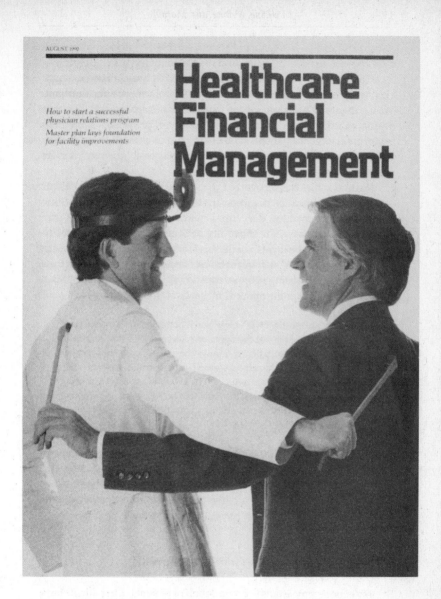

AUGUST 1990

Healthcare Financial Management

How to start a successful physician relations program

Master plan lays foundation for facility improvements

Figure 1-3

7

cians considerable discretion. Patients entrust physicians with enormous power, expecting loyalty and independent judgment in return.

However, the power of doctors is subject to abuse. Patients cannot very well monitor, control, or sanction physicians for abuse of trust. Most patients lack the knowledge to understand technical choices or to evaluate the competence of doctors. Moreover, physicians sometimes perform services for patients who are in pain or anxious, outside their presence, or unconscious. When supervision is possible, it may interfere with the physicians' performance.[12]

Medical ethics has recognized the special vulnerability of patients and the moral obligation of physicians to act in their best interest. Since the time of Hippocrates, the central canon of medical ethics has promoted the patient's welfare above all else. It emphasizes that physicians have duties to: (1) be loyal to patients; (2) act in their patients' interests; (3) make their patients' welfare their first consideration, even when their own financial well-being is opposed; and (4) keep patient information confidential.[13] The philosopher Hans Jonas stated the ethos:

> In the course of treatment, the physician is obligated to the patient and to no one else. He is not the agent of society, nor of the interest of medical science, the patient's family, the patient's co-sufferers, or future sufferers from the same disease. The patient alone counts when he is under the physician's care. . . . [H]e is bound not to let any other interest interfere with that of the patient in being cured. . . . We may speak of a sacred trust; strictly by its terms, the doctor is, as it were, alone with his patient and God.[14]

Indeed, the heroic image of physicians inspires professionals in other fields. One legal scholar advises that lawyers should be as loyal to clients as doctors are to patients.[15] Similar analogies have been drawn by securities brokers.[16] But can this ethos alone protect patients in the face of the conflicts of interest physicians face today?

What Are Conflicts of Interest?*

Society expects physicians to act on behalf of patients. But patients have multiple and sometimes inconsistent interests.[17] And like other people, physicians have interests and commitments that can motivate them to

*Appendix A discusses the concept in greater detail.

act in ways that may not favor patients.[18] When the interests of physicians and patients diverge, there is greater risk that physicians will abuse the trust of patients. Physicians have a conflict of interest when their interests or commitments compromise their independent judgment or their loyalty to patients. But conflicts of interest are not the same as conflicting interests. Multiple interests may pull people in different directions. But unless such interests compromise known *obligations*, no conflict of interest exists.

As defined in law, conflicts of interest are distinct from breaches of obligation. Although law or ethics may require one to not enter into conflict-of-interest situations, this is only a measure to prevent acts considered wrong in themselves.[19] Conflicts of interest can influence action, but they are not acts and do not ensure disloyalty. They do increase the risk that physicians may abuse their trust. The least serious possible breach entails professional neglect: a compromised physician might not perform at his or her customary high level of competence, diligence, or effectiveness. At worst, physicians may knowingly exploit their position or harm patients. Extreme disloyalty obviously presents the more dramatic danger and is easier to identify. Situations that compromise independence, loyalty, or judgment, more subtly or even unintentionally, occur more frequently—and are harder to recognize. Yet even compromised clinical judgment can bias physicians' advice and imperil patients.

Some observers use the term *potential conflict of interest* to refer to what I call a *conflict of interest* and restrict the term *conflict of interest* to *actual acts of disloyal behavior*. But according to standard legal usage, conflicts of interest have the capacity to cause harm; the injury may not yet have occurred. To label such situations as merely *potential* would mitigate the very real risk involved. And calling a breach of trust a conflict of interest obscures the fact that physicians have violated their obligations.

There are two main types of conflict of interest:
1. conflicts between a physician's personal interests (often financial) and the interests of the patient and
2. conflicts that divide a physician's loyalty between two or more patients or between a patient and a third party.[20]

However, some authorities (and dictionaries) elide the fine distinctions.[21] Others define conflicts of interests exclusively as personal financial interests.[22] But personal interests *and* divisions in loyalty can compromise a physician's commitment to patient welfare. I distinguish between them as different *sources* of risk for patients. In this I follow prevailing legal usage.[23]

Conflicts of interest are ubiquitous; their gravity is hard to assess. Some are trivial and can be dismissed. But there is no simple means of determining whether a physician's known obligations are compromised. In each case, we must rely on our interpretation of the facts to pass judgment.

Identifying a conflict of interest is only the first step in analyzing risks for patients. Questions follow: How strong or direct are the conflicts? What is the probability of inappropriate behavior? What kinds of risk are posed? How serious might the consequences be?

Financial Conflicts of Interest

Although physicians have many different kinds of conflicts of interest, the focus here is on their financial conflicts of interest.* These are some of the most glaring conflicts doctors face; they highlight, even serve as a test case for, conflicts of interest in general. Also, society has long addressed the financial conflicts of interest of other professionals, which permits fruitful comparisons.

A prime example of a financial conflict of interest is a practice known as self-referral, that is, when physicians refer patients to medical care facilities in which they have a financial interest.[24]

Consider the case of a physician with financial ties to a nursing home who is treating patients in a hospital. The physician decides when patients should be discharged and may recommend nursing care at his or her own facility. When doctors can earn money from patient referrals, this may bias their judgment about the patients' needs or the most appropriate provider. Financial ties can compromise physicians' loyalty to patients. The financial incentive may prompt physicians to discharge patients from hospitals earlier than is advisable or to refer patients to nursing homes unnecessarily. The physician might also refer patients to his or her own nursing home, rather than to another that may in fact be preferable for the patient.

In some self-referral situations, the interests of the physician and patient will actively conflict with each other: the doctor would benefit financially by having the patient in his or her nursing home, while the

---

*Appendix B discusses conflicts of interest that arise from their divided loyalties.

patient would be better off elsewhere. Of course, other scenarios are possible: even though a physician earns money by self-referral, his or her choice may be ideal for the patient. But in both situations, the physician retains a financial stake, and professional judgment is compromised.[25] By definition, physicians who self-refer always have conflicts of interest. They are not neutral arbiters.

Most physicians do not take advantage of their patients for the sake of pecuniary gain, but financial incentives may bias their judgment. For despite the increased reliance on science and the greater efficacy of modern therapies, great uncertainty continues to pervade medicine. Many therapies are not validated or well tested. The medical community is only beginning to develop standard protocols for medical practice. There is a large gray area in medical practice within which physicians legitimately choose how to treat patients. Within this range, many medical choices are probabilistic, entailing a wide array of treatment options.[26] It would be surprising if, within this zone, financial incentives did not affect clinical judgment.

The Changing Context of Medicine

In this century, and particularly since World War II, medical practice, organization, and finance have undergone vast transformations. These have heightened existing conflicts of interest and created new ones.

Medicine as Commerce

One of the main changes Eli Ginzberg termed the *monetarization of medicine*.[27] Medicine, once a quasi-eleemosynary institution, has become an expensive article of commerce. Until the 1930s, charity was a major source of capital and operating budgets for hospitals. Interns and residents, as well as nurses, received only token wages. Until the twentieth century, doctoring involved little more than the labor and advice of a practitioner, with minimal training, using tools that were carried in a black bag. Even hospitals used relatively modest equipment and required minimal capital. Whereas professionals in business, banking, law, and government had traditionally made decisions managing substantial sums of other people's money, medicine, until recently, did not. Fewer opportunities for profit making and financial conflicts of interest occurred. Those that did involved less money than they do today.

With the development of modern medicine, the money economy penetrated nearly all facets of the medical care system. There was more work to be done, and it cost more. Medical education grew more rigorous, and required longer and more costly training. Medicine developed an array of powerful, expensive tools and equipment. The range of effective medical procedures, diagnostic tests, pharmaceutical products, and medical equipment burgeoned. Physicians relied more heavily on capital-intensive equipment and diagnostic tests. These changes increased the cost of medical services—and, as a result, physicians' clinical decisions affected larger sums of money. Doctors enjoy greater financial security now than in the past, which may reduce the pressure on them to earn income. But they also can earn much more money by recommending services, which may offer novel temptations.

Changes in technology and the cost of medical care illustrate the commercialization of medicine. For example, X-rays became widely used in the 1930s. But new technology—ultrasound in the 1960s, computerized tomography (CT) scans in the 1970s, and magnetic resonance imaging (MRI) in the 1980s—provided superior, more expensive diagnostic imaging. These technologies have proliferated. Over 5,000 hospitals have CT scanners or direct access to them. Estimates list between 2,000 and 2,200 MRI scanners in the United States now, and some observers believe there will probably be 4,000 to 5,000 within 5 years.[28]

A simple X-ray machine now costs as little as $20,000 to $30,000. Fees paid by patients or insurers run from $50 to $100 for typical work. Ultrasound equipment costs between $60,000 and $200,000. Fees paid for producing ultrasound images run between $200 and $300. CT machines provide clearer images than X-rays and allow physicians to see soft tissue, three-dimensional reconstructions, and axial views. But CT machines are more expensive, costing between $350,000 and $1 million. Reimbursement for performing a CT scan can range from $300 to $600 per scan. MRI avoids the use of radiation and provides images superior to those of CT scans in many cases, also at a price; machines cost between $650,000 and $2.1 million. Providers are typically reimbursed between $400 and $800 for performing scans, although charges may run as high as $1,200.[29]

Parallel developments have marked nearly every area of medicine. Today's operating room involves more complicated and expensive technology: lasers are now used for cataract surgery and cholecystectomy (gallbladder removal), and lithotripters for breaking up kidney stones and gallstones without surgery. Our major metropolitan hospitals are capital-intensive institutions employing thousands of people and furnishing an array of related services and providers—truly a "medical-industrial complex."[30]

The growth of medical technology has helped to spur specialization. At the beginning of the century, approximately 70% of physicians were general practitioners; in the United States today, nearly 70% are specialists and many work in subspecialties.[31] Specialization promotes expertise and more proficient practice. But it also weakens the bond between patient and physician. In the past, physicians frequently knew patients and their families over a lifetime, creating a bond that increased physician loyalty. Patients could gauge the conduct or at least the reputation of physicians over a long period of time. Today, lifelong patient-physician relations are rare. Medical care, frequently delivered through large organizations, is often fragmented. Patients commonly consult specialists for a single problem and may never deal with them again. Many patient-physician encounters—especially those involving specialists—are more akin to anonymous transactions than to long-standing relations built on trust.

Third-Party Payment

The rise of third-party payers has also exacerbated conflicts of interest. Until 1929, patients in the United States paid physicians entirely out of pocket.[32] Many patients could thus pay only modest fees. Sometimes physicians set lower fees for the poor, did not charge, or could not collect fees owed. In other cases, they simply did not treat those who could not pay. But almost all patients knew budget constraints. Direct payment limited the amount of money that physicians could extract from patients by recommending and performing unnecessary or marginally useful services.

From the 1930s to the 1950s, the nation developed a system of private, employment-based, voluntary health insurance that paid physicians and hospitals through third-party payers, such as Blue Cross and Blue Shield, private health insurers, and prepaid group practice. In 1966, the federal government added to this private insurance network by creating Medicare and Medicaid, two health-financing programs targeted to pay for the medical care of the aged and the very poor.

Third-party payment was an enormously beneficial change. It allowed people who could not otherwise afford it to receive medical treatment. Thanks to private or public insurance, most patients could receive medical care for a single illness costing more money than a middle-income worker earned in a lifetime.[33] But third-party payment also had perverse effects, precisely because it insulated doctors and patients from budget constraints. Doctors worried less about the cost of services—or their value in relation to cost. Patients did not need to monitor the cost of medical services vigilantly.

In addition, the rise of third-party payers spawned a new kind of conflict of interest in which a physician's loyalty is divided between patient and payer. Third-party payers are intended to reimburse physicians and patients for all appropriate medical care for which patients are insured—but in fact, they now seek to limit the services physicians provide. Although government programs and nonprofit insurers are dedicated to securing coverage for patients, they must limit their expenditures, and commercial insurers seek profits. In recent years, payers have helped to redefine the standard of medical care through their reimbursement policies and protocols. And the trend is to do less, rather than more, especially when uncertainty prevails about the efficacy or cost effectiveness of medical care.

Folk wisdom tells us that "he who pays the piper calls the tune." Payers control reimbursement, wielding significant influence over physicians' clinical choices. When paid by third parties, doctors may serve the interest of payers, not patients.

Health maintenance organizations (HMOs), which combine medical insurance with provision of services, offer a prime example of how payment can divide physician loyalty. HMOs offer comprehensive care in return for a set premium and then render the services through their own doctors. In HMOs, insurer and physician are bound by organizational and financial ties, so control over physician behavior is made easier. Many traditional indemnity insurers now offer analogous policies to "manage care." Both HMOs and indemnity insurers with managed care policies review the clinical decisions of physicians, require preauthorization for hospitalization and other expensive medical services, and will not pay physicians unless they deem the medical services appropriate. They even offer financial rewards for using resources frugally. The net effect of these policies is to transform the doctor into a "double agent" committed to patients but beholden to third-party payers.

Increased Supply of Physicians

An increase in the number of physicians has compounded the danger of conflicts of interest. Until the mid-1960s, most health manpower experts believed that a doctor shortage existed.[34] There was more than enough work for physicians, and the doctor shortage obstructed access to medical services for many people. In response, the federal government subsidized the construction and expansion of medical schools in the 1960s and 1970s to increase the physician supply. The number of physicians rose from 140 per 100,000 in 1950 to 200 per 100,000 in 1980 and 237 per 100,000 in 1990.[35] Between 1960 and 1980, the number of physicians rose by more than 70%.[36] Although the distribution of physicians is uneven, and some areas and groups are still underserved, many labor economists now cite a glut of physicians. By the early 1980s, health policy scholars were writing books about the coming surplus and speculating on how federal policy should respond.[37] Today, some physicians must compete for patients or provide more services to those they have simply to maintain their income.

Changes in Hospital Payment

Traditionally, hospitals charged third-party payers fees based on their costs. Hospitals therefore had an incentive to increase the number of services they provided and to extend the patient's length of stay. Medicare payments for inpatient hospital care increased from $4.2 billion in 1970 to $39.7 billion in 1984.[38] In an effort to control medical care spending, Medicare, which is the largest purchaser of hospital services, changed its hospital payment system in 1983. Under the new Prospective Payment System, Medicare pays hospitals a set fee per patient based on the patient's principal diagnosis on admission. Medicare uses a system of approximately 486 Diagnosis Related Groups (DRGs) to classify the condition of patients. It reimburses hospitals for each patient based on the average cost of treating patients within that DRG. With this arrangement hospitals now have an incentive to limit their expenditures, since they keep any amount by which the DRG payment exceeds their costs but are responsible for costs that exceed the DRG payment.[39]

In fact the system is more complex. There are adjustments in DRG payments for regional costs and for costs of teaching hospitals; for patients with unusually high expenses, Medicare will chip in 60% after the expense of treatment exceeds a designated level (150% of the DRG payment). But despite various adjustments, hospitals fare better if they use resources frugally. Critics charge that the system encourages hospitals to discharge patients "quicker and sicker," with patients or their families bearing the burden of paying for or dispensing nursing care.[40]

Although there are many anecdotes about the negative effects of the DRG payment system, the weight of evidence suggests that there have been no significant changes in the health status of Medicare patients as a result.[41] This may be due in part to the separation between hospital and physician payment. Physicians, who make the clinical decisions that affect hospital resource use, are paid separately from hospitals based on the services they provide, or by salary if employed by hospitals. Still, the new system has led hospitals to put pressure on physicians to change their clinical decisions about patients' admission, discharge, and resource use in the hospital. They have sought to link the financial interests of doctors to those of hospitals through a variety of incentive programs, subsidies of private practice, and joint ventures.

Physician Investment

The physician as investor is not a new phenomenon. Some doctors owned pharmacies in the past; many owned hospitals. Subsiding in mid-century, this practice has grown in recent years, but in new forms. In 1925 physicians owned—either individually or through partnership—2,397 hospitals with 62,674 beds, approximately 32% of all hospitals but only 7.5% of all hospital beds.[42] The extent of physician ownership declined during and after the Depression. By 1952, there were only 1,305 proprietary hospitals with 51,005 beds. But the nation's supply of hospitals and beds had grown, so the percentage of physician ownership had, in effect, declined to only 19% of the hospitals and approximately 3.3% of the beds.[43] The decline in ownership became more pronounced in the 1960s, when the Hill Burton Act promoted hospital expansion. By 1968 less than 11% of hospitals were proprietary.[44]

Today, however, physician ownership of and investment in hospitals and other medical facilities are on the rise, galvanized by new financing arrangements.[45] A typical way to arrange such physician ownership is for a large hospital chain to maintain a controlling share of the facility and sell the rest through limited partnerships, syndication, or separate corporations. Hospitals also form joint ventures with physician groups, co-owning ancillary medical facilities such as outpatient surgical centers, diagnostic imaging centers, and home health care programs. Since the overwhelming share of patients' payments is assured through third-party payers, the investment is fairly safe. And by investing through limited partnerships or corporations, doctors limit their liability and operational responsibility.

Physicians find opportunities to form joint ventures with many other providers too. They have entered into joint ventures with diagnostic imaging centers, clinical laboratories, medical equipment suppliers, free-standing surgical centers, nursing homes, pharmacies and other providers of ancillary services. Physician investment is widespread and increasing. Physicians have a financial stake in 25 to 80% of ancillary medical facilities, depending on the region and the kind of facility.[46] And there is compelling evidence that when physicians have a financial interest in ordering services, they recommend them more frequently.[47]

Loss of Autonomy

Together, all of these changes have reduced the independence and autonomy of doctors. In the past, physicians worked mainly on their own. Today, they are increasingly employed by or affiliated with HMOs, hospitals, or group practices. In 1989 more than one third of U.S. office-based physicians were affiliated with HMOs.[48] Group practices have also grown in size and number. In 1965, only 4,289 group practices employed 28,381 physicians. In 1986, 26% of nonfederal doctors providing patient care were employees.[49] By 1988, 16,579 group practices employed 155,628 physicians. The percentage of doctors working in groups increased from just over 10% of nonfederal physicians in 1965 to nearly 33% in 1991.[50]

Even when not employed by others, physicians are often tied economically to the interests of hospitals and other providers or third-party payers. These arrangements link the physician's financial well-being to that of these groups—or, at least, to their good will. They offer physicians financial incentives, expecting to generate patient referrals or use of their firm's products. Hospitals have sought to increase patient admissions and induce physicians to economize their use of resources by subsidizing their private practices and offering perks. Pharmaceutical companies and other medical product suppliers have paid physicians kickbacks for using their products. More often, "gifts" are offered as part of product promotion. Hospitals, HMOs, and other so-called managed care providers reward physicians who use resources frugally. In all these situations, physicians generate income for themselves or third parties through clinical decisions supposedly made on behalf of patients.

The Role of the Federal Government

The federal government has unintentionally exacerbated conflicts of interest. It spurred the development of private third-party insurance by giving employers tax benefits for offering health insurance to employees. Federal government policies also increased the supply of physicians, which increased competition for patients. In addition, federal policies have contributed to the problem in two other important ways.

First, federal policy used financial incentives for physicians to help implement Medicare and Medicaid policies. In an effort to cut down on expensive hospital care, incentives have promoted outpatient care and home-based care, thereby encouraging physicians to participate in lucrative new arrangements. Federal policy has explicitly allowed and implicitly encouraged HMOs to use physician incentives to help control the volume of medical care. The government assumed that most health policy problems could be handled by adjusting incentives for providers.

Considered in isolation, the approach may not seem unreasonable. But these policies were implemented without any sense of the negative effects they would produce, and with inadequate counterchecks. Such policies legitimized self-interested behavior in physicians and compromised the patient-centered ethos. Government policy disregarded the possibility of physicians' conflicts of interest even though in other domains, such as business, law, and government, the problem was recognized and countermeasures were taken.

The second way government has increased physicians' conflicts of interest stems from its inaction. The financing of medical capital was left largely in private hands. This is not the bent of governments in Western Europe, where the state is the main investor in medical capital. In the United States, the default left physicians as prime candidates for the role of investors. With resources to invest, incomparable knowledge of the field, and the ability to control the flow of patients and the use of medical services, doctors are well able to determine whether an investment is profitable. Allowing them to play a central role despite the obvious conflict, government has only recently established an institutional regulatory mechanism to address these problems; and rather than address the core problem, they have focused on glaring abuses. As we shall see, until recently, to the extent that physicians' conflicts of interest were addressed at all, it was by the medical profession. But the profession did so only indirectly.

2

The Medical Profession's Response: 1890-1992

Will the peddling of patients prove permanently profitable? ... Can the general practitioner always land his patient in the net of the specialist who will charge the largest fee and share it most liberally? Can the transaction be repeated with the same patient or any of his friends? Will the patient so referred ever return to the general practitioner at all? Will not the specialists, instead of regarding the patient as leased, regard him as transferred in fee simple, and be shrewd enough to see that the way to recoup is by himself referring the patient to the next specialist, and so on until the patient can no longer be "referred" (sold) or is not worth "referring"?[1] (*Journal of the American Medical Association*, 1898).

When the physician's commercial interest conflicts so greatly with the patient's interests as to be incompatible, the physician should make alternative arrangements for the care of the patient[2] (American Medical Association, 1989).

Unlike other professionals such as lawyers, financial professionals working in business, and public servants, physicians did not even address financial conflicts of interest explicitly in their ethical codes until the 1980s, and the term *conflict of interest* was not part of medical discourse. Even the new field of bioethics—a growth industry that has infiltrated the medical school and the liberal arts curriculum—has neglected physicians' conflicts of interest.

This chapter looks at the history of physicians' conflicts of interest and the organized profession's response, examining two influential groups with differing perspectives: the American Medical Association (AMA) and the American College of Surgeons (ACS). They offer a window on the views of physicians in the United States.

Although early codes of ethics do not use the term *conflict of interest*, medical association reports discuss financial issues such as payment of commissions, fee splitting, dispensing of drugs, and ownership of medical facilities. These practices exemplify conspicuous conflicts. If the organized profession were to address any conflicts of interest through self-regulation, one would expect it to address these. Its response is thus a test case. Because the record does not yield good quantitative data, we cannot measure the extent of these activities. But we can indicate the evolution and range of various commercial practices, how they have evolved, and how the response of organized medicine has changed. Moreover, these core conflicts are analogous to many financial conflicts of interest discussed today, such as physician self-referral.

Between the 1890s and the 1950s, the AMA first ignored fee splitting and other questionable commercial practices, then denounced them, but was never able effectively to enforce its policies. From mid-century until 1991, as new, more extensive and sophisticated commercial practices emerged, the organization's public stance weakened even though these conflicts did not diminish and may even have become more serious.[3] Its guidelines were chipped away, and the few clear prohibitions in its codes were abandoned in favor of subjective standards. The AMA revised its ethical codes to allow practices previously forbidden. The ACS was more outspoken, but also lacked the means to enforce its ethics. And faced with new legal strictures against fee splitting and professional approbation, physicians developed substitutes: financial incentives for patient referrals. These took many forms, but basic conflicts of interest remained.

Since the 1980s, a debate has ensued both within and without the medical profession over the apparent clash between medicine as an expensive article of commerce and as a profession. Partly in response to public concern and proposed federal regulations, the AMA developed conflict-of-interest guidelines in 1986 that said that doctors should disclose referrals to facilities in which they invested. In 1989 Congress enacted prohibitions (which took effect in 1992) on physician self-referral to clinical laboratories, but only for Medicare patients.[4] In 1991 the AMA's Council on Ethical and Judicial Affairs strengthened its previous position and declared that most physician self-referral was inappropriate. However, the AMA's House of Delegates actively opposed this position in June 1992 and only lent official support after considerable debate in December 1992.

The AMA and other medical groups still maintain that government intervention is unwarranted, and it does not believe there is a need for public, enforceable standards. It favors approaching these issues through voluntary ethical codes and relying on the discretion of individual physicians. Yet this history shows that over the last century, the profession never developed a normative or regulatory framework to address conflicts of interest effectively and is unlikely to be able to do so in the future.

Conflicts of Interest and the AMA and ACS Response: 1890 to 1950

When the AMA was established in 1847, its members were state medical societies, medical colleges, hospitals, and other regional institutions, all of which sent delegates to the founding conference. Today, individual physicians are AMA members, but only medical societies and medical specialty associations are represented in the House of Delegates, the policymaking body. Constituent organizations are autonomous and not required to adopt AMA policy.[5] But physicians who are members of the AMA are instructed to follow the Principles of Medical Ethics as standards of conduct.[6] Within the AMA, the Judicial Council, established in 1873 (renamed the Council on Ethical and Judicial Affairs in 1985), interprets the Principles.[7] It also hears appeals for members disciplined by local and state medical societies.

The AMA adopted its first code of ethics at its national conventions in 1846 and in 1847.[8] It affirms that physicians should act in the interest of their patients, not own patents on surgical instruments or medicines, and shun unnecessary visits to patients to avoid being suspected of interested motives.[9] Although the code elaborates the physicians' "duties" to patients, much of the code concerns proper relations between physicians. The first AMA code was voluntary, adopted by local medical societies if they wished. But in 1855, the AMA decided that member state medical societies must adopt the code.

Codes of ethics perform multiple functions. Some historians suggest that the AMA has used its code to "discredit interlopers," to boost the profession's prestige, to stave off attacks, and to discourage external regulation.[10] Codes may have helped the medical profession to reduce external competition, to promote an oligopoly status, and to protect prominent physicians against challenges.[11] Nevertheless, codes also establish norms that can protect individual patients. They articulate organizational policies and official standards of conduct, and they show how the organized profession frames issues.[12] Reports on difficulties in enforcement provide evidence of actual practices.

Fee Splitting and Other Commissions: Definitions and Variations

Fee splitting in the United States started in the 1890s, when physicians began accepting payments from apothecaries and medical supply firms for prescribing their merchandise. The practice, Donald Konold argues in his history of the medical profession's regulation of ethics, became prevalent among general practitioners and surgeons after 1900.[13]

Early in the century, the AMA came to regard fee splitting as the heart of a group of related, improper commercial practices—including paying *commissions*, *drumming*, and *steering*. It also looked askance at doctors owning pharmacies, dispensing or patenting medical products, and advertising. It condemned these practices until the 1950s.

The term commissions is roughly equivalent to the contemporary term *kickback*, that is, payment by one party to another for having referred business or otherwise produced income for the payer. A 1913 report of the AMA's Judicial Council defined commissions as "'rake offs,' or pro rata moneys sent for referring patients or for favors received, and not for medical and surgical services rendered by the receiver."[14] Fee splitting constitutes a commission, but refers in particular to payments made by physicians to one another. Early on, the AMA defined fee splitting as "the sharing by two or more men [sic] in a fee which has been given by the patient supposedly as the reimbursement for the services of one man alone."[15] Subsequent definitions equated fee splitting with commissions.[16] Starting in the 1950s, some medical articles started to use the term *kickback* for fee splitting and commissions.[17] Drumming consisted of obtaining patients by agents, sometimes by fraud and other deceptive means.[18] Typically, drummers were paid a commission by physicians. Hotels and resorts would at times receive payments directly from physicians to recommend them to clients. Proprietors praised the virtues of their resident physician and disparaged the names of any others, or resorts would permit drummers to frequent their lounges, posing as guests. Physicians relied on news agents, bar keepers, clerks, medical students, priests and preachers, and "traveling men" as drummers.[19] Steering was akin to drumming. Physicians who referred patients to colleagues were called steerers, but the term was also applied to lay people—in the employ of physicians—who performed the same function.

Doctors sometimes use the term *fee splitting* to refer to any situation in which a commission is paid or in which physicians engage in self-referral. This less precise way of speaking reflects a correct intuition: the boundaries between these different practices are hazy. Although the medical profession has not used the term *conflicts of interest* until recently, some doctors sensed the issue. More recently, the medical profession has drawn distinctions between various practices, but these often obscured the underlying problem.

The proceedings of the AMA's House of Delegates from 1900 through the mid-1950s indicate the AMA's awareness that commissions thrived in many forms. Classic fee splitting occurred as payment by one physician to another for referral of patients. Another commission practice consisted of so-called stock ownership, which paid physicians returns in proportion to the amount of work they referred to a clinic or laboratory.[20] A further variation consisted of appointing and paying physicians as "associate directors" of a medical clinic in return for their referral of patients.[21] AMA reports noted that doctors received rebates from optical companies[22] and other payments from manufacturers of mechanical aids in return for recommending products.[23] Surgeons and physicians sometimes demanded commissions from manufacturers of surgical appliances.[24]

The Prevalence of Fee Splitting

In 1899, G. Frank Lydston, a prominent Chicago physician, published an exposé of fee splitting and commissions in the *Philadelphia Medical Journal.*[25]

Lydston recounted that at a social gathering he had asked the wife of a colleague whether her husband's practice was going well. She replied that it was, but that most of his income came from the 50% commission he received from patient referrals. She suggested that Lydston should split fees as well, since all the other surgeons did.

Lydston was surprised to learn of the practice. To test its prevalence, he wrote letters to "nearly all the representative surgeons" of Chicago, posing as a rural general practitioner who offered to refer patients in return for a 50% commission. He then published a sample of the replies, removing the names. Lydston reported that over 60% accepted the practice, although some responded by bargaining over the percentage to be paid. And at least one surgeon said that he would pay the 50% commission in return for the referring physician's "assist[ing] in the operation." Lydston felt that this was a greater evil than accepting fee splitting outright, evidently because it was a subterfuge. In a follow-up article, Lydston wrote that drummer doctors were ethically superior to those who merely took a commission, because they were at least honest about what they did.[26]

Fee splitting outraged Lydston. He thought that the deception of patients was wrong. He suggested that the profession should resolve the issue and, if fee splitting were deemed ethical, it should be acknowledged and all physicians should participate on equal terms. Lydston noted that fee splitting occurred not only among physicians. Undertakers, "the postmedical adjunct to the profession," he reported, sometimes paid 25% commissions to physicians who steered business their way. Lydston concluded on a glum note:

> 'Tis but a step to the undertaker's—a short step indeed from some commission men's operating tables—so let us arrange for a fixed standard of percentages all around.[27]

In a follow-up article in 1900, Lydston charged that "cases in which operation is unnecessary are being operated on" for a divided fee.[28] He claimed that he could prove that such cases were "auctioned off to the highest bidder." The charge that fee splitting led to unnecessary surgery was repeated by many others in later years.

The AMA surveyed prominent physicians in 1912 to determine the extent of secret commissions and found that it existed in every state, although its prevalence varied by region.[29] The report identified three ways in which commissions were paid: (1) by surgeons to physicians for referring patients; (2) by pharmacists or medical and surgical appliance suppliers to physicians ordering their supplies on behalf of patients; and (3) by hospitals and sanatoriums to physicians who admitted patients. Rebates were so widespread, the report noted, that many hospitals openly offered commissions in circulars; physicians would routinely inquire whether they were to receive 15% or 20%.[30] Thirteen percent of the physicians surveyed believed that receiving secret commissions was justifiable, 9% were doubtful, and 77% considered it inappropriate.[31]

In 1914 the AMA's Judicial Council again investigated reports of fee splitting by sending a survey to medical suppliers. The council found that many surgeons and other physicians demanded commissions from suppliers of surgical appliances, such as artificial limbs, trusses, and belts. According to the council, the practice was pervasive—and disgraceful.[32] Letters received by the council from suppliers described the practice as "graft" and "radically wrong and deceptive." One letter scoffed at the medical profession for the discrepancy between its professed standards and practice. Concluded the medical supplier: "As long as the majority of physicians ask [sic] for commissions, . . . it is impossible for us to consider that medical ethics are against this custom."[33] Some firms opposed paying commissions but competitive pressures prevented them from ending the practice. They blamed the medical profession for demanding payments in secret while publicly denouncing commissions.

The Judicial Council ruled that physicians who demanded commissions from medical suppliers were "analogous to a man demanding commission from the buyer and seller of a piece of property [a practice which] . . . is not tolerated legally." And the council added:

> Physicians cannot be partners in the business house of instrument makers nor honorably act as their sale agents when dealing with their own individual patients, and cannot, therefore, ethically partake of the profits of the manufacture and sale of their goods. They cannot, therefore, honorably receive a secret rake-off from the instrument maker for goods sold to any patient.[34]

According to the AMA, the situation had not improved by 1924. A report of the Judicial Council opens: "Whispered reports and even open statements to the effect that the practice of fee-splitting prevails in many places have been heard with increasing frequency during the last year to two."[35] The report makes provisions for situations in which county medical societies support so many fee splitters that it is impossible for them to enforce the AMA ethical standards. When this occurred, the state councilor was obligated to alert the state board of councilors and to revoke the county medical society's charter, establishing a new one in the name of a physician well known for being ethical.[36]

In 1930, the AMA Judicial Council reported a new practice: physicians were becoming members of cooperative diagnostic laboratories and receiving payment in proportion to the amount of work they referred.[37] It declared the practice unethical. In later years, the AMA declared that profits from diagnostic clinics should be paid only to those who performed services.[38] In the late 1930s, the Judicial Council cited "widespread complaints" concerning the division of fees between hospitals and doctors, and rebates and commissions between ophthalmologists and opticians. The council had condemned the practice earlier but had no power to control these abuses.[39]

Fee splitting did not subside during World War II. AMA reports noted that articles in the popular press exposed rebates to physicians and called on local medical societies to take appropriate action against physicians who violated the AMA Principles of Medical Ethics.[40] No evidence exists of effective countermeasures. Quite the contrary. The Moreland Commission, set up to investigate workmen's compensation graft in New York in 1944, heard testimony that kickbacks to physicians, ranging from 15% to 50%, were pervasive.[41] The testimony indicated that physicians, both private practitioners and those working for workmen's compensation, received kickbacks from surgeons, X-ray labs, sellers of surgical appliances, opticians, and specimen labs.

The Initial Professional Response

A vigorous debate ensued within the profession on whether fee splitting and other commissions were acceptable. Defenders claimed that these practices did not affect their recommendations. They also argued for its necessity, stating that general practitioners could not receive fair fees because patients did not understand the value of their work, whereas surgeons could extract whatever the market would bear. In their view, general practitioners merely used surgeons to collect fees for work general practitioners had performed in diagnosis and care before or following surgery.[42]

Those opposed claimed that fee splitting often led referring physicians to shop for the highest payer, even soliciting bids by mail.[43] Such practices, they claimed, are inconsistent with promoting the patient's interest because they prompt referring physicians to ignore medical skill or qualification.[44] Critics charged that fee splitting led to unnecessary surgery.[45] Surgeons opposed to fee splitting contended that if general practitioners wanted more income they should have the courage to demand higher fees directly and they should educate patients about the value of their services.[46]

Well-publicized corruption in public and private affairs in the late nineteenth and early twentieth centuries undoubtedly reinforced the lenient attitudes toward these practices. Yet many physicians considered fee splitting plain graft.[47] One who discussed fee splitting in 1906 under the title "Graft in Medicine," attributed its prevalence to corruption that had "touched every department of social and governmental life."[48] He pleaded for physicians to join the "revolt against dishonesty."

However, the medical profession's objection to fee splitting is cast in a different light when compared to other ethical code provisions regarding interference by colleagues. In the early twentieth century, physicians viewed the "stealing" of patients by colleagues as the most serious ethical violation. This concern was reflected in medical codes as late as the 1970s in provisions on treating patients under the care of another physician, precedence when several physicians are called to treat a patient, criticism of other physicians, and social calls on patients of another physician.[49] Objections to fee splitting may have initially revealed greater concern with "unfair" competition among physicians than with patient welfare.

In 1900 the AMA House of Delegates considered a resolution stating that receiving or giving commissions or dividing fees under any guise was unethical, and that members found guilty should be expelled. But the House rejected the resolution, convinced that the AMA would not be able to resolve the truth in such cases.[50] In 1902, however, the House of Delegates resolved that members of a county medical society proven guilty of fee splitting *without* patient knowledge be held guilty of misconduct and that the county medical society be allowed to expel them.[51] And a year later the AMA issued a revised code of ethics, declaring it unprofessional to pay, receive, offer, or solicit commissions in return for recommending patients.[52] The AMA explicitly removed itself from the business of policing its members by declaring that its revised code was merely an advisory document, and maintained this policy until 1913.[53] Supporters of the code believed it preferable to appeal to professional ideals and honor—not to enforce standards outright. Some advocated education as a remedy for unethical behavior. Others proposed friendly counsel to any doctor who "made mistakes." One medical journal editor suggested that character alone should be the foundation of ethical conduct.[54]

A dramatic case indicates the laxness of the AMA and local medical societies in enforcing prohibitions against fee splitting. In 1904, two Chicago physicians again exposed the prevalence of fee splitting. They sent letters to 100 doctors in Chicago saying that they wished to bring a wealthy patient to that city for a consultation and requesting a 25% commission. Many accepted and the responses were published in the *Chicago Daily Tribune*. The Chicago Medical Society responded by disciplining the physicians who exposed the fee splitters, not the physicians who accepted the offer.[55]

Nonetheless, efforts to stop fee splitting continued, and were strengthened during the Progressive era by President Theodore Roosevelt's campaign against corruption in public and private life.[56] At least one physician called Roosevelt's speeches a positive step against fee splitting.[57] The subject was discussed frequently in medical journals.[58]

In his 1906 AMA presidential address, William Mayo described fee splitting as a "crying evil."[59] Yet the AMA took no significant action. In its 1912 report, the Judicial Council said fee splitting led physicians to make referrals based on income received from referrals, not on the qualifications of surgeons, thus tempting physicians to operate unnecessarily. According to the report, it was immaterial whether the physician was paid for each referral for medical supplies or earned the difference between wholesale and retail price. In both cases, the physician exploited patients by charging them without providing services. The AMA reiterated this view in 1912.[60]

Following the 1912 report, the AMA tried to regulate ethical conduct,[61] threatening to expel members found guilty of *secret* fee splitting, either with other physicians or with medical suppliers.[62] Fee splitting was reckoned acceptable so long as it was disclosed.[63] Once again, however, enforcement was left to local medical societies, which were generally unwilling or unable to discipline physicians.[64] Some explicitly *condoned* the practice.[65] State medical societies rarely decertified local medical societies for failing to uphold standards. As Oliver Garceau, a political scientist writing about AMA discipline noted, "A voluntary association cannot afford to contribute too lavishly to its own dismemberment."[66]

The American College of Surgeon's Fight Against Fee Splitting

The ACS, founded in 1913 in order to raise the clinical and ethical standards of surgery, took a more active stand against fee splitting than the AMA. Members had to sign an oath pledging to shun "unwarranted publicity, dishonest money-seeking and commercialism" and to "refuse utterly all secret money trades with consultants and practitioners."[67]

The ACS tried to eradicate fee splitting. From 1918 to 1952, as part of its hospital standardization and accreditation program, it required the staffs of hospitals wishing certification to sign resolutions pledging not to split fees. This met with resistance. Even the ACS found it hard to stop fee splitting—and critics charged that some of its members accepted fees.[68] In 1924, the Eclat Society, an organization of young surgeons, accused the ACS of not disciplining all fee splitters and overlooking fee splitters in its own hospital standardization program. The ACS regents denied that they could identify any fee splitters but admitted that some members had deliberately disregarded the pledge.[69] In later years, ACS officials admitted that fee splitting flourished in spite of their efforts.[70]

Although the ACS had judiciary committees that reviewed complaints and expelled members who were found to split fees, the names of these members were not published and this diminished the deterrent. Fee splitting was also hard to police because the ACS had no institutional framework to identify fee splitters. Evidence sufficient to expel members proved hard to come by.[71]

The ACS took a stronger stance against fee splitting than the AMA. The difference may have reflected a different moral vision. It is also possible that fee splitting affected surgeons' interests more directly: the most typical case of fee splitting was payment from surgeons to referring general practitioners. Professor Rosemary Stevens suggests that the more prominent surgeons within the ACS membership opposed fee splitting because they had sufficient referrals without financial inducements, unlike surgeons who were less well known.[72]

The Immediate Postwar Situation

One journalist called the prewar efforts to deal with fee splitting by pledges, codes, and laws only as effective as prohibition during the 1920s.[73] However, the years immediately following World War II saw a renewal and a consolidation of efforts to eliminate fee splitting. Starting in 1946, the Surgical Society of Columbus, Ohio, required members to submit their tax return books and office records for annual auditing to ensure compliance with their pledge on refraining from splitting fees. In two magazine articles a journalist affiliated with the ACS reported that these methods all but eradicated fee splitting in Columbus, and also reduced the volume of unnecessary surgery.[74] Even in that city there were holdouts. The Internal Revenue Service (IRS) helped to enforce the ban. It had reportedly allowed split fees as a necessary deductible business expense until 1946 when the local surgical society wrote to them that the practice could no longer be considered "necessary" because it had all but ceased to exist. Apparently, Columbus was the first city in which the IRS did not allow split fees as a business expense.[75]

In 1947, an AMA committee on rebates followed the example of the Columbus Surgical Society, recommending that local medical societies employ auditors to examine randomly 10% of their membership as a way to enforce AMA policy against accepting rebates.[76] There is no indication in AMA reports that this advice was followed, and the plan was not mentioned in official reports again. It seems that the efforts of the Columbus Surgical Society were atypical. The assistant director of the ACS wrote in 1948 that the practice of fee splitting was still widespread and "almost universal ... in some communities."[77] He attributed it to the "letdown in moral sensibilities which seems frequently to follow war," and suggested that it would be useful to enlist the aid of the Better Business Bureau and government agencies in enforcing fee-splitting prohibitions.[78] A journalist surveying physicians in six cities reported their claim that between 50 and 90% split fees. Eventually even the surgical society in Columbus stopped its auditing program that had been instrumental in enforcing its anti-fee-splitting policy. Records explaining the change are unavailable, but a 1992 publication commemorating the society's 100th anniversary states it moved to a system of spot audits when auditing fees became expensive and eventually stopped "because of escalating costs and lack of need."[79]

The AMA reiterated its policy against fee splitting in its 1947 Principles of Medical Ethics, which, unlike previous versions, included a single section on paying commissions, patenting appliances, receiving rebates on prescriptions, and sale of appliances.[80] Combining these topics into one discussion suggested that the AMA thought these practices were closely related. However, it is debatable whether the medical profession adhered to the new standards. That same year, the AMA Judicial Council reported having received many inquiries about rebates from suppliers, and added:

> By far the largest number of requests for information or for approval were received from ophthalmologists who have submitted every conceivable plan to circumvent the section of the Principles of Medical

Ethics concerning rebates.... The Council has the impression that these or similar plans are at present openly used in various parts of the country. Nevertheless, the Council is constrained to advise all members of the Association that, no matter how prevalent these practices may have become, they are still unethical. Another scheme presented to the Council would permit doctors owning the stock of a drug company to refer their patients to this company and divide the profits from the sale of the drugs....[81]

The Commercial Transformation: 1950s to 1980

Changing Conditions and Practices

The 1950s brought changes in medical care finances and physician practices that were reflected in the organized profession's policies. At the beginning of the 1950s, the AMA maintained and even strengthened its official stand on fee splitting and related commercial practices. By the end of the decade, however, its official stand had weakened: practices were deemed ethical that had not been so regarded before. Conflicts ensued within the medical profession, but they were eventually forgotten, if not resolved, and the profession addressed fee splitting less frequently, sidestepping the problem of enforcement by again placing the onus on individual physicians.

Why was it that the organized medical profession all but stopped discussing fee splitting and commercial practices by the end of the 1950s? And why did the AMA actually weaken its stance? It seems reasonable that the profession would discuss fee splitting less if the practice diminished. But if fewer physicians split fees, why would the organized profession back away from its traditional anti-fee-splitting stance rather than adopt a stronger ethical posture? The two phenomena are at odds.

At least four factors could account for the discrepancy. Increased income security may have caused fee splitting to diminish. So, too, might have legal changes, such as the IRS policy disallowing the deduction of split fees as business expenses and state laws rendering fee splitting illegal. The development of new ways of structuring economic incentives for referrals might have reduced fee splitting. Finally, shifting ethical standards may have caused the organized profession to discuss fee splitting less often. Let us consider these possibilities more closely.

In the 1950s, the medical profession grew in prestige and financial power. Private health insurance, which had begun in the 1930s, boomed during World War II and the years afterward. With the spread of health insurance coverage to a substantial segment of the population, physicians found a secure source of payment. The Hill-Burton Act of 1946, bolstered by increased funding in the 1950s and 1960s, encouraged hospital construction and also supported physicians by providing them with modern workshops. A doctor shortage meant more than enough work for most physicians. These conditions reduced pressure on physicians to make ends meet. Fee splitting was thus less necessary—or less urgent.

Changes in law could have deterred fee splitting as well. Between 1914 and 1953, 22 states passed statutes making fee splitting illegal. Wisconsin led the way with legislation that made fee splitting a misdemeanor punishable by forfeiture of the diploma of any surgeon who gave a commission.[82] These state laws might have reduced the incidence of fee splitting, although the AMA claimed they did not.[83] In addition, the IRS continued its policy, which began in Columbus, Ohio, in 1946, prosecuting physicians who deducted fees as "necessary business expenses." The policy was enforced more generally in the 1950s. The position of the IRS was that such payments went against public policy and therefore could not be considered legitimate business expenses. One lawsuit, appealed to the U.S. Supreme Court, held that public policy against fee splitting had not been established in North Carolina, so disallowance of the deduction was unwarranted there.[84] In response, the ACS offered to testify before Congress, saying that fee splitting violated medical ethics and thus public policy.

Legal restrictions on fee splitting may also have spurred the growth of alternative practices. For example, one way to bypass the disallowance of deducting split fees for business expenses was for surgeons to hire referring physicians as assistants.[85] New institutions also performed similar referral-generating functions. Medical schools launched practice plans that fed patients to their hospitals and physicians. Hospitals developed programs to encourage physician loyalty and referrals.

Despite these four factors that might have caused fee splitting to diminish, it did not disappear. The ACS and others attested to it as a continuing problem in the 1950s and 1960s.[86] Substantial evidence from congressional investigations documents physicians paying and receiving kickbacks since the early 1970s.[87] With the inauguration of Medicare and Medicaid in 1966, the federal government gathered data and monitored the behavior of providers, including Medicare and Medicaid fraud, exposing the prevalence of kickbacks (the new term for fee splitting and other commissions). Scandals led to federal legislation prohibiting kickbacks in the Medicare program in 1972. When this legislation proved insufficient, the definition of kickback was expanded, and the legislation was strengthened in 1977, 1980, and 1987.[88]

Because fee splitting apparently did not cease and similar new practices emerged, one might infer that the AMA spoke about it less because ethical standards changed, making splitting fees a less serious, perhaps insignificant, breach. When the profession first condemned fee splitting and commissions, strictures also existed against advertising and profiting from patents on medical devices. Some medical ethics scholars now believe that enforcement of the latter was unethical because it restricted market competition.[89] The restrictions were lifted after a series of antitrust and consumer protection lawsuits were filed against the AMA in the late 1970s and settled in the 1980s.

Today government policy promotes competition in medical markets and uses financial incentives to back goals. Many hospitals discount prices for firms or HMOs which refer a high volume of patients to them. Also, many payment schemes link doctors' income to their clinical choices and referrals. HMOs use physician risk sharing to reward the frugal use of referrals and diagnostic tests. Physician investment in medical facilities creates incentives for doctors to refer patients. Viewed in this context, prohibitions against fee splitting could appear anachronistic. At any rate, from the 1960s on physicians were less likely to agitate against fee splitting, denounced as "evil" in the past.[90] The line between the permissible and the impermissible grew fine indeed.

Pressure for Change Splits the Organized Medical Profession

In 1952, the AMA Judicial Council noted increasing requests "for interpretations of principles of medical ethics ... which reflect desire to increase income through devious means," including physician ownership of pharmacies and ophthalmologists employing opticians.[91] Paul Hawley, director of the ACS, declared that some doctors were attempting to "re-code medical ethics in a way which will legitimize practices which have, for many years, been regarded as inimical to the interests of patients, and so are condemned."[92]

From 1953 on, AMA members made several proposals to amend the Principles of Medical Ethics in ways that chipped away at fee splitting and commercial restrictions.[93] Ophthalmologists sought permission to sell eyeglasses. Several other resolutions would have allowed physicians to dispense drugs. One proposal would allow doctors in group practice to divide income according to a *percentage* arrangement, presumably allowing income from referral within a practice to be shared.[94] A journalist observed that some physicians even advocated allowing fee splitting.[95]

Despite pressures to liberalize the Principles of Medical Ethics to allow previously forbidden commercial practices, the AMA maintained its code provisions against fee splitting and related practices early in the 1950s. As the decade progressed, however, the AMA defined fee splitting more narrowly, and passed judgment more softly and less frequently. It also attempted to silence members who opposed fee splitting and abandoned its traditional hostility to physicians as entrepreneurs who engage in self-referral. Although it is hard to say what produced this change, a special report by the AMA on the causes of fee splitting in 1955 observed that fee splitting was driven by economic circumstances and was not easily stopped. "Little hope" remained, said the committee, "of ending the practice with plans imposing more oaths, rules, restrictions, CPA audits, and inspections."[96]

The ACS responded differently to these pressures; it launched an anti-fee-splitting campaign, often clashing with the AMA. The ACS issued two reports on fee splitting in 1951, and in 1952 waged a publicity campaign that included round-table discussions with the ACS regents and the press on ethics and fee splitting. As part of this campaign, Dr. Hawley, an AMA member and director of the ACS, gave an interview to *U.S. News and World Report;* he said that fee splitting was prevalent and led to unnecessary surgery. The same claim was reiterated in the medical and popular press.[97] Colliers published an article in 1953 called "Why Some Doctors Should Be in Jail."[98] *The Bergen Evening Record,* a newspaper of Hackensack, New Jersey, declared, "Fee-splitting has been like venereal disease was a few years ago; it existed, but nice people did not talk about it."[99]

The response of AMA members to the ACS campaign was swift and vehement. The Chicago medical society initiated disciplinary proceedings against Loyal Davis, a prominent member of the ACS, for speaking out against fee splitting without obtaining their permission.[100] AMA members introduced 11 resolutions condemning the Hawley interview.[101] These resolutions, many prefaced with angry denunciations, attacked Hawley and the ACS and called for disciplining or censuring Hawley and others.[102] Other resolutions called for "controlling public expressions of [AMA] members," and also called on the AMA to mount a publicity campaign showing that AMA members were opposed to fee splitting and "reassuring the public that, although a single infraction of medical ethics is serious, still, such unethical practices are the exception rather than the rule," a statement contradicted by earlier AMA reports.[103]

The AMA Committee on Legislation and Public Relations deferred action on the resolutions against Paul Hawley, stated that few doctors violated the Principles of Medical Ethics, and referred the matter to the Judicial Council. The Judicial Council never responded explicitly. However, a 1954 Judicial Council report mentioned the publicized discussion of fee splitting and "recommend[ed] a moratorium from the constant discussion of `principles' about fees. . . ."[104] Although not an official policy, the statement reflected AMA practice. Until the 1980s, fee splitting was neglected, except for reports complaining that ACS public statements on fee splitting harmed the profession.[105]

The AMA and ACS also differed on whether to support state anti-fee-splitting laws. The AMA had officially supported such legislation in 1948.[106] However, it reversed itself in 1953 when the ACS proposed that the AMA Board of Trustees urge its House of Delegates to support state legislation against fee splitting in states that had no laws. The AMA did not support such efforts, saying that legal prohibitions had not accomplished anything.[107]

The AMA's Retreat from Prohibitions

The pressure for change led the AMA to reinterpret and redraft its Principles of Medical Ethics. To be sure, it purported to preserve fundamental values. But in revising its principles, the AMA permitted practices previously prohibited by eliminating strictures against physicians who dispensed medical products, owned medical facilities, and entered into joint ventures with medical suppliers and providers. To see the change one need only contrast the AMA restatement of its traditional position in the early 1950s with the positions it took after 1955.

For example, a resolution in 1950 required that the Council on Medical Education expel any hospital from its approved list if the hospital discovered that a staff physician had engaged in unethical conduct but did not remove the physician.[108] In 1952, the Judicial Council declared that physicians may not serve as associates in clinics *and* receive compensation for referring patients to the same clinics.[109] In 1953, the Judicial Council proclaimed it unethical for physicians to have a financial interest in pharmacies or to profit from the sale of devices or remedies they prescribed.[110]

In 1954 the House of Delegates adopted revised Principles of Medical Ethics, which were more stringent than ever. The principles deemed unethical "any inducement (for referral) other than the quality of professional services."[111] These inducements included not only split fees but also loans, favors, and gifts. The prohibition was not limited to *secret* payments but included any "emoluments with or without the knowledge of the patient."[112] In addition the principles also stated that it was unethical for physicians to "engage in barter or trade in appliances or devices or remedies prescribed for patients."

As time passed, these positions were whittled away: first in 1955, to allow dispensing of drugs; in 1957, to allow physicians to dispense drugs and devices if it was "in the best interests of the patient"; in 1959 and 1961, ownership of pharmacies was permitted "as long as there is no exploitation of the patient."[113] The AMA did not explicitly give carte blanche to physicians; some dispensing could be regarded as unethical. But how to distinguish ethical from unethical? No guidance or explanation was given.

In 1957, the AMA revised and shortened its Principles of Medical Ethics. The 1912 version's 3,000 words, comprising 48 sections, were reduced to 500 words and 10 sections. The 1957 principles weakened standards. For example, the earlier principles had stated that physicians should limit their professional income to medical services. The 1957 version allowed services "rendered under their supervision." This change permitted physicians to hire allied health professionals, like physical therapists, and to profit from referring patients to these colleagues working in their office.

Despite the injunction to act in patients' interests and to not exploit them, the new standard constituted a retreat from previous policy. In the past, clear rules delineated proper and impermissible conduct. The new standards left individual doctors to their own consciences. Although the language of the new policies may sound impressive, in effect it allowed a low standard of conduct. No other professional group has declared it to be ethical to exploit clients or to act contrary to their interests. By allowing doctors to judge their own conduct, the changes reversed previous AMA policy.[114]

Alternatives to Fee Splitting

Let us now consider in more detail the innovations in practice that emerged during this period as alternatives to fee splitting. The three main ones were employing referring physicians, practicing itinerant surgery, and changing institutional and medical practices.

Employing Referring Physicians. As early as 1899, G. Frank Lydston had described the practice of referring physicians assisting in surgery as a cover for fee splitting.[115] Although the ACS maintained its public opposition to the practice, the AMA was swayed by its supporters in 1960.[116] Proponents of the practice argued that it was different from fee splitting—and ethical—because the payment would not be secret, and physicians would only be paid for services they performed. In 1952 a physician named W. L. Downing even promoted the practice as a way to *eliminate* fee splitting. He argued that if surgeons

> utilize the general practitioner in caring for [their] surgical patients, use him . . . in diagnosis, counseling, operative assistance and care and charge a joint fee and divide it equitably with their full knowledge, "fee-splitting, secret division for mere reference" will soon be a thing of the past.[117]

Apparently, Dr. Downing's advice was followed. In Massachusetts in the late 1950s, Blue Shield developed fee schedules to pay 15% of the surgical fee to compensate physicians who assisted in surgery and 15% to pay physicians who performed follow-up care.[118] This plan accommodated interests pushing for fee splitting, although it regulated the practice. Presumably, surgeons would use the "deduction and allocation" procedure only when they could not perform after-care, or when they performed the surgery away from their main hospital, where they would have staff to assist. In such cases, paying referring physicians to assist in surgery might be deemed a necessary exception. However, it was unlikely that these procedures could be confined to the exceptional cases. The ACS opposed the Massachusetts "reform," saying that it "greatly restricts the application of the traditional definition of fee-splitting."[119] Robert Meyer, executive assistant director of the ACS, said that kickbacks had been replaced with similar practices, particularly hiring referring physicians as surgical assistants who performed pre- and postoperative care.[120]

Itinerant Surgeons. The other practice akin to traditional fee splitting that started around 1960 was *itinerant surgery*: the custom of calling a distant surgeon to perform surgery while leaving the pre- and postoperative care to those who called the surgeon. Itinerant surgery provided additional work for participating surgeons and for the hospitals that provided the patients and called in the surgeon. The ACS argued that in most circumstances itinerant surgery promoted poor quality of care because surgery was not coordinated with postoperative care; surgeons were not available for consultation afterward; competent surgical teams and assistants did not work together; and local community hospitals that engaged in the practice did not develop their own staff of surgeons.[121] Although "itinerant surgery" subsided, in the 1980s the practice reemerged under the rubric of *outreach surgery.*[122]

Instituting Changes in Medical Practice. For-profit medical schools were widespread in the nineteenth century, and commercial ties distorted their educational functions; they did not train physicians adequately. After the *Flexner Report* in 1910, which promoted medical schools as scientific and educational institutions, medical schools were reluctant to become the base for so called faculty-practice plans—under which faculty practiced part-time in affiliated hospitals and clinics.[123] In the mid-1950s, however, the exponential growth of medical school faculty-practice plans constituted an increasingly important source of revenue for medical schools and their affiliated hospitals.[124] Between 1960 and 1985, the number of faculty practice plans increased almost twenty-fold, from 6 to 118. Faculty-practice plans provided a steady flow of patients to hospital affiliated surgeons, thus dispensing with the need for surgeons to pay kickbacks to clinicians for referrals.

Hospitals, of course, are not immune from using kickbacks to get physicians to admit patients, even today.[125] Starting in the 1950s, however, hospitals evaded kickback restrictions with functional equivalents: financial incentives for referrals. An example shows how past practices were mimicked. In the 1940s some surgeons developed *feeders* by paying doctors just starting a practice 110% of their fee for referrals initially and then, over time, reducing the rate until it reached the standard 50% split.[126] The surgeon subsidized young physicians with a loss-leader, and achieved long-term loyalty and referrals.

Similarly, in the mid-1950s, hospitals established ties with practitioners that subsidized their practices and prompted them to refer patients. They provided physicians in private practice with office space in buildings in or near the hospitals, often with subsidized rent. The use of such incentives—moderate at first—took off after the creation of Medicare and Medicaid in 1966 increased hospital funding. When physicians had incentives to admit patients to a hospital, affiliated surgeons reaped the benefit: they received a steady flow of patients without having to pay for them.

By the late 1970s, many hospitals guaranteed up to three years' income for physicians in private practice as part of so-called recruitment programs. They also loaned doctors money at subsidized rates, paid for office space or administrative expense, invited physicians to invest in joint ventures that gave doctors a stake in hospital outpatient or diagnostic facilities, and offered other perks. Later, some hospital chains even sold shares to local physicians so they would have a stake in the hospital's financial profits.

The AMA's Response

As new ways of organizing medical practice made it possible for physicians to earn income from their referral decisions and bypass traditional fee splitting, the AMA continued to retreat from its earlier official condemnation of physician ownership and self-referral. Until 1980 the Judicial Council still stated that physicians should limit professional income to medical services they provided or supervised.[127] Yet in 1965, the Judicial Council said it was proper for physicians to invest in nursing homes or similar facilities, provided patients could choose their doctor.[128] In 1969, a resolution was introduced that would have declared it unethical for physicians to own stock in firms that owned or operated hospitals to which physicians could steer patients.[129] The House of Delegates directed the matter to the Judicial Council, which concluded that physician-owned hospitals provided benefits to patients and that it was improper to declare a class of physicians unethical by a resolution without investigation of all the facts and circumstances. The lack of AMA restrictions effectively encouraged physicians to form joint ventures with hospitals and benefit from referrals to hospital facilities and clinical decisions that cut costs.

In 1976, the AMA entertained resolutions that would require the House of Delegates to adopt ethical guidelines relating to physician ownership of expensive diagnostic technology.[130] After studying the matter, however, the AMA decided not to develop specific guidelines. It approved physician ownership, stipulating only that "physician ownership of equipment should not involve abuse or exploitation of the physician-patient relationship."[131]

The Ethics of Markets: 1980 to 1992

After Ronald Reagan's election as president in 1980, the federal government promoted greater use of market competition in the medical care sector. The use of market forces was seen as a way to reduce medical care spending that would be more effective than regulatory controls.[132] Once again, the AMA revised its Principles of Medical Ethics by eliminating code provisions that regulated competition among physicians or addressed other commercial issues. Their move to revise was in reaction to court decisions in the late 1970s and early 1980s that ended the professional exemption from antitrust liability and to the chilling effect of private antitrust suits brought by disciplined physicians against the ACS.[133] The 1980 AMA Principles dropped the injunctions against fee splitting and earning income outside of services performed. No mention was made of other economic issues, such as dispensing drugs and appliances, ownership of pharmacies and other providers, or deriving income from patents. Today's Principles contain no statement on the issues that were a focus of the AMA ethical concerns for nearly 80 years. Antitrust law now prevents the AMA from restricting advertising and certain other commercial practices. It does not require that the AMA abandon all of its prior ethical positions; nor does it prevent the AMA from developing comprehensive conflict-of-interest policies.[134]

The AMA may contend that its policy has not changed, because many of its previous positions can be found in opinions published by its Council on Ethical and Judicial Affairs. However, the fact that the AMA removed portions from the principles diminishes their importance; the reassigned parts are no longer treated as fundamental. Furthermore, as the AMA revised its ethical opinions, some were dropped or circumscribed.

These revisions helped to undermine values previously accepted. As hospitals began using financial inducements to secure physician compliance with their economic goals, older fee splitting restrictions appeared to be antiquated. In 1984, the Joint Commission on Accreditation of Healthcare Organizations (Joint Commission), which had taken over the ACS hospital accreditation program in 1952, eliminated its stipulation that hospital bylaws require physicians to pledge not to split fees. This policy, initiated by the ACS in 1918 as a means to promote both quality of care and professional ethics, had been neglected since the commission's assumption of control of the hospital standardization program in 1952 because the commission's focus was on standards of technical performance. From 1952 to 1983 the commission included anti-fee-splitting requirements in its model bylaws but did not require that hospitals adopt such policies. When the Joint Commission stopped writing model by-laws in 1983, it reinstated the anti-fee-splitting requirement as a standard. Yet the following year, the commission dropped the standard and stopped trying to guide ethics.[135]

In this climate it was easy to develop other means to receive patient referrals that bypassed classic fee splitting and instead relied on self-referral. Physicians who would potentially refer patients were offered limited partnerships in ventures with physicians, hospitals, and other providers. Self-referral was more subtle than a kickback. Referring limited partners did not make money for each referral; these physicians did, however, have a financial stake in the enterprise and earned income if it turned a profit. They avoided kickbacks but were subject to similar referral incentives.

In the 1980s, the medical profession and the public alike became increasingly concerned over the growth of for-profit health providers and the role of the physician as an entrepreneur. Arnold Relman, then the editor of the *New England Journal of Medicine*, called attention to "The New Medical-Industrial Complex."[136] The first prominent physician to declare that physicians *had* conflicts of interest, he argued that the medical profession needed to develop ethical guidelines.[137] He also suggested that physicians should not be entrepreneurs, or at least not engage in economic self-dealing transactions or sell collateral services or products that they prescribe.[138] The Institute of Medicine produced two volumes on for-profit medicine.[139] Dr. Relman and economist Uwe Reinhardt engaged in a series of public dialogues and published letters on the business and professional aspects of medicine; the language of conflicts of interest entered medical discourse.[140]

The AMA Conflict-of-Interest Guidelines

In response, since 1984, the AMA's Council on Ethical and Judicial Affairs has issued numerous reports and opinions addressing conflicts of interest, culminating in 1986 with conflict-of-interest guidelines and a major report that defined AMA policy through 1991.[141] The reports show that although the AMA still publicly opposed splitting fees and payments linked directly to referrals, it replaced rules that used objective standards to delineate proper from impermissible conduct with vague prescriptions and subjective standards.

The 1986 AMA conflict-of-interest guidelines adjured physicians to act in their patients' interests to resolve all conflicts on the patient's behalf; and to make arrangements for alternative care when doctors' interests are incompatible with those of their patients.[142] However, the AMA did not establish criteria to guide this behavior. They allowed, perhaps even indirectly encouraged, physicians to enter situations fraught with conflicts of interest, placing the burden on doctors to act properly.[143] Physicians who wondered whether they should change their behavior did not have guidance in an extensive or systematic set of rules, examples, cases, or a bureau, such as the American Bar Association provides lawyers, to give advice on conflicts of interest.

The 1986 AMA guidelines relied almost exclusively on disclosing conflicts to patients, except for recommending some protections already legally required. For example, the AMA allowed physician referral to facilities in which they invest requiring only an "ethical obligation to disclose his ownership. . . . to his patient prior to admission or utilization."[144] Rather than discourage physicians from entering into joint ventures that create conflicts of interest, the AMA produced a manual explaining how such arrangements can be structured.[145] The only restriction: the doctor must act in the patient's interest. Each doctor was left to determine the patient's interest, using his or her subjective impressions.[146]

Supposedly, disclosure allows patients to choose between their own physician's facility and an independent one, but it may protect physicians more than patients.[147] Disclosure helps to insulate physicians from liability.[148] Patients, however, are rarely able to evaluate the information, and they do not have significant new options; the advice their physicians provide is still compromised. Conflicts of interest can affect a physician's assessment of whether a medical service is needed—not just who should provide it. Bias in recommending a particular facility is only part of the problem. The more fundamental threat: ownership compromises the doctor's assessment of whether the service is needed.

The AMA's own studies confirm that its disclosure policy is not effective. A 1989 survey of members found that nearly one-third admitted that they did not comply with AMA ethical disclosure guidelines.[149] Furthermore, in areas where we have more experience with disclosure— such as informed consent—results are also disappointing. Physicians are supposed to disclose the risks and benefits of proposed medical therapies, but studies show that compliance is low and that full disclosure rarely occurs. Even when information is accurate, it is not always accessible.

The AMA conflict-of-interest guidelines did not prohibit physicians from performing any role, entering into any situations, or engaging in any transactions not already of dubious legality. AMA opinions stated that it was unethical for physicians to split fees or receive payments for prescribing a product or making a referral. But kickbacks are now prohibited by 36 state laws, as well as by the federal Medicare and Medicaid fraud and abuse statute.[150] The organization stated that when physicians refer patients to a facility in which they have a financial interest, they must allow the patient to choose an alternative. Patients have this right by law. The AMA opposed direct hospital incentive payments to physicians under Medicare to reduce medical services. Such payments are illegal for Medicare patients.[151] Where the law was silent, the AMA shunned restrictions and opted for laissez faire.

The AMA guidelines are, in effect, voluntary. The organization has no procedures for monitoring compliance or for investigating professional misconduct. The strongest sanction the AMA can impose is to revoke membership, a power rarely exercised and not particularly onerous since membership is not necessary to practice medicine; less than one-half of American physicians are members.

Moreover, the AMA itself is unlikely to revoke membership for violation of its ethical codes; it leaves that to state medical societies. The AMA will revoke membership for only the most egregious wrongs: if physicians have been convicted of fraud or a felony involving professional misconduct or moral turpitude; if their licenses have been revoked by a state medical society for incompetence or unprofessional conduct; or if they have been discharged from the armed forces or government employment for incompetence or unprofessional conduct.[152] However, the AMA relies on other groups to notify it of disciplinary actions, and this may not occur. The AMA, which conducts copious annual surveys on physicians' practices, incomes, and other issues, does not even release data on the number of members it has dropped.[153]

In effect, the AMA leaves enforcement of its guidelines and principles to state medical societies and licensing boards. Yet a 1983 AMA survey found that most state medical societies had not disciplined any members in the last five years.[154] To the extent that physicians are ever disciplined, licensing boards oversee it. These boards follow laws set down in state statutes. In general, they focus on medical incompetence or gross fraud and abuse, but most states also have provisions that allow discipline for "conduct unbecoming of a physician," which can be interpreted to include ethical infractions.

Recent Developments

By 1989, Representative Pete Stark's (D-Cal.) efforts led to federal legislation that prohibited physicians from referring Medicare patients to clinical laboratories in which they invested and required reporting of other self-referral.[155] The AMA opposed the legislation while the ACS supported it. Representative Stark made clear his desire to extend such restrictions in the future. Numerous empirical studies have now documented the extent of physician ownership and shown that when physicians have a direct financial interest in referrals this affects the volume of their referral.[156] Furthermore, an appellate court decision in a lawsuit brought under the Medicare and Medicaid fraud statute made clear that many existing physician-owned ventures risk legal liability for physician self-referral.[157]

Only then, in December 1991, did the AMA modify its stance. The AMA still declared that self-referral could be ethical and desirable, but it went on to say that the medical profession needed to maintain its professionalism and declared that the practice of self-referral to physician-owned facilities was "presumptively inconsistent" with the physician's obligation to patients where adequate alternative facilities existed.[158] Although this position made AMA policy conform to emerging legislation while staving off greater prohibitions, it still left loopholes. Physicians could still self-refer if they deemed the existing facilities were "not adequate" in terms of number, quality or location and alternative financing was not available. No effort was made to define what distance a patient would have to travel, or how different a facility would have to be, before it was deemed not equivalent or not suitable as an alternative. Equally important, the AMA has no mechanism to enforce the new policy.

How does one explain the AMA's recent switch? Although some groups within the AMA oppose self-referral as an end in itself, quite possibly the move is a political stance to stave off federal regulation and promote physician autonomy. One AMA report suggests as much. After discussing federal legislation first proposed in 1988 by Representative Stark that would regulate physician self-referral, the report proposed committees to oversee the ethics of joint ventures between physicians and hospitals, ventures in which physicians self-refer. The report states, "The Board of Trustees believes that increased promotion of ethical guidelines by the profession will discourage unethical conduct ... and obviate the pressures for federal intervention."[159]

In any event, the anti-self-referral ethical guideline was weakly supported and the AMA may not be able to maintain this position. State medical societies actively opposed the guideline, which suggests that enforcement will be minimal.[160] Moreover, powerful groups within the AMA initially opposed the guideline and proclaimed a different policy. In June 1992 the AMA House of Delegates passed a resolution that declared physician self-referral appropriate so long as patients were told of the ownership and the existence of alternative facilities, the position rejected by the Council on Ethical and Judicial Affairs.[161] The split on self-referral between the House of Delegates and the Council on Ethical and Judicial Affairs reflected a divided organization. In December 1992, after 6 months of public debate, the House of Delegates reversed itself and supported the restrictive self-referral policy of the Council on Ethical and Judicial Affairs.[162] The House of Delegates committee proposing the new resolution noted that a strong policy was needed to counter threats of "overly restrictive legislation." It also underscored that the guidelines allowed exceptions.

The AMA's position on self-referral in the future remains uncertain. In December 1992 delegates in favor of allowing self-referral stated that a restrictive position would reduce membership. Dr. Cheryl Winchell noted that the Maryland state medical society had supported state legislation restricting self-referral but that local medical societies in two communities hired lobbyists to oppose it. Commented Dr. Winchell, "If we think we are in touch with rank and file physicians when we take these high-handed, holier-than-thou ethical stands, we are sadly mistaken."[163]

Medical subspecialty groups also have codes of ethics, but like the AMA, they can't ensure compliance. Even the ACS, which championed the fight against fee splitting, is ambivalent on other conflicts of interest. Their principles declare that "professional income should come from professional services, and not from the sale of drugs, appliances, spectacles, etc." Yet it allows physicians to sell such products to patients "when it is in the best interest of the patient, and there is no exploitation of the patient."[164] The ACS policy makes individual doctors the arbiter of whether they meet these amorphous criteria.

Bioethics*

The response of professional medical organizations like the AMA and ACS to conflicts of interest reflects the views of their members. These organizations, however, do not adequately represent the diverse views or actions of all physicians. Moreover, some people argue that these organizations are trade associations, and that one should look to the field of medical ethics, or *bioethics*, for guidance. Yet the field of bioethics has addressed conflict-of-interest issues only partially and tangentially and, like professional associations, has emphasized individual physician discretion and self-regulation. In the late 1950s and 1960s, medical ethics, which had once been the exclusive preserve of physicians, became an area of public concern. Theologians, philosophers, social scientists, and legal scholars became involved and helped to launch the field of bioethics, which eventually became part of the curricula of universities and medical schools. But its initial growth was due to a mix of theologians challenging traditional medical ethics, protest movements of the 1960s, and scandals that led to federal regulation of clinical research.

A leading figure was Joseph Fletcher, who in 1954 challenged the medical community's paternalism by examining medical ethics from the point of view of the patient.[165] He was ahead of his time. By the 1960s, many groups were challenging the idea that experts should make decisions for them. A disaffected public bucked authority figures and sought empowerment. This trend, which has affected institutions as diverse as the family and government, also affected medicine, particularly clinical research.[166]

Regulating Clinical Researchers

A movement to hold clinical researchers accountable developed when the medical and popular presses revealed a series of scandals. Researchers had risked the health of human subjects by performing dangerous experiments on them without their consent. Dr. Henry Beecher's revelations in the *New England Journal of Medicine* in 1966 constituted one of the turning points. Beecher detailed the circumstances of 22 experiments from over 100 similar cases he had found.[167] Some

---

*Appendix C elaborates on bioethics and medical school education.

were conducted in major teaching hospitals, others under the aegis of the U.S. armed forces, still others with the approval of state boards of mental health. They included withholding medical treatment from patients who were ill to test the effects of disease; exposing patients to hepatitis; injecting cancer cells into patients' bodies; introducing catheters into patients' hearts; and other dangerous actions without any conceivable benefit to the subjects. Moreover, researchers had performed these experiments without the informed consent of the subjects.

Beecher concluded that disregard for the rights of patients was widespread and that unethical medical conduct was common. His suggested solution was to educate physicians and raise their consciousness. Beecher and many physicians thought it was preferable to rely on the integrity of researchers rather than subject them to regulation. Others outside the profession thought differently. Reformers claimed that researchers were less interested in patients' welfare than in the advancement of science—and, all too often, in professional advancement and fame.

Members of Congress and public groups pressured the National Institutes of Health (NIH) to do something. After all, they funded most clinical research in the United States. In 1966, the NIH established guidelines on research involving human subjects (and later regulations) for all institutions receiving federal funds for such research.[168] These guidelines set up a system of peer review under federal standards. They required that institutions set up Institutional Review Boards (IRBs) to review research proposals. Most of the IRB members could be peers, but they also included some lay representatives. IRBs are required to bar research that does not meet federal guidelines. They are supposed to evaluate the potential value of the proposed research and the risk to experimental subjects, and have procedures in place to ensure that researchers obtain the informed consent of subjects.

The IRB framework was the first public policy designed to deal with physicians' conflicts of interest. The regulations are directed at physicians simultaneously performing conflicting roles as clinicians and researchers. They presuppose that physicians who are trying to advance science may act improperly, even if in pursuit of noble ends. Yet they ignore physicians' financial interests that create conflicts of interest in research. Only recently has the federal government considered guidelines for researchers' financial conflicts of interest.[169]

The NIH regulations recognize that individual clinical researchers have conflicts of interest, and so restrict their discretion; the regulations rely on researchers as a group to police themselves, although they do require IRBs to have two members unaffiliated with the institution. Furthermore, when IRBs were established, reformers assumed that research is a special case, and that conflicts of interest do not pose problems in the delivery of medical care. In light of the organized medical profession's history, this assumption appears unfounded. Regulation of research ethics is not yet matched by equivalent regulatory oversight of physicians' conflicts as entrepreneurs and as sellers of medical services or products.

Teaching Bioethics

By the late 1970s, IRBs had become institutionalized and had generated interest in the ethics of clinical research and medicine. The federal government had sponsored several important commissions to study ethical problems in biomedical research, medicine, and health policy. The National Commission for Protection of Human Subjects was formed in 1974.[170] The President's Commission for the Study of Ethical Problems in Medicine and Biomedical and Behavioral Research, formed in 1979, issued the last of its reports in 1983.[171]

These actions by government helped promote the growth of research on medical ethics and created a climate in which bioethics became a serious topic of intellectual inquiry and debate. Starting in the late 1960s, institutions developed for the study of bioethics.[172] Universities offered medical ethics courses in medical schools, departments of philosophy and religious studies, and law schools. The literature blossomed: there were numerous anthologies, handbooks, textbooks, specialized journals, and an encyclopedia.[173]

Medical schools now include ethics and humanities in their undergraduate curricula and in internship and residency programs. Some even offer postgraduate fellowships in ethics.[174] Although some groups have proposed standards, these programs vary widely.[175] They deal with the nontechnical or nonscientific aspects of medical decision making and introduce the humanities and social sciences into medical education, focusing on the discretionary choices faced by physicians in the absence of definitive clinical standards.

Main Themes in Bioethics

Bioethicists tend to view traditional codes of medical ethics as parochial, involving more etiquette than ethics. Its scholars do not rely heavily on the authority of medical codes.[176] Their work is grounded in ethical theory. In examining medical decisions others often view as purely technical, they identify and clarify the values at stake.[177] In this way, bioethics represents a major transformation of past medical ethics.

As in any field, bioethics scholars have a diversity of approaches and opinions. But there are also central tendencies. Bioethicists, on the whole, share one important characteristic with traditional medical ethics: until recently, they tended to focus on individual patient-doctor issues rather than institutional or social issues. They have also been more concerned with deciding what is right than on developing or examining institutions to hold individuals accountable. As a result, they have emphasized the choices of individuals. Such an approach encourages the view that ethical issues need to be resolved by individuals, albeit guided by ethical theory, case studies, and moral reasoning. Not surprisingly, many social issues are seen through the prism of individual choices and analyzed accordingly. Bioethics also pays scant attention to how physicians' personal conduct or financial interests can compromise their judgment or loyalty to patients. As yet, that has not struck many bioethics scholars as intellectually interesting. Until recently, conflicts of interest were not recognized as a problem for ethical analysis.[178] This approach coincides with the organized medical profession's long-standing resistance to public regulation of medical practice.

Bioethicists often assess individual moral dilemmas. They portray physicians as neutral decision makers examining the pros and cons of difficult clinical choices. The assumption is that critical analysis can resolve dilemmas. A typical approach would have physicians promote patient welfare by refining their ethical analysis, combined with practical experience in patient care. Textbooks present difficult cases, and students are asked to resolve the problems and to justify their decisions.[179] Rarely is a doctor's financial interest depicted as the source of a problem.[180]

A new trend in medicine is the creation of medical practice standards and the surveillance of physicians by third-party payers and government regulators. Much of medical ethics resists this trend. Rather than promote standard practices, bioethics scholars often embrace the idea that physicians and patients should make ethical decisions on their own, although doctors now have the option of consulting hospital ethics committees for unusually hard cases. Scholars often advocate shared decision making between patients and physicians, but these matters are usually treated as private decisions and rarely as public policy issues.[181]

Some bioethicists, of course, differ, arguing that certain decisions should be made by communities, that physicians must accept and become involved in social policy, that physicians must fulfil a "covenant" that binds them and limits individual discretion, or that the physician must be a "partner" in medical ethics rather than the key decision maker.[182] Other authors have stressed tensions between physician self-interest and altruism.[183] There are also many bioethicists concerned with rationing and other issues of social justice.[184] But as important as these countertendencies are, they do not diminish the strong tradition that emphasizes individual choice, clinical decision making, and analyses of what the morally correct approach is, rather than collective mechanisms to deal with ethical problems.[185]

Bioethics and Self-Referral

The limitations of addressing conflicts of interest through bioethics can be illustrated by a hypothetical case commentary on physician self-referral published in 1990 in the *Hastings Center Report*, a leading bioethics journal.[186] A short summary explains that a general practitioner had an opportunity to invest in a free-standing radiology center. If the physician invested, he would earn a pro rata share of the profits based on the money he invested. The case study states that the promoter tells the physician that similar ventures have produced an 80% return annually after two years. He also makes it clear that profits will depend on the total number of referrals the center receives. The question the journal asks the two authors to comment on is this: "What should Dr. A do? Are there any legal and ethical limits on physician investments of this sort?"

Dr. Robert Berenson argues that this investment is ethical, while Dr. David Hyman argues that it is not. Both authors are knowledgeable about conflicts of interest and have written thoughtfully on the problem.[187] The point here, however, is not to argue the merits of their positions or the particulars of the case, but the way the issue is framed by the journal. The journal poses the question as one that should be decided by individual physicians. An ethical problem arises; the physician must resolve it. Such an approach is certainly appropriate for many problems, but when applied to social or policy questions, it truncates inquiry by individualizing ethical issues.

What is ethically permissible should not always be decided solely by each professional, nor should social issues always be seen through the lens of individual patient-physician relationships. Indeed, there may not always be satisfactory solutions at the level of a case. Instead, many issues should be regarded as part of the fabric of *social* ethics and decided as a matter of public policy. When social or commercial practices, such as self-referral, pose risks for the public, perhaps these practices should be restricted as a preventive measure. Framing the issue as a collective rather than an individual issue suggests different solutions. We need to examine the social implications of self-referral. Depending on the consequences of the practice, it may be appropriate to develop policies that limit the individual choice of physicians. Treating these issues primarily as matters of individual ethics frames them in a way that impedes society from taking effective measures to resolve the problem.

Conclusion

Physicians' financial conflicts of interest arising from fee splitting, self-referral, entrepreneurship, and other commercial practices are not new. The organized medical profession has faced these issues, although only indirectly and partially, for over a century.

Unlike other professionals who are subject to extensive conflict-of-interest regulation—such as government employees, lawyers, and certain financial professionals working in business—physicians have addressed these issues largely on their own and have been subject to minimal regulation by state and federal laws or even by professional codes. But professional self-regulation has not been particularly effective. The AMA addressed these issues primarily by relying on professional norms, individual discretion, and subjective standards. For many years the ACS explicitly condemned fee splitting. But both organizations lacked an effective means to hold physicians accountable. In the mid-1950s, the AMA weakened its code to placate its members. Despite the AMA's contention that its code and principles of ethics promote the interest of patients, both were amended to reflect the economic interests of physicians.

Nor has the new discipline of bioethics shed light on conflicts of interest. It has neglected these issues. The field has also focused discussion on what is right rather than on mechanisms to hold physicians accountable.

Although existing evidence does not indicate whether fee splitting decreased or increased, it certainly has persisted despite professional self-regulation, and new variations arose that posed similar conflicts. Moreover, from the mid-1950s on, the organized medical profession tolerated, and sometimes even encouraged, substitutes for fee splitting that are at the heart of today's debate about physician self-referral and conflicts of interest.

In the past, conflicts of interest arose mainly from medical practices and were left to be resolved largely by the medical profession. Today, however, physicians face new conflicts of interest—as well as the old—many of which are spawned by policies and financial inducements of third party payers, government, and providers. As we shall see in the following chapters, the deference to the medical profession and lack of accountability that was the rule in the past emerged as more of a problem when medicine became big business and social business.

PART II

Current Problems and Institutional Responses

■

3

Incentives to Increase Services: The Range of Existing Practices

A primary care internist can increase his or her net income by a factor of almost three by prescribing a wide but not unreasonable set of tests. The term *not unreasonable* is a reflection that the use of such tests is so common as to be almost standard practice; yet some clinicians would argue that few of the tests are actually necessary[1] (Harold S. Luft).

Financial Arrangements That Create Conflicts of Interest[2]

Conflicts of interest in fee-for-service medicine are significant and intractable. Coupled with insurance, they have spawned a great deal of overuse of medical services.[3] In reaction, third-party payers have developed alternative ways of paying physicians that do not provide incentives for increasing services. These include salary, capitation payment (a set fee per patient for a fixed period of time), and risk-sharing plans that hold physicians financially responsible for the volume of services they provide. But fee-for-service payment still dominates our medical care system. Eliminating fee-for-service payment would require major changes in the organization of medicine that would be politically difficult, and this form of payment does provide some benefits for patients and society.

Closely related to, but distinct from, fee-for-service practice are a range of other financial incentives to physicians. The six most important are as follows:

1. Paying and receiving kickbacks for referrals.
2. Income earned by doctors for referring patients to medical facilities in which they invest (physician self-referral).
3. Income earned by doctors for dispensing drugs, selling medical products, and performing ancillary medical services.
4. Payments made by hospitals to doctors to purchase physicians' medical practices.
5. Payments made by hospitals to doctors to recruit and bond physicians.
6. Gifts given to doctors by medical suppliers.

These six kinds of income produce the same built-in incentives to overtreat as fee-for-service practice. They encourage physicians to provide services and products from which they personally benefit. Evidence increasingly suggests that these practices frequently lead to overuse of services, increase the risk of harm to patients, and channel competitive energies into unproductive areas.

Health care policy and law can easily distinguish these payments from fee-for-service practice and treat them separately. Most physicians do not depend on such payments for a major portion of their income. Fee-for-service practice can exist without them. Moreover, unlike fee-for-service medicine, the practices associated with these six kinds of payment lack social value. The benefits they bring can be produced by other means with less risk of harmful effects.

The six practices have differences. The incentive to produce services is stronger or more direct in some than in others. The source and nature of the payment vary. But these practices resemble each other. With kickbacks, physicians earn money based on a mere referral; the link between a consultation or a procedure and payment is direct. When physicians refer patients to facilities in which they own an interest, they are paid indirectly, based on the level of their investment; but like kickbacks, such payments create a financial incentive to refer patients. When physicians dispense products, they are paid for providing a service or product, just like other providers and like fee-for-service practice. When physicians receive payments from hospitals, it increases their loyalty to the hospital, creates dependence, and may compromise loyalty to patients. In the case of gifts, physicians receive income with no explicit requirements in return, but the gift may influence judgment, create indebtedness, and lead to reciprocation.

Existing policy and medical ethics have distinguished among these six practices, most often discouraging kickbacks and tolerating or even encouraging other practices. From a conflict-of-interest perspective, however, all constitute a common phenomenon and create similar risks for patients. Institutional providers and medical suppliers wishing to promote their own financial interests can and do draw on all six. Firms often use several arrangements simultaneously. When prevented from using one, providers and suppliers can often achieve nearly the same end with another. For patients who depend on physicians to act in their interests, all six practices corrode the bond between them and doctor.

The Maze of Financial Incentives

Kickbacks for Referrals

Kickbacks, usually frowned upon, are not always illegal. Physicians can both pay and receive them. They can produce income for other doctors or institutional providers (such as hospitals) by referring patients to them or by using their services or products, and thus can extract a kickback in return. In other situations, physicians may pay kickbacks to others in exchange for receiving referrals of work or patients. Kickbacks occur in numerous settings and in many different ways. Now illegal in the Medicare-Medicaid programs and in many states, the practice persists, and so does litigation attempting to define what inducements count as illegal kickbacks.[4]

Hospitals. One blatant example of kickbacks is "selling" patients to hospitals. The special relationship between hospitals, physicians, and patients permits this. Physicians in private practice are generally not hospital employees but are affiliated, and have *privileges* to admit patients.[5] Frequently they obtain admitting privileges at more than one hospital and decide whether, when, and where to admit a patient. Although rarely acknowledged, the power of physicians to admit patients gives them leverage over hospitals. The 1986 testimony of a physician at a trial of Russell Furth, a hospital administrator who had been prosecuted under the Medicare fraud and abuse statute (sometimes also called the anti-kickback law) for paying him kickbacks, lays out the issue.

> Generally patients go where I told them to go. And, I can admit to any hospital that I want to for any reason I want to. I don't have to justify that to anybody. I can admit there because I don't like the color of the carpet, or I don't like my parking spot there [sic]. . . .[6]

The cross-examination of this doctor's colleague is also revealing.

> Q: *That's really the doctor's major source of power in the hospitals, isn't it; threatening to pull their patients?*
> A: Well . . . it is the power they have over hospitals. That's the only power.
>
>   . . .
>
> Q: *Hospitals run only on patients, don't they?*
> A: That's right.
>
> Q: *Without the doctor there is no patient?*
> A: That's right.
>
>   . . .
>
> Q: *Have you ever pulled any of your patients from a hospital because you have been unhappy with the hospital?*
> A: Yes.[7]

By directing admission of patients to hospitals, physicians control hospitals' revenues. Currently, most hospitals have excess capacity—too many beds for the available number of patients—so they compete for patients. Fewer patients cut hospital revenue, but not the hospital's high fixed operating costs. Therefore, hospitals—nonprofit as well as for-profit—depend on physicians to admit patients to remain solvent. If a hospital provides poor quality of care, physicians can pressure hospitals to improve their performance by admitting patients to another hospital. But physicians can also extract personal benefits, including money, for themselves. Some hospitals pay physicians to admit patients even though this is often illegal.[8]

Testimony in the trial of Russell Furth illustrates how these schemes can evolve.[9] Furth was the administrator of Pasadena General Hospital near Houston; the hospital was owned by American Healthcare Management, Inc. (AHM). When Furth was appointed administrator in the spring of 1985, the hospital was losing money because physicians were referring their patients elsewhere. Some, like Drs. David Spinks and Jerry McShane, two physicians who owned a thriving local clinic, had received monthly checks from the previous owners of the hospitals without an explicit arrangement for referrals. They were told that the checks were for "supporting the hospital." When the hospital was sold, the checks stopped, and Drs. Spinks and McShane started referring patients elsewhere. But they started admitting patients again when AHM approved Furth's plan to pay kickbacks to physicians for admitting patients.

Furth, who was indicted under the Medicare and Medicaid fraud and abuse statute, which prohibits payments that induce referrals, admitted having paid kickbacks but claimed that no Medicare patients were involved.[10] Spinks and McShane were granted immunity from prosecution in return for testifying against Furth. Their testimony, and tape recordings of their discussions with Furth, provided details of the transactions.

At a meeting in the spring of 1985, the physicians and Furth agreed to a kickback scheme. The hospital agreed to pay Spinks and McShane $70 for each patient they admitted to the hospital.[11] In an attempt to avoid legal difficulties, the kickbacks were disguised as consulting fees.[12] In the first month after the agreement, their admissions rose from 0 to 14 patients. In the second month, both doctors together admitted 82 patients.[13] Court testimony shows that the pressure to admit benefited the hospital, not the patients. Before AHM executives paid a visit to Pasadena Hospital, Furth had met with Spinks and McShane in an effort to boost the patient census. Furth warned them about the visit, saying it would be good if they could admit patients "around Tuesday."[14]

Another kind of hospital/patient kickback scheme is that used by Methodist Hospital in Minneapolis.[15] The hospital, a non-profit corporation, entered into a written contract under which it paid $2.5 million to the Park Nichollet Medical Center in return for the center's referring 90% of non-Medicare patients requiring specified medical services over a three- to five-year period. These services included CT scans, radiation therapy, home health care, and certain surgical procedures, all lucrative medical treatments. Here the payment was based on referring the patients as a group, rather than on an individual basis.[16]

Still another kind of kickback arrangement was devised by Ohio General Hospital, also a nonprofit hospital.[17] The hospital agreed to make a $75,000 "loan" to six physicians in the Madison Clinic. But the physicians didn't have to repay the loan. They could agree, instead, to admit 75% of their patients to Ohio General Hospital over a five-year period. The negotiated arrangement followed a decrease in hospital admissions and an explicit warning. Bill Stoerkel, one of the physicians, had informed the hospital board several months before that he was reluctant to admit patients to the hospital because of substandard conditions. Yet at the same meeting, he told the board that getting "some financial help makes one feel better that the board is standing behind you." The hospital noticed that this warning was backed ominously by action: in the four months before making the agreement, Dr. Stoerkel had decreased his admissions to the hospital by 50%.

Pharmaceutical Firms. Kickbacks are also paid to doctors in return for generating revenues for pharmaceutical manufacturers and other medical suppliers. In the 1970s, some pharmaceutical firms awarded "prizes" to doctors for prescribing or ordering drugs. Pfizer gave physicians rebates for prescribing Diplovax polio vaccine. The prizes received depended on the volume purchased. For purchasing 100 doses of the vaccine, physicians received a textbook on microbiology or one on baby care. Greater purchases entitled them to electronic calculators, a deluxe office chair, a portable cassette tape recorder, a physician's bag, or a refrigerator.[18] But these explicit kickbacks were discontinued. It seems the firms became embarrassed by them.

More recently, kickbacks from pharmaceutical firms have been disguised as payments for drug validation studies or marketing studies.[19] Wyeth-Ayerst Labs, a pharmaceutical division of American Home Products Corporation, developed a frequent-flyer program to encourage physicians to prescribe Inderal LA, a drug for treating high blood pressure, angina, and migraines.[20] Physicians received a two-week supply of the drug to start patients off, and a prescription pad with their name and the name "Inderal LA" printed on each prescription. All the physician had to do was sign the prescriptions for patients and spend a minute filling out a form for the firm's marketing study, noting the patient's age, sex, condition for which the drug was prescribed, previous medication, medication taken with Inderal, and the dosage prescribed.[21] In return for completing the marketing questionnaire and starting each patient on the drug, physicians received 1,000 point-miles on American Airlines. For prescribing the drug to 50 patients, physicians received a free plane ticket to any location in the United States. If physicians prescribed even greater quantities of the drug, they received additional points and could use them to fly outside the continental United States or to receive additional plane tickets. If they preferred, they could receive diagnostic equipment or textbooks instead.

Although the so-called Patient Profile Program was described as "a program designed to obtain medical data and other important information," the data requested and reported consisted merely of simple information about the patients of participating physicians, information that had no scientific value. It was only a cover. The pamphlets physicians received focused almost entirely on the benefits accrued from participating. Pamphlets listed cities to which participating doctors could fly and various medical conferences and recreational events they could attend. Also included were photographs and descriptions of medical equipment they could receive, such as a Littmann stethoscope or a Baumanometer wall unit.

In a report based on the information supplied by physicians, Wyeth-Ayerst stated that 20,068 physicians enrolled and 10,477 remained active for a year before the program was discontinued.[22] In Massachusetts, 347 physicians participated, and 76 received flight benefits.[23] A study by the company predicted that the program would produce millions of dollars of profits from increased drug sales. But when press reports caused bad publicity and a Massachusetts grand jury subpoenaed their records, American Home Care Products negotiated a settlement releasing them from liability in return for ceasing the program and paying Massachusetts $195,000 in restitution.[24]

In another case of disguising kickbacks, Janassen Pharmaceutica, a subsidiary of Johnson & Johnson, used continuing medical education credits to market drugs. Credit was offered to doctors who simply reviewed a monograph, or prescribed a drug, and reported on its results.

Pacemakers. Congressional investigations in 1982 and 1985 revealed that cardiac pacemaker manufacturers were paying kickbacks to doctors for installing their devices.[25] Many of these abuses could be verified only by expert evaluations, but some abuses were flagrant—such as the installation of two pacemakers in one patient. The congressional committee heard testimony indicating that kickbacks contributed to the then current 30 to 50% rate of inappropriate pacemaker utilization, a program costing Medicare approximately $2 billion in 1982. The average per capita rate of pacemaker installation in other Western developed countries in the 1980s was less than one-fifth that of the United States.

In some instances, between $150 and $450 in cash was tendered openly for each pacemaker a physician implanted.[26] In other situations, the cash tendered was under the pretext of clinical evaluation or consultation.[27] Frequently, these evaluations were not performed; the information was not used by the company, and the fee paid greatly exceeded the usual compensation for clinical evaluations.[28] More typical were disguised kickbacks in the form of in-kind benefits. These included stock or stock options and the provision of ancillary equipment such as programmers, analyzers, transtelephonic transmitters, receivers, and miniclinics—equipment valued at between $200 and $2,000.[29]

A flagrant example surfaced in the trial of Dr. Felix M. Balasco. Balasco was convicted of accepting kickbacks from pacemaker manufacturers and for conspiracy, extortion, and fraud under the Medicare and Medicaid fraud statute. The story that emerges from the trial transcript, the government legal memorandum, and the judge's sentencing memorandum is sordid.[30] Evidence presented at the trial indicated that between 1979 and 1983, Balasco received $238,000 in kickbacks from two firms (Telectronics and Pacesetter Systems) for implanting 474 pacemakers.[31]

Before 1979, Balasco used several different manufacturers' pacemakers, implanting six to ten units a month. But in early 1979, Balasco negotiated a kickback scheme with Telectronics under which they would pay him $250 for each of their pacemakers that he implanted.[32] Following the agreement, Dr. Balasco increased the number of Telectronics pacemakers he implanted, and for a while used them exclusively. But marketing representatives from Pacesetter Systems, a competitor, approached Balasco and asked that he use their brand. After negotiation, they agreed to pay him $400 for each pacemaker he implanted.[33] In 1981 Dr. Balasco told Telectronics sales representatives that he was being paid $400 by another company to implant their pacemakers and asked that they match the price. In response, Telectronics invited him on a company-paid trip to St. Martin.[34] Subsequently they matched the $400 price.

To cover up the kickbacks, the companies devised a ruse. They claimed that Balasco was paid for training cardiologists to use the pacemakers, paid as a consultant for the company, and paid as a clinical researcher conducting validation studies of the pacemakers. But Balasco never trained physicians, never performed consulting work, and never performed clinical research.[35] The validation forms, supposedly the basis for payment, consisted of boxes to be checked indicating whether his patients had expired, their pacemakers had failed, or the pacemakers were still implanted. Moreover, Dr. Balasco completed these forms only partially—and only after he had already received many payments. At the trial, a Telectronics marketing department employee testified that the forms were created so that physicians could provide "token information . . . in return for remuneration." She said the firm used the term *validation payment* as a more savory alternative to *kickbacks*.[36] An employee of Pacesetter wrote a research paper, using Dr. Balasco's name, to make it appear that Balasco was conducting research for the company.[37] Another Pacesetter employee testified to having written letters referring to the payments as consultant fees as "a coverup for just paying a doctor."[38]

In a sentencing memorandum, the prosecution produced evidence that the kickbacks resulted in Dr. Balasco's implanting pacemakers unnecessarily. Between 1981 and 1986, Balasco filed 158 Medicare claims for reimbursement for implanting pacemakers. Forty-nine claims were initially denied as medically unnecessary on prepayment review. Balasco accepted 10 of these denials but appealed 38 others. He lost 19 of his 38 appeals. The other 19 were still undecided at the time of the trial sentencing. In addition, between 1981 and 1983, Blue Cross/Blue Shield denied 10 of Dr. Balasco's 49 claims for pacemaker battery change for lack of medical necessity. Evidence suggested that he altered medical records, substituting cardiograms of other patients to justify his claims.

Ophthalmology. Congressional investigation of ophthalmology and optometry practices under Medicare provides another case study of kickbacks.[39] Many manufacturers of intraocular lenses, instrumental in cataract surgery, paid ophthalmologists kickbacks for using their product. A 1988 congressional committee survey of ophthalmologists showed that this practice was common. The cost of the lens was paid by the patient or the insurer (often Medicare), but the physician who chose the lens—usually the one who performed the surgery, but sometimes the optometrist who refers the patient for surgery—received the rebate. When optometrists received the kickbacks, they requested that the ophthalmologist use the manufacturer's lens for each patient they referred to surgery. Ophthalmologists often obliged because doing so ensured them a source of referrals.[40] Congressional investigations have found cases in which physicians who were paid kickbacks implanted lenses in patients when their vision was 20-20. The same congressional committee estimated that $1.2 billion in Medicare funds were wasted in inappropriate cataract surgery. A 1988 report by the Inspector General indicates that surgeons who referred patients back to referring optometrists enjoyed twice the volume of business of those who did not.[41]

Sometimes lens manufacturers pay physicians cash rebates for each lens ordered. Manufacturers also may offer volume discounts to ophthalmologists who can bill Medicare the standard fee, pocketing the difference.[42] Or they may provide in-kind benefits, such as equipment and supplies or merchandise credit.[43] One company offered a microscope and a phacoemulsification machine, worth $135,000, to those who purchased 1,260 lenses. Another provided similar equipment valued at $94,000 to physicians who signed a three-year contract for the lens purchase. Some firms offer credit toward the purchase of equipment, a practice they call *green-stamping*. More routine kickbacks are arrangements under which, for each lens purchased, physicians receive such items as postoperative kits or ancillary medical supplies valued at about $100. Lens manufacturers have offered services as payment for referrals. These services have included producing a customized videotape explaining cataract surgery for office use and sponsoring attendance at conferences. Other kickbacks paid to induce physicians to use a particular lens include stock in the firm and use of resort condominiums, cars, boats, and related facilities,[44] as well as designing and building a surgical suite in return for long-term contracts.[45]

Ophthalmologists sometimes pay kickbacks to optometrists for patient referrals. Some ophthalmologists have made cash payments of $100 to $500 and offered other in-kind benefits to optometrists, using as a pretext the optometrists' provision of postoperative care.[46] A more subtle practice, called *ping-pong referrals*, has optometrists referring patients to ophthalmologists who perform cataract surgery and then refer the patients back to the initial optometrists for follow-up care.[47]

There often is no need for this care. The optometrist will order visual field tests, fundus photographs, or other unnecessary procedures—or merely examine the patient and bill for the exam.[48] The ophthalmologist refers patients back to the optometrist to reward the optometrist for the referral and to guarantee a source of future referrals.[49] In a similar practice, ophthalmologists hire referring physicians as assistant surgeons.[50] The link between referral and these hirings suggests that payment is made for referrals.

Optometrists and ophthalmologists sometimes come to explicit understandings about ping-pong referrals. Appendices to Senate hearings include correspondence in which optometrists either promised reciprocal referrals or threatened to cut off referrals unless ophthalmologists referred back patients.[51] Other correspondence shows that ophthalmologists solicited referrals by writing letters and making phone calls telling optometrists that their surgical patients would be referred back to the initial referring physician for follow-up care. Sometimes physicians in these referral networks are far apart, which requires patients to travel great distances. Referral arrangements have been linked to poor patient care. Many cases have been documented where surgeons failed to examine the patient before surgery *and* neglected the patient afterward. Other records reveal inappropriate surgery.[52]

Clinical and Physiologic Laboratories. Laboratories have frequently used kickbacks to get referrals for diagnostic testing.[53] Virtually every physician has opportunities to use diagnostic testing in the normal course of practicing medicine. The case of *U.S. v. Greber* illustrates how routine tests can be turned into a source of kickback income.[54] In *Greber*, a doctor owned a company called Cardio-Med, Inc., that provided physicians with holter monitors to record cardiac activity. Physicians would prescribe the monitor for their patients and choose Cardio-Med. The physicians would use Cardio-Med's monitor and send the recording to Cardio-Med for processing. Cardio-Med billed Medicare for its diagnostic services. It then paid each physician who used its services 40% of the charges it billed Medicare (but no more than $65). Allegedly, the fee Cardio-Med paid to physicians was made in return for the physicians' interpreting the tape that recorded cardiac activity and for explaining the results to patients. But at trial, evidence was presented that Cardio-Med, and not the referring physician, usually interpreted the recording. Additionally, patients paid physicians on their own for their examination. The court convicted Greber for Medicare fraud, but physicians receiving kickbacks were not even tried.

Another example of such kickback subterfuges is *U.S. v. Hancock*.[55] In *Hancock*, two chiropractors sent samples of blood and tissues for testing to Chem-Tech Laboratory in Fort Wayne, Indiana along with Medicare forms. Chem-Tech billed Medicare and allegedly paid handling fees to the chiropractors for sending the samples and interpreting the results of the tests. But the court found that these fees paid for referrals.

A lawsuit brought in 1988 by the U.S. Attorney in the Eastern District of Pennsylvania confirms that this practice continues.[56] Based on evidence obtained from only one clinical laboratory, the Justice Department sought compensation for kickbacks paid to nearly 400 physicians. Before filing the suit, 300 physicians settled out of court and paid three times the kickbacks they received; 25 others made partial payment and are negotiating a payment schedule.

The abuses have been documented most thoroughly in the Medicaid program, where "Medicaid mills," often owned by physicians, were routinely paid kickbacks by clinical labs of 30%, and often as much as 50%, of the billings.[57] Government investigators set up Medicaid clinics and representatives of clinical labs rapidly contacted them, offering rebates, volume discounts, equipment, and salaries for nurses and receptionists. The most common device was to "rent" part of the offices to serve as a collection station for lab samples and have lab personnel draw blood. Such rents often totaled several thousand dollars a month, even when physicians paid less than $500 in monthly rent.[58]

Allied Health Professionals. Many allied health professionals rely on physicians for referrals and pay kickbacks to get them. The Medicare program and many states do not allow physical therapists to treat patients without a physician's referral. Medicare also requires a physician to develop a plan for the physical therapy treatment and that patients receiving physical therapy treatment periodically see a doctor.[59] These provisions make physicians gatekeepers to physical therapists. Some physicians use their leverage over patient referrals and reimbursement to extract kickbacks.

Sometimes these arrangements are disguised. Physical therapists renting office space from a physician may pay much more than the market rate, with the understanding that the physician will refer patients to them.[60] But explicit arrangements also exist. The case of Walter Ford is instructive. In a lawsuit brought in Georgia, Ford alleged that in 1978 William Cabot, M.D., contacted him and offered to refer all patients needing physical therapy to him at the Austell Physical Therapy Center in Austell, Georgia, in return for being paid 45% of the fees received. In his complaint, Ford says he accepted the offer, set up an office just a few blocks away, and paid Cabot $217,463 under this arrangement between

September 1978 and September 1982.[61] When a new state law made this practice illegal, Ford says he stopped paying the kickbacks—and he received no more referrals.

Physician Investment and Self-Referral

Physicians have numerous opportunities to invest in medical care facilities. Those discussed here have three common characteristics: (1) the physician earns money only if the facility is profitable; (2) the physician can enhance the venture's profitability by referring patients, ordering equipment, or using the facility's services; and (3) the physician, acting as a clinician, either chooses or recommends the services that the facility provides.

When these conditions exist, physician investors often risk some of their own funds and receive a pro rata share of the profits based on the amount invested, rather than a fee for each referral or service performed. Still, such physician investors reap benefits by referring patients, ordering tests, or purchasing products, so they may use or recommend services that promote their financial interests rather than their patients' interests. In the past two decades, such activities thrived despite the Medicare and Medicaid antikickback statute. But as we shall see in Chapter 4, recent lawsuits and new legislation are now attempting to reduce such practices.

One common form for physician investments is *limited partnerships*.[62] A general partner manages the facility and provides most of the capital, either personally or through bank loans. Physicians, each investing between $5,000 and $15,000, become limited partners. Limited partners do not participate in day-to-day management of the facility; their return or loss is based on the facility's profitability. If the business fails, they bear no financial responsibility beyond their financial investment. And if the provider acts in a negligent manner, limited partners are protected from potential tort liability.

Because of the organization of such partnerships, limited partners will earn income if the facility earns a profit—even if they make no referrals. Likewise, limited partners lose their investment if the facility becomes insolvent, even if they refer many patients. There is no certainty that referrals will produce income. Nevertheless, physician limited partners have a strong incentive to make referrals, since it increases the partnership's revenues and will increase the likelihood and amount of their profit as well. It is not surprising that physicians traditionally recruited to become limited partners were typically able and expected to refer patients. Usually the ventures will be profitable only if limited partners refer their patients. This fact is often explicit in the prospectuses used to solicit investors.

In the past, many physician investments met the three conditions in theory only. In practice, the general partners or other parties loaned them most of the money they invested. Sometimes firms made distributions based on expected earnings or on criteria other than actual profits. Physicians who made large numbers of referrals (or were likely to) were sold multiple shares of limited partnerships to increase their incentive to refer. Such arrangements were, in effect, kickback arrangements using limited partnerships as an organizational means. Although the partnerships thrived, many physicians and others considered them disreputable. The medical trade press has reported on these ventures sometimes portraying them as imbued with greed (Figure 3-1). Yet other physician investments did meet the three requirements listed above and were considered legitimate. Proponents of physician ownership often distinguish between these two kinds of investment, arguing that public policy should target the abuses of the second kind and permit legitimate physician investments. Some practitioners believe that recent legal developments have discouraged ruses and that most recent investments avoid such deceit.[63]

Through limited partnership agreements (or stock ownership), physicians can invest in a wide range of medical facilities, including laboratories for clinical and diagnostic testing, home health care centers, imaging centers, nursing homes, durable medical equipment suppliers, and pharmacies. Physicians often invest in facilities to which they can easily make referrals. Nephrologists can own dialysis centers; general dentists may own the practice of dental specialists, such as periodontists or orthodontists.[64] These facilities are diverse, and so are the ways in which they can be financed. But a common element in all of them is that physician investors can promote the enterprise, and their own financial interest, by using its services.

A report by the Inspector General of the Department of Health and Human Services on investments by doctors participating in the Medicare program indicated higher than expected rates of physician ownership of health care facilities.[65] In 1987, 12% of physicians paid by Medicare owned or invested in medical facilities to which they referred patients. Referring physicians owned, wholly or partly, at least 25% of indepen-

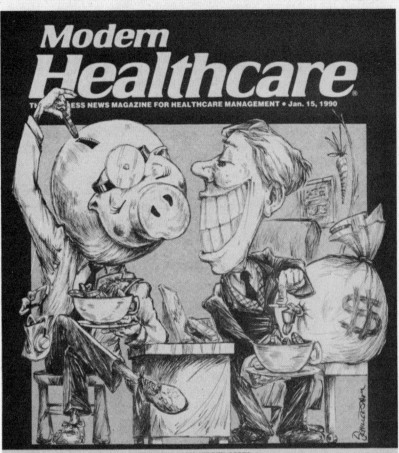

Figure 3–1

dent clinical laboratories and 27% of independent physiological laboratories to which Medicare payments were made. Doctors who invested in clinical labs provided patients with 45% more services than Medicare beneficiaries in general.[66]

Physician ownership may have been even greater then. The Inspector General testified that these statistics were "conservative" estimates because they only counted direct physician ownership and excluded ownership through family members or parent companies.[67]

In 1991 the Florida Health Care Cost Containment Board found that Florida had an even higher rate of physician investment in medical facilities.[68] Many facilities are owned by corporate entities that are themselves owned exclusively by physicians. The organizations often form pyramids or corporate shells that disguise the extent of physician ownership. Lawyers and management consultants created these intricate arrangements to help disguise the identity of the investors and owners.

Over 80% of the direct owners of health care facilities in Florida are physicians. But total physician ownership is greater because approximately 7% of medical facilities are owned by professional associations made up of doctors or other health facilities which may themselves be owned in whole or part by doctors. And between 40 and 46% of all physicians practicing in Florida have invested in joint ventures. Ninety-one percent of physician investors in medical facilities practice in specialties that allow them to make referrals to facilities in which they invest. The extent of physician investment varies among types of facility and medical specialties. The centers in which ownership is most concentrated are diagnostic imaging centers (93% owned wholly or partly by physicians), radiation therapy centers (78% so owned), ambulatory surgery centers (76% so owned), and clinical laboratories (60% so owned).[69]

In Florida serious problems were associated with doctor-owned clinical labs, diagnostic imaging centers, and physical therapy and rehabilitation centers: they performed more tests per patient and often charged more than other facilities. For example, physician-owned clinical labs performed nearly twice the number of tests per patient as labs not owned by physicians and charged over twice as much per patient. Contrary to the claims of proponents, they did not increase access to underserved groups. They were not located in rural or underserved areas and provided fewer services to Medicaid patients than nonphysician-owned facilities.

A follow-up study by Jean Mitchell and Elton Scott, Florida Cost-Control Board researchers, revealed that physician-owned joint ventures generated between 39% and 45% more visits per patient than other physical therapy facilities. Gross and net revenues in physician-owned physical therapy ventures were between 30% and 40% higher than centers without physician investors. Yet physician-owned centers employed fewer licensed physical therapists and assistants and used less labor per patient than other physical therapy centers.[70]

And in a third study, Mitchell and Jonathan Sunshine found that Florida physicians participating in joint ventures prescribed 40% to 60% more radiation therapy services than is the norm for radiation facilities in the rest of the country. Their costs were 40% to 60% higher, too. And the self-referring physicians in Florida spent 18% less time with each patient during treatment than the national norm.[71]

Many ventures that seek physician investors tout the financial rewards to physicians or explain that referring patients will bring profits. The MR Cooperative, a leader in assembling joint ventures for MRI and other imaging centers, reports candidly: "The most economically successful Centers are those where a large number of referring clinicians share in the economic risks and rewards."[72] One of the projects they helped to establish, the Nashville Imaging Center, originally projected returns of 400%, but later adjusted its projections to 100% because such high returns were not believable to potential investors.[73]

The letters soliciting physician investors are revealing. One begins: "You can increase your income significantly by merely referring your radiology studies to your own facility which *has cost you nothing*."[74] Another letter states, "C.P. Rehab Corp West *will* talk about increased revenues and profits of $15,000-25,000 annually per physician merely by sending your patients to your own facility."[75] Another letter starts, "Dear Doctor: Would you pass up the opportunity to increase your office revenue by an amount of anywhere from $35,000 to $200,000/year after a relatively minimal investment?"[76] And another letter closes with this thought: "With American Pain & Stress, Inc., you, as the physician and investor, control the revenues and net profits of the clinic by referring your patients to your facility."[77]

Clinical Diagnostic Services. Nationally, in 1987, more than 25% of independent clinical labs were partially or entirely owned by physicians who referred patients to them.[78] Patients of physicians who invested in clinical laboratories received 45% more lab services than

Medicare patients in general.[79] The Inspector General estimated that this increased use of lab services in 1987 cost Medicare $28 million in lab services.

Some clinical laboratories require that physicians who become limited partners refrain from patronizing other laboratories for clinical tests.[80] Others are organized to provide medical services exclusively for physician-investors. One example is Physicians Diagnostic Associates of Huntsville, Ltd., in Alabama. The center was planned as a limited partnership to provide investors with "a diagnostic center to utilize as an extension of their private practice of medicine." Only physicians with their principal practice in Huntsville were allowed to invest. The center provides diagnostic testing and evaluation, such as CT scanning, nuclear medicine, ultrasound, cardiography, breast diagnostic testing, and general laboratory and other services. Purchasing partnership interests provides investors with income and a tax shelter.[81]

MRI of Elizabeth, New Jersey, another limited partnership, illustrates one way physician ownership of medical facilities can be organized.[82] Dr. Jerome Molitor, a radiologist at the Alexian Brothers Hospital in Elizabeth, promoted the investment. He owned a professional corporation, MRI of Elizabeth, Pennsylvania, that performed MRI scans and billed patients or their insurers for this service. Dr. Molitor established MRI of Elizabeth Associates, L.P., to finance the purchase of MRI equipment and manage his business. He became the general partner and solicited 25 limited partners from among his colleagues in the fields of neurology, orthopedics, and internal medicine. The partnership bought the equipment, created the facilities to store it, and hired staff to manage its operation and the business side of the venture. Each limited partner invested $25,000 and agreed to assume a pro rata share of the liability on a lease of the equipment.

An investment this large might have been considered a substantial risk for investors. But the investors were able to promote the center's success by referring patients. In fact, they had a direct incentive to do so. Dr. Molitor paid the partnership $416 for each MRI scan he performed.[83] This per-scan payment was in addition to other unspecified fees he paid the partnership in return for its providing the equipment and performing business services. The limited partners knew that each patient they referred would produce revenue for the partnership, the profits of which would flow to them. The private placement memorandum distributed to interested investors made this clear, and projected scan rates and earnings. The memorandum projected that the facility would do 2,448 scans in 1987 and that the rate would increase each year until 1989, when it would level off at 3,456 scans per year.[84] The prospectus anticipated that each investor would recoup his or her $25,000 investment in about two-and-a-half years, receiving a payout of about $228,000 over 10 years.

Hospitals. Hospitals are only too aware that physicians control their flow of patients and can often create ambulatory surgical facilities, imaging centers, and other facilities that compete with hospitals. To avoid competition, hospitals often undertake joint business ventures with physicians. These joint ventures help them to maintain or increase hospital admissions or referrals to hospital-affiliated services. In such joint ventures, the hospital joins with either its medical staff or referring physicians and forms a limited partnership. The partnership then provides a service. Both the hospital and the physicians earn income from the service. The services provided vary. The partnership may operate an ambulatory care facility, purchase medical equipment and rent it to the hospital, sell durable medical equipment, or provide imaging or other diagnostic services. Usually the investing physicians do not provide the service, but they can increase their income by referring patients to the facility that does. The partnership's profits are divided between the hospital and the physicians.[85] In addition to the direct income earned by hospitals from such ventures, they acquire physician loyalty and patient admissions to the hospital.

The proposed financing in 1988 of a new surgical unit by the Lancaster Hospital Corporation in California, a subsidiary of the Paracelsus Healthcare Corporation, illustrates one way hospitals and physicians form joint ventures. Lancaster Hospital sought between 9 and 35 physicians practicing in California to invest $10,000 each in new medical and surgical equipment and refurbished surgical and gastrointestinal facilities. Investors would share any profits from the surgery center. The hospital was seeking only between $90,000 and $350,000 to finance the unit, a small sum for a corporation of its size. But it chose not to use its own funds or loans, and instead solicited funds from local doctors. The subscription agreement specified that the only investors accepted would be local physicians. Investors would not be able to transfer their ownership to others, and the corporation retained the right to reject any potential physician investors.[86] The hospital would also have the right to terminate the investment contract if the physician's license to practice medicine was revoked in California. To ensure that ownership and the incentive to refer patients would be distributed among numerous parties, no investor would be allowed to purchase more than four investment contracts.[87]

But financial details show what was really proposed. Under the terms of the contract, the investment is quite safe. If in the first year of operation the surgical center had generated the same operating revenues as in the previous year, investors would get back $10,900—$900 more than they had invested. And if conditions remained the same, they would reap an additional $10,900 for each year the surgical center remained in existence. If revenues increased—which was likely, since the center was refurbished with new high-tech equipment dedicated to expensive procedures—the profits for physician investors would increase as well. Moreover, the contract allows the investors to be paid on a quarterly basis.[88]

If Lancaster Hospital had merely wanted to obtain between $90,000 and $350,000 in capital for equipment, this would seem a strange way to get it. Assuming that the maximum 35 physicians invested $10,000 each in the facility and the revenues matched those of the previous year, the hospital would pay out $381,500 to the physicians in the first year, more than the amount of capital it sought to raise through the joint venture.[89] And if conditions stayed the same, the hospital would pay the physician investors the same amount each year. Since the center would annually pay out more than the capital initially received, the plan makes economic sense only if the physician investors gave the hospital something else in return. That something is patient referrals, which generate revenue.

National Medical Enterprises (NME) provides another example of hospital-physician joint ventures. NME, a hospital chain that owns or leases more than 129 hospitals and 366 long-term care facilities, developed a plan in 1989 to shore up the Jo Ellen Smith Medical Center and Meadowcrest Hospital, two facilities it owned in New Orleans.[90] In the years before the plan, the hospital occupancy rate was dropping, causing a loss in revenue. Patients were more frequently admitted to one of the hospitals' seven other competitors.[91] The rate had been 66% in 1984; by the beginning of 1989, it was down to just over 46%. NME hoped to turn the situation around by inviting between 100 and 200 physicians affiliated with the hospital to become limited partners and share hospital profits.

NME conducted interviews with affiliated physicians to test the possibility of sharing hospital profits with them. They found that "the medical staff would significantly alter their admitting patterns if they held the class A units" that the corporation was considering offering them.[92] In fact, based on these interviews and on information about other hospitals, management believed that if 100 or more physicians joined the limited partnership plan, the average daily census at both hospitals would rise by 20%, from 168 patients at the beginning of 1989 to 202 patients in 1990.[93] And when the rate increased, the hospital projected that its adjusted net revenues would rise from just over $62 million in 1989 to over $80 million in 1990 and $88 million in 1992.

The plan would work as follows: physician investors would each contribute $15,000. In return, they would be guaranteed an 8% return on their investment, regardless of hospital revenues.[94] But if the number of patients increased as projected, physicians would receive additional income that would more than double their original investment in two years.[95] And physicians would continue to earn similar income in subsequent years if conditions remained the same. Although selling the limited partnership shares to physicians would raise between $1,350,000 and $2,700,000, NME did not plan to use the money to purchase new equipment or refurbish the facilities to make the hospitals more attractive. Instead, the funds would be used as "working capital" for the partnerships.[96] The physician investors would share this capital with NME if the assets were ever sold. As the prospectus frankly stated, the "principal purpose" of the offering was not to raise capital, but "to provide local physicians with an opportunity to be investors in the ownership of the hospital."[97]

With increasing frequency, hospitals sell partial ownership to physicians who can admit patients. National firms, such as Republic Health Corporation, syndicate hospitals and sell shares to local physicians. Typically, the firm owning the hospital sells a partial interest to a limited partnership made up of local physicians.[98] In another variation, the partnership leases the hospital. In both cases, physician owners have a financial interest in increasing hospital admissions and making clinical decisions regarding treatment and discharge, strategies intended to increase the hospital's profits.

Once physicians become investors, the profitability of a hospital can change dramatically. One hospital had sustained a $155,000 annual loss. But it turned this loss into a $1.2 million profit two years after selling a 49% share to physicians through limited partnerships.[99] Another case study of three hospitals showed that patient admissions increased between 20 and 100% following the sale of ownership interests to physicians by the hospitals.[100]

Nor are such deals unusual. The Columbia Hospital Corporation, a for-profit hospital chain, now the sixth largest hospital management firm in the United States, was structured to rely on physician ownership from the start.[101] Private investors Richard Rainwater and Richard Scott acquired 14 financially distressed hospitals in 1987. They closed two and brought in local physicians as investors in the remaining 12 to encourage patient admissions. The El Paso hospital group in Texas typifies Columbia's practices. This group has 140 doctor partners in two hospitals and three outpatient facilities. Physician partners have reportedly earned a 25% return on their investment. Competitors say that the physician investors admit patients to their own hospitals, except for uninsured patients, whom they send to the non-profit hospitals. In 1992, hospital admissions were down 2% for the United States as a whole, but rose by 5% for hospitals that Columbia owned for over a year. Columbia's net revenues rose by 44% in the first nine months of 1992.

Most people associate hospital-physician joint ventures with for-profit corporations. However, non-profit hospitals also seek joint ventures with physicians. In fact, the National Council of Community Hospitals (NCCH), an organization representing over 100 non-profit hospitals and hospital systems in more than 30 states, urged the U.S. Department of Health and Human Services—which was drafting regulations to interpret the Medicare fraud and abuse statute—not to prohibit joint ventures between hospitals and physicians. NCCH officials believed that

> the real world consequence of a hospital's funding a joint venture in an ancillary medical facility is that most patients served by the venture will be admitted to the hospital making the investment, and that is the hospital's hope, expectation, and understanding.

They added that the legality of such arrangements should not be affected by "the explicitness with which the understanding is stated ... [or] the particular terms of the joint venture." NCCH went on to recommend dividing profits between the hospital and the physicians, based on factors other than the financial investment each group makes, because it will often be in the hospital's interest to pay physicians a "premium." Since this premium is not offered in return for capital or services, it is most certainly made in return for referral of patients. By way of clarification, NCCH has noted that hospitals that provide financial assistance to physicians should be able to require doctors to admit patients "as a condition."[102]

Home Health Care. Hospitals are not the only institutions that seek joint ventures with physicians to encourage referrals. Home health care agencies, which compete with hospitals in providing care, do the same.[103] Most patients in home health care agencies arrive there after a stay in a hospital. And the role of the hospital's attending physician is crucial, since the physician decides when to discharge a patient and often recommends a home health care agency. The agencies, naturally, are eager to ingratiate themselves with physicians.[104]

One home health care provider, T^2 (pronounced "T-squared") Medical Management, Inc., now manages over 24 companies that provide intravenous treatment at home in the southeastern United States. The manner in which T^2 established and managed Tri-State Home Therapeutics, Inc., in Cincinnati, Ohio, exemplifies one way these ventures are arranged.[105] T^2 set up Tri-State as a corporation. T^2 then sought between 15 and 35 investors to purchase shares at $15,000 each. And investors found that they had an attractive option: Tri-State arranged with a local bank to lend their investors funds. Investors could borrow $14,900 from the bank at 1% above the prime interest rate and relend this sum to Tri-State on the same terms. Investors would put up only $100 of their own funds to purchase the stock, and could repay their loan from the payments Tri-State made on its loan. The corporation's ability (or inability) to repay its loans posed their only risk.[106]

T^2 narrowed its field of investors to physicians in the Cincinnati area.[107] The prospectus's discussion of marketing makes it clear that T^2 chose physicians because they could refer patients. "The Organizers believe that a physician will be more likely to refer patients to the Corporation if the physician owns an interest in the Corporation."[108] Furthermore, the promoters acknowledged that referrals from physician investors were necessary for the firm to succeed. "The ability of the Corporation to compete successfully with the other entities [competing firms] will depend upon the Corporation's ability to secure a large number of referrals from physician-investors."[109]

The prospectus discusses ethical considerations and justifies the importance of physicians as sources of business, declaring that "potential investors should be aware that the Corporation's potential profitability is based, in part, on use by investor physicians."[110] According to the prospectus, there can be no guarantee that physicians will make such referrals because "physicians must base their choice of a medical service provider for their patient with the needs of the patient in mind." The same paragraph notes that physician investors face a potential conflict of interest, but concludes that a physician recommending services must be "the ultimate judge" of whether the provider recommended is appropriate.

Another common practice of T² is to buy back the stock of physician investors after a few years offering substantial profits to physicians who sell. But there is a catch. T² purchases the partnership interests of doctors paying mostly with T²'s own stock and physicians must agree not to sell the stock for at least two years. Doctors selling their partnerships therefore still have an interest in referring patients to the home health care facility.

As a result of these practices, T² has prospered. It is now a publicly traded firm worth over $500 million, ranked by *Forbes* as one of the nation's 18th fastest-growing enterprises and treating more than 3,000 patients a day nationwide. The company has branched out and now owns subsidiaries providing radiation, diet treatment, outpatient intravenus services. These, too, have physician investors who send patients.

T² claims that they offer high quality care at lower prices than competitors. But Dr. Deborah Chollett, director of the Insurance Research Center at Georgia State University, says there is no significant cost differential. And if use of services is greater due to physician self-referral, then any savings in cost of service would be canceled out.

Some patients have claimed that their doctors, who invested in T², were aggressive almost to the point of insisting that they use T² as a provider. Julia Lippman, who needed intravenous feeding as part of her treatment for cancer, claims that her doctor, Stanley Winokur, told her in February 1990 to cancel arrangements she had with another home health care provider. He refused to be responsible for her treatment unless she used Georgia Home Therapeutics, a subsidiary of T², she claims. As a result, Ms. Lippman had to find another doctor to supervise her treatment.[111]

Pharmacies. Physicians have also invested in local pharmacies and pharmaceutical repackaging firms and steered business their way. In the mid-1950s and 1960s the practice thrived and attracted considerable attention. The Senate held hearings on physician ownership of pharmacies in 1964 and 1967 and considered amending antitrust legislation to prohibit the practice.[112] Although the ownership of free-standing pharmacies has waned since the 1960s, it is now on the rise again in new forms.

Between 1990 and 1992, Medical Associates of America has established 33 pharmacies through joint ventures with physicians in at least 14 states and the District of Columbia. By the end of 1993 they plan to open another 60 to 70 pharmacies. The organization that provides the management services for the pharmacies is a national firm. But the pharmacies themselves are small, closely held corporations, each with no more than 35 owners. Of these, typically 30 are local physicians, the other five are individuals working in the management company or independent investors. What accounts for the rapid growth of Medical Associates' pharmacies? They receive about 60% of their business from patients sent by physician investors who share the profits. Information on profits is not publicly available but the pharmacies reportedly each have yearly gross revenue of over $1 million.[113] Physicians have occasionally profited from similar practices, namely by dispensing drugs and other products from their own offices.

Dispensing Drugs, Selling Medical Products,
and Performing Ancillary Medical Services

This classic conflict is noted in a Daumier caricature (Figure 3-2): a doctor stands under a sign that reads "free consultations." Holding out two bottles of medicine to his patient, he says:

> For Heaven's Sake, Don't take this sickness lightly.... Believe me, drink water, lots of water. Rub the bones of your legs. ... And come to see me often.... That won't impoverish you.... My consultations are free. Now, you owe me 20 Francs for these two bottles (This includes 10 centimes deposit on each container).[114]

Although the medical and pharmacy professions have traditionally been separate, there is a long history of physicians dispensing drugs and other products. Pharmaceutical products have become much more important in modern medicine, as their therapeutic power is enormous. The volume of drug use has greatly increased; so have prices and variety. These trends worsen the problem of physician dispensing.

According to one estimate, nearly 25% of U.S. physicians dispensed drugs in 1947; this figure dropped to 10% by 1965 and to near zero in the late 1960s.[115] But in the early 1970s it rose again. Today all but five states allow physicians to dispense the pharmaceutical products they prescribe.[116] A 1988 survey of state regulatory officials found that they believed 5% of physicians were dispensing drugs, but that the number was growing.[117] Joy Thompson, a market analyst for Marshall & Co. of

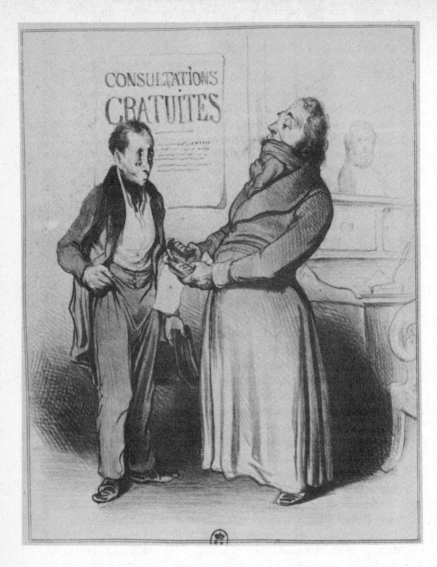

Figure 3-2

Atlanta, predicted in 1991 that another 10% of the market will shift from pharmacies to doctors' offices within seven years.[118] The potential for further growth is enormous. In Japan, physician dispensing is much more common; not surprisingly, Japan's per capita consumption of pharmaceutical products is one of the highest in the world, even higher than in the United States.[119] Today there are more drugs on the U.S. market than in the past, and thus more money to be made through dispensing. Since 1963, the Food and Drug Administration has approved 455 new drugs.[120] Sales of pharmaceutical products in the United States rose from $1.2 billion in 1954 to nearly $43.5 billion in 1991.[121]

One force responsible for the increase in physician dispensing is the growth in the 1970s of the pharmaceutical repackaging industry. Repackagers buy drugs wholesale, repackage them in individual prescriptions ready for dispensing, and resell them to physicians. The drugs arrive in sealed containers with built-in dispensing records and warning labels. The physician can avoid the time-consuming process of supervising the packaging of the drugs, simply adding the patient's name and any instructions, then reselling the sealed packages to patients.

Pharmaceutical repackagers aggressively market themselves to physicians and tout the extra income that dispensing can generate. One advertisement directed to physicians reads, "How to Earn $52,000 This Year with No Investment." Another asks, "Why pass the buck? Every time you sign a prescription, it's like writing a check to the pharmacy."[122] Yet another reads, "Each script you write is like a check to the pharmacy; why not write that check to your practice instead?"[123]

Physicians can also sell from their office other products they recommend. For example, the Nutritional Institute of Maryland sponsors a diet plan in which physicians sell diet powder to patients and monitor their health.[124] Participating physicians buy the powder diets from the institute and resell them at twice the price. The institute estimates that physicians who enroll 15 new patients a month and follow them for an average of 3.8 months will earn $62,000 a year from the sales. These physicians can also earn approximately $6,000 per patient for performing diagnostic lab tests to monitor the patient's health.

Physicians often recommend and perform certain clinical tests within their offices—simple blood and urine analyses, electrocardiograms, X-rays—that are usually performed by others. This kind of collateral activity is much more common than dispensing drugs or other medical products and increases with financial incentives.[125] It rose in the 1980s as new technology made it possible to perform more tests economically in offices. From 1984 to 1988, the cost of laboratory services for Medicare more than doubled, from $936 million to $1.9 billion.[126] While costs doubled, lab services were shifting from hospital to outpatient settings. As the volume of lab tests grew, so did the volume performed by physicians within their own offices. Lab services accounted for nearly 25% of the items paid by Medicare carriers from 1985 to 1989. They accounted for nearly 50% of the increase in Medicare payments to physicians during this period. The increase in Medicare laboratory services reflects the growth of lab services ordered by physicians for the country as a whole.[127]

Patients rely on physicians for neutral advice on whether they need a drug or test and, if so, what kind. But doctors engaged in these activities have an interest in recommending the products they sell and the tests they perform. In the case of pharmaceutical products, this can cause them to recommend drugs more frequently than may be desirable or to prescribe a product that they have on hand when an alternative would be more appropriate. This latter problem is likely to occur because most physicians who dispense drugs carry only between 25 and 50 drugs.[128] Physicians who prescribe inappropriate drugs already constitute a major problem; this practice is the most common basis for disciplining physicians by state licensing boards.[129] If physician dispensing increased, it would add an incentive to prescribe (especially for a limited range of drugs) that would exacerbate the problem.

Hospital Purchase of Physicians' Medical Practices

At the opposite end of the spectrum from physicians who serve as entrepreneurs are physicians who appear to be masters of their own practices but are employed by others. This situation occurs when hospitals purchase a physician's medical practice and employ the physician to maintain it.

Once a hospital owns a practice and employs the physician, it has a new means of encouraging admissions. The hospital can dismiss physicians or alter their compensation, depending on admission rates. The terms of sale may specify that the physician must refer all patients needing hospitalization to the purchasing hospital. Some hospitals have suggested that such arrangements should be immunized from liability under the Medicare and Medicaid anti-kickback statute.[130]

Hospital marketing experts have strongly recommended that hospitals purchase primary care practices.[131] Some suggest that hospitals create a primary care network to attract referrals. The rate of hospitals purchasing physicians' primary care practices in 1988 ranged from just over 9% of hospitals in the Southwest to over 32% in the Midwest.[132] Most have purchased only a few practices. But in the late 1970s, a few hospitals moved aggressively and formed a network by purchasing practices and clinics.[133] Experts advise this tactic as an "unbeatable strategy for securing tens of thousands of future referrals" and cite case studies to prove it.[134] The tactic, they say, is worthwhile despite high up-front costs. One hospital paid over 300% of the gross practice revenues to cover good will. They also paid for the assets and accounts receivable.[135]

Most clinics lose money after the hospitals assume control, but their loss is more than made up by increased income to the hospital from new admissions. For example, one hospital paid over $7 million to purchase a network of 34 primary care physicians that continued to lose money. But the hospital still made a 26% return on its investment.[136]

Federal regulators now regard hospitals' purchase of a practice combined with employing the former physician owners to run it as a disguised kickback, so the practice may be declining. However, there appears to be no legal risk when hospitals purchase retiring physicians' practices as part of *succession planning* to avoid losing a source of referrals, and Jackson and Coker, a national physician recruiting firm, says this practice is increasing.[137] Typically, hospitals arrange for retiring physicians to reduce their workload gradually and train a younger colleague to take over the practice. The hospital acts as a broker, purchasing the practice and eventually selling it to the new physician. The retiring physician will encourage patients to accept the younger colleague as their physician when he or she stops working. The younger physician will then admit the patients to the hospital that brokered the sale and owned the practice before the transfer.

The problem with straightforward ownership of physician practices is that patients may look on the doctor as an independent practitioner, rather than as an employee with loyalties to the hospital. That risk is diminished but still present when the hospital transfers the practice through a purchase and resale. The new physician has purchased the practice from the hospital and serves the community through its good graces. The terms of the sale are likely to be favorable to the physician, with the implicit understanding that the physician will refer patients. And patients are unlikely to guess that the hospital is providing physicians with incentives to increase admissions or to discharge Medicare

patients quickly, or is acting in ways that promote the hospital's financial interest rather than the patients'.

Hospital ownership of a physician's practice is the starkest example
of physicians working for hospitals while providing patient care in a
private practice. Here, physicians are in the hospitals' pocket. More
common are practices, often called physician recruitment and physician
bonding, through which hospitals use financial incentives to induce
physicians to act in the hospitals' interests.

Hospital Payments to Recruit and Bond Physicians

Physicians and hospitals have an interdependent, sometimes even
symbiotic, relationship. Relations between the two are complex, often
drawing on organizational loyalties and ties not reducible to financial
relations; and close coordination between them can certainly provide
benefits to patients. Still, many financial ties between physicians and
hospitals promote referrals. Frequently, hospitals recruit physicians to
be affiliated and practice in the vicinity. These physicians do not actually
operate as employees. They carry on a private practice and are granted
admitting privileges at the hospital. A survey indicates that hospitals
target recruitment of specialists, who tend to admit the most patients.[138]

In 1988, a nationwide survey conducted by Jackson and Coker found
that 95% of the hospitals surveyed made use of income guarantees to
recruit physicians.[139] Eighty-eight percent of the hospitals reimbursed for
relocation expenses and provided practice start-up assistance; 52%
provided free office rent; and 36% offered interest-free loans.[140]

Hospitals that guarantee physician practice income make up the
difference between what physicians earn and the guarantee. Typical
guarantees vary between $50,000 and $120,000 in net income. In a 1987
Jackson and Coker survey, 33% of the hospitals paid out over one-half of
the income they guaranteed to make up for lack of physician earning in
the start-up phase. The remainder paid lesser amounts.

Hospitals often guarantee the physician's income in private practice
for several years. Usually these guarantees are based on sums that
physicians are likely to earn once their practices are fully developed. But
in some cases, hospitals offer premiums to ensure a change of loyalty.
One hospital in the Midwest offered physicians a three-year contract at
150% of their current income to lure them away from a competing
hospital. Physicians typically have to return part of the payment if they
leave the region within a few years.[141] In the past, such income guaran-

tees were often explicitly in return for patient admissions. Recently, hospitals have relaxed this requirement, but the quid pro quo is implicit. A memorandum from Jackson and Coker tells why:

> The most obvious benefit [of physician recruitment] is incremental admissions which would occur as the natural result of relocating the physician to the community; however, to require or provide an incentive for the physician to admit patients to the hospital would be clearly illegal.[142]

While some experts insist that they are unaware of explicit agreements limiting physicians' freedom to participate in the physician recruitment or bonding programs of two or more competing hospitals, recruiting firms and hospitals frown on this divided loyalty. Such practices are "unethical," says Mark Bryant, a former Jackson and Coker executive.[143] Informal limitations on accepting financial aid from more than one hospital help hospitals maintain a loyal source of referrals. They also limit physicians' discretion to recommend hospitals or physicians to patients.

Recruiters and consultants urge planning to determine market conditions.[144] They have developed statistics on average hospital revenue generated through patient admissions by physicians in each specialty. Hospitals can recruit physicians with reasonable expectations of what they will get in return. But many hospitals plan only by "the seat of their pants." This can lead to disaster. On average, it costs about $100,000 to recruit a physician through a recruitment firm, once the costs of income guarantees, relocation expenses, interviews, and so forth are figured in. But perhaps as many as one-quarter of these recruitment plans fail. Either they do not generate the revenue expected or the physician leaves the community.

What remains unspoken is how patients are affected when hospitals recruit without adequate planning. Presumably, physicians without enough work to occupy them will have strong incentives to perform unnecessary or marginally useful services. The financial pressure for physicians and hospitals to generate revenue may lead to gratuitous hospital admissions or other medical services.

Sophisticated hospitals don't stop at recruiting physicians as part of a general plan to develop staff based on market conditions. They also employ bonding programs that seek to wed doctors to the hospital. These programs cultivate loyalty in local physicians both on and off

the staff.[145] Some hospitals loan physicians money to start or expand a
practice, and they may make loans conditional on referral.[146] Other
programs use other diverse incentives to earn physicians' loyalty. These
range from sponsoring seminars and workshops for physicians, operating referral services, helping doctors in private practice to market and
advertise their services, developing referral programs with physicians
in private practice, helping doctors with retirement planning, and
establishing joint ventures with them.

Bonding programs work by "meshing the interest of key admitters
and the hospital" and by "expanding the number of key admitters by
changing loyalty of low admitters and/or recruiting new physicians,"
says Charles Woeppel, vice president of Jackson and Coker.[147] Bonding
programs, according to Frank Perez, CEO of New England Memorial
Hospital in Stoneham, Massachusetts, are based on the "premise that
you must be willing to give the customers [i.e., the physicians] what they
want."[148]

In 1987 the Health Care Advisory Board, a private research organization with over 550 member hospitals, reviewed 24 different bonding
strategies. The board recommended physician bonding as one of the best
ways to help hospitals grow, since each new bonded physician can
generate between $200,000 and $240,000 a year for a hospital.[149]

The Health Care Advisory Board contrasts strategies that entail
financial incentives with ones it calls "legal handcuffs": programs that
use contractual requirements that obligate physicians to admit 100% of
their patients to a designated hospital. Legal handcuffs appear attractive
but are often hard to enforce—or illegal. So instead, the board recommends that hospitals promote admissions by using financial incentives,
seeding new practices, and promoting existing ones.[150] Its case studies
indicate that such tactics are effective. One hospital that helped seed new
practices explained the increased patient admissions quite frankly:
"The success of the program is due to the fact that the physicians 'owe us.'
We haven't been disappointed yet."[151]

Hospitals and private practitioners often keep track of who refers
patients to them and reciprocate with ping-pong referrals.[152] Another
bonding technique is for hospitals to refer patients to doctors who refer
patients to them. Some hospitals operate referral services for physicians
in their bonding programs. The hospital will provide the names of the
physicians to patients who ask for a referral. In return, the physicians
admit their patients to the hospital.

Some bonding consultants claim that their programs can increase hospital revenue by 5 to 12% within the first year.[153] Many are so sure that bonding programs increase hospital admissions that most of their payment is contingent on success. Jackson and Coker, for example, will charge an initial fee for designing a medical staff plan. But over 7/8ths of the company's earnings are contingent on a percentage of increased hospital revenue following the introduction of the bonding program. Typically, Jackson and Coker receives 6% of the increased revenue, as is the custom in the industry.[154]

Among the newest hospital bonding strategies is *massive contract management*. The idea is simple. Hospitals will take over many of the management functions for physicians in private practice. These functions can include billing and collections, accounting, computer processing, tax compliance and auditing, medical records management, management staffing, purchasing and inventory management, practice marketing, malpractice insurance, and health insurance. The hospitals provide these services as "more than [a] 'favor' to physicians seeking assistance."[155] The heading of a consulting report describing the tactic explains hospitals' ulterior motives:

Hospital Hidden Agenda: Penetrate Score of Family Practices, Become "Indispensable Man" for Physician; Professional Management Boosts Physician Income, Strengthens Hospital's Hold on Practice[156]

Once physicians are controlled by hospitals, they are beholden and can no longer make independent clinical choices for patients. Instead of serving patients alone, such physicians serve two masters.

The seedier side of some recruitment and bonding programs can be explained with documents from a successful unfair trade practices and antitrust lawsuit. The suit was brought by Dr. Henry Jones and his Monroe Medical Clinic in Louisiana against the Hospital Corporation of America (HCA), the North Monroe Community Hospital, and the North Louisiana Clinic.[157] Dr. Jones was chief of staff of North Monroe Community Hospital until he resigned in 1985 because he disagreed with HCA's management practices.[158] He contended that HCA used unfair trade practices —including sending his patients to other doctors, luring his colleagues away, and subsidizing competitors—in an effort to ruin his medical practice after he complained of HCA's unethical conduct. HCA, which owned the North Monroe Community Hospital, established a program to recruit physicians and subsidize their practices in order to enhance their loyalty. According to the deposition of Dr. Lee Roy Joyner, who worked for the North Louisiana Medical Clinic when the events transpired, HCA struck a bargain in 1984 with the North Louisiana Medical Clinic, an internal medicine practice located near the St. Francis Hospital in downtown Monroe. HCA offered to loan the clinic money for construction of a new office building if the clinic moved to the grounds of the North Monroe Community Hospital. HCA also offered to assume and pay off the clinic's $500,000 mortgage on the existing building, which required a $15,000 monthly payment. HCA loaned the clinic funds at 12% a year on a 20-year mortgage to finance the new building and gave the clinic an option to purchase additional space for $1 per square foot. To make up for any loss of income in the clinic in the initial period after the move, as well as any revenue loss from the absence of a heart catheterization program promised by the hospital, HCA paid the physician group approximately $1 million over a three-year period.[159] HCA also provided the clinic with free dictating transcription services and other amenities.

HCA allegedly promised not to interfere with the physicians' practice. But soon after the loan contract was signed, the hospital administrator, Pat Grady, exerted pressure on physicians to admit their patients. At the time of the loan, the hospital had a daily census in the 20s. HCA told the clinic that its breakeven point was 45 patients. The census went up to the 40s after the loan agreement because the clinic started admitting patients at North Monroe instead of St. Francis.[160] But soon the census dropped again. Following a weekend when hospital occupancy was in the 20s, Grady sent each physician a memo asking them to admit patients.[161] It read, "Admit patients to North Monroe. Help me." The doctors objected to Grady's interfering with their practice of medicine, but he responded by telling them that the bottom line was 45 patients, and that sooner or later it would have to be met.[162] HCA used its loan and its ability to refer patients to the clinic from their emergency room as leverage over the clinic. In response to the clinic's request, HCA granted a deferment on loan payments for one year, but decreed that future deferments would depend on whether the clinic helped the hospital to achieve an occupancy rate of at least 80%.[163]

The next hospital administrator, Arlen Reynolds, used similar approaches. He started attending the clinic's business meetings because he believed the hospital and clinic shared similar interests, namely, to "get as many patients as possible in the hospital."[164] He also encouraged the North Louisiana Clinic to buy the practice of a local physician who primarily served Medicaid patients; he then subsidized the office rent. The plan was to refer these patients to HCA for lucrative lab services but to admit all Medicaid patients to the competing St. Francis Hospital, skimming off the lucrative privately insured and Medicare patients for North Monroe Hospital and reducing St. Francis's revenues by filling the hospital with Medicaid patients, who paid less. Moreover, by admitting the Medicaid patients, who were mostly black, to St. Francis, HCA hoped to discourage privately insured, middle-class white patients from seeking services there and thus attract them to North Monroe Hospital.[165] Reynolds informed the physicians which medical procedures were paid highest by Medicare and which were paid least. He told clinic physicians that patients needing highly profitable medical work should be admitted to North Monroe; those needing medical procedures less well reimbursed by Medicare should be admitted to St. Francis Hospital.[166] The bonding and recruitment payments thus became enmeshed in a larger scheme.

The jury awarded Dr. Jones $600,000 in damages. Both parties have appealed the award: HCA to have it overruled, Dr. Jones to have it increased.[167] The HCA-North Louisiana Clinic situation is an unusually blatant example of hospital pressure exerted to gain patient admissions. Whether or not one believes that these practices are typical, the case illustrates the general problem. Everyone involved in physician recruitment and bonding programs admits that the aim is to encourage physicians to admit patients. The large sums of money paid are clearly intended for some reciprocal return. As Dr. Joyner testified, this was understood by all parties.[168] Dr. David Raines, a physician who turned down the financial inducements HCA offered, states the issue well:

> There is no way you can take something without obligation, . . . they were going to help us with our building, make our rent payments. . . . I think it obligates you, if someone gives you something—especially if you are a person who likes to repay your debt. . . .[169]

Dr. Marshall Leary, who negotiated the terms of the Clinic's move with HCA testified at trial, that his colleagues could retaliate if they were not paid. "We could stop admissions to the hospital."[170]

Gifts from Medical Suppliers

Without a physician's prescription, many pharmaceutical products cannot be sold. Even when a prescription is not needed, physicians exert control over the use of medical products by their advice. Thus, gifts from suppliers to doctors present a conflict of interest for all doctors but are compounded for any doctor who dispenses drugs and other medical products.

Product marketers regard physicians as a focal point in sales. They use "gifts" to generate good will. Detail men—that is, drug company sales representatives—find it easier to engage physicians over a dinner, or when inviting them to a conference at a resort, or after presenting, gratis, an item of value. Over the last three decades, pharmaceutical sales representatives have given gifts to most practicing physicians, but they often concentrate on influential physicians who can help set a clinical trend.

Senate hearings on the marketing practices of pharmaceutical companies held in December 1990 indicated the scope of gift giving by industry to physicians.[171] The Senate Committee on Labor and Human Resources asked 16 major pharmaceutical firms to supply data on their promotional practices. These companies spent more than $165 million in 1988 on such promotional practices as gift giving, lavish trips, and cash payments.[172] This represents a significant increase from the 1974 Senate survey, which revealed that the same firms spent only about $40 million.[173] The 16 firms represented a major part of the pharmaceutical industry, but not all of it. The industrywide figure for promotion is undoubtedly larger. Moreover, the data did not include income spent by foreign affiliates.[174]

The giveaways included direct gifts, symposia, samples, and reminder items bearing the product's or company's name. All were given to physicians for marketing purposes. All somehow benefit physicians. No quantitative data are readily available for gifts from other medical suppliers, but the practice thrives among them as well.

Spencer King, a former sales representative for a drug company, explained his practices in the 1974 Senate hearing on promotion of pharmaceutical products:

> One of the most difficult things in selling drugs to a doctor is to actually get into his office to see him and once inside, to get him to listen to what you are saying. His receptionist is often the key to this situation. To win

her over we were supplied with several giveaways including perfume, pens, and scratch pads. We also received adequate supplies of giveaways for the doctor himself.[175]

Another approach of sales representatives is to build bonds with physicians by taking doctors out to dinner, explains King:

> The object, of course was to sell the drug, and also to get to know these people better so that we could talk to them about our products the next time that we saw them.[176]

In addition to befriending physicians in order to gain their trust, sales representatives provided incentives to purchase products. In the early 1970s, kickbacks—in the form of prizes—were used:

> To persuade a doctor or pharmacist to use your brand of generic drug required some extra enticing. At Pfizer, we sometimes sponsored contests and offered prizes for those who bought our generic drugs. If the doctor ordered a certain amount of penicillin, he could pick a prize off a certain page of the catalog. The value of the prizes increased as the amount of the order increased. This was a very effective way of gaining business.[177]

But kickbacks could be illegal, so medical suppliers have resorted more often to gifts and samples, especially in recent years. Hearings in 1974 indicated that in 1973, 20 pharmaceutical companies surveyed gave away 12.8 million gifts and 45 million reminder items, and distributed over two billion free drug samples.[178] Several people testified that many physicians traded drug samples at pharmacies for other products for their personal use. Others sold the samples. More commonly they used the samples in a more traditional way—to start patients on a drug that would need to be refilled, thus generating future sales at a pharmacy.

Some physicians have long recognized the influence of gifts. Roger J. Bulger, M.D., then the executive officer of the Institute of Medicine, testified in 1974 that the use of free gifts "plays a significant role in determining the subsequent influence of the detail man on the physician and his prescribing practices," and he advocated eliminating free gifts and free samples.[179] And Dr. Douglas Waud, writing about pharmaceutical company gifts in 1992 described them as "the essence of good bribery."[180] But these have been the views of a minority. From 1960 until December 1990, the AMA took no position on gifts, merely reiterating its position against fee splitting, or what was called "receiving gifts in return for prescribing a particular company's product."[181] In fact, the AMA pooh-poohed evidence of the practice. Speaking for the AMA, Dr. Morton Bogdonoff testified in 1974 that "these business practices have been limited to a handful of manufacturers and recipients."[182] He withdrew the statement when confronted with evidence by Senator Ted Kennedy of widespread use of gifts, based on pharmaceutical company-supplied data.

The Range of Gifts. Today, physicians still receive an enormous range of gifts from pharmaceutical firms and other medical suppliers, despite a new AMA ethical stricture that would restrict the practice.[183] A 1992 survey of nearly 1,000 physicians by the Inspector General of the Department of Health and Human Services found that pharmaceutical firms offered gifts or payments at least once in the last year to 82% of physicians, with an average annual value of $727 per physician.[184]

One gets a sense of the practice from chronicling the range of gifts physicians have received in recent years.[185] Starting in their first year of medical school and continuing throughout their careers, they receive such gifts as medical bags and stethoscopes.[186] Expensive gifts, however, often go to influential physicians in private practices.[187] Firms give away note pads, pens and pencils, mugs, posters, notebooks, binders engraved with the recipient's name, medical bags, tourniquets, medical textbooks, reflex hammers, flashlights, through-stick holders, knot-tying kits, Woods lamps (a lamp with a magnifying glass used for examining lesions), goneometers,[188] review texts,[189] anatomical drawings, and slide transparencies.[190] Firms will often give physicians in private practice business cards or samples of medicine, or pay the salary of nurses in a clinic.[191] One company provided physicians with a gold-plated name plaque mounted in a walnut frame.[192]

Firms also give away items that are not associated with the practice of medicine. These have included sewing kits, automobile repair tools, canvas beach bags, alarm clocks, garden gloves, work goggles, winter scarves, binoculars, dashboard sun shields,[193] bicycle helmets, hats, golf balls with a drug logo, tennis balls, rulers, mugs, shirts, socks, towels, tie tacks, clip boards, games, candy, tickets to shows, dinners, and weekend getaways.[194] Pharmaceutical and skin care companies often give physicians free samples of their products for personal use. Some entertain residents with boat trips or dinners.[195]

Some firms sponsor the costs of attending national specialty meetings or seminars. In addition to paying for registration, transportation, hotels, and meals, they may provide cash to offset "expenses."[196] Supplementary enticements may include thermoses for holding liquid nitrogen, valued at nearly $500, or perfume.[197]

Drug company representatives will often make their pitch to interns and residents over "doughnut rounds": company-sponsored luncheon seminars held at hospitals, medical schools, or restaurants.[198] Such meetings may or may not be devoted to an evaluation of the firm's products. The sponsor may distribute brochures and product information. Other promotional practices are a bit unusual. At a luncheon given at the Case Western Reserve Medical School in Cleveland, $5 and $10 bills were distributed to the first residents who could correctly answer questions about the firm's product.[199]

Another trend is to pay doctors to attend a dinner. In one medical school, a company paid residents $500 to attend a dinner seminar on their drug.[200] But payments of $100 to $200 are more typical.[201] In fact, such dinners have become increasingly important; specialized firms now organize and run them. A leader in this business estimates that over 175,000 physicians in the United States took part in promotional dinners in 1989.[202] The practice is growing because physicians find the dinner and cash more agreeable than the customary office sales pitch. The president of one company noted that dinner meetings increased sales from about 80% of physicians who attended them.[203]

Many pharmaceutical companies sponsor "scientific symposia" to promote their products.[204] Usually the firm sponsoring the symposium will devote the meeting to its products or to a medical condition treatable with them. The meetings are often located and scheduled so that they can be combined with vacations in places like Paris, Venice, Hawaii, Palm Springs, Monte Carlo, and Acapulco. Frequently firms will invite not only a physician but also the physician's spouse or a "guest." Entertainment is provided: golf, cruises, sailing, concert tickets. Some firms offer gold coins, cash prizes, and honoraria to physicians who attend.[205]

Ciba-Geigy sponsored a weekend scientific symposium about the drug Valtarin on Marcos Island off the coast of Florida. The company provided transportation, hotel accommodations, meals, two receptions with an open bar, a dinner dance, and other entertainment for 150 physicians and their spouses. Three-and-a-half hours on a Saturday morning were taken up with scientific presentations; the rest of the weekend was free. G. D. Searle scheduled a conference in Los Angeles just before the Super Bowl and handed out free tickets. The symposium was to examine one of Searle's drugs for high blood pressure. Smith Kline French paid physicians all expenses and $500 in cash to attend a San Francisco conference about one of its antibiotic drugs. Some firms will even pay for additional vacation days at conference sites.[206]

One prominent physician has testified that he and his colleague resisted the overtures of a sales representative from Ciba-Geigy to use a new estrogen patch called Estraderm. But the rep continued to pursue the doctor's colleague, inviting him and his wife to a symposium in the Caribbean to learn about the drug. They went, stayed at first-rate hotels, were served lavish meals, and snorkeled. The doctor even attended some lectures on Estraderm. Following the trip, he prescribed Estraderm as the drug of choice to patients who needed estrogen.[207]

Other medical suppliers also offer gifts to physicians. For example, pacemaker manufacturers have held meetings and entertained physicians to get them to implant pacemakers. Gifts for users have included vacations in the Caribbean, fishing trips in Alaska and the Gulf of Mexico, meetings held to coincide with the Indianapolis 500, gambling junkets to Las Vegas, trips to ski resorts, and travel to Australia and Europe.[208] Some clinical laboratories also provide gifts to physicians who use their services: surgical gloves, gowns, refrigerators, specimen collection kits, or equipment used to generate revenue.[209]

The Unity of Conflicts of Interest

Though the financial, organizational, and legal structures of these six practices differ, the conflicts of interest are similar. All offer physicians self-serving incentives to generate services and channel referrals. When providers cannot indulge in one practice, they often can use another. This suggests that public policies should not focus on one practice alone, such as kickbacks; to do so would only encourage doctors and providers to gravitate to other practices and conflicts of interest, with similar results.

Consider the case, described earlier, of physical therapist Walter Ford. Mr. Ford paid Dr. Anthony Cabot 45% of his fees as kickbacks for patient referrals over a four-year period. But later, fearing legal liability and the stigma of kickbacks, the men "formalized" their agreement by setting up a limited partnership arrangement.[210] Ford was the general partner. The limited partners were Cabot and his colleague Sylvia Urratia, and both of their wives as custodians for their children. The limited partners collectively made a capital contribution of $3,000 and had no further liability. Ford, who performed the work, received 55% of the income.[211] The remaining 45% was divided among the limited partners, who referred patients.[212] Converting the kickback scheme to a limited partnership agreement changed little in the relationship but made it legal.[213] Cabot made referrals to Ford and received income from doing so.[214]

Another example of how physician self-referral arrangements can merge into kickbacks comes from the comments of a lawyer in response to the federal government's notice that it intended to create "safe harbors" from prosecution under the Medicare fraud and abuse law. Attorney Joanne B. Erde started with a conventional limited partnership arrangement to provide durable medical equipment and then sketched out variations closer to kickbacks.[215] First, physicians would become limited partners in a medical equipment firm to which they referred patients and then were reimbursed a pro rata share of the profits. Erde then asked whether it would be legal if physician limited partners invested only $500 each, while a general partner set up the remaining capital. In her third scenario, a medical equipment supplier served as a general partner and charged the limited partnership for services rendered.[216] In a final variation, Erde proposed that individual physicians establish separate arrangements and telephone lines with a medical equipment supplier who would bill each physician group for services rendered and reimburse the referring physicians for the money collected from their patients. The first two arrangements dilute the incentive to refer, while in the second two the relation between profit and referral is more direct.[217] Yet in all four situations, physicians may make referrals for profit. The four different arrangements are but variations on a theme.

One lawyer devised a plan to link physician ownership of equipment and rental arrangements to allow payments similar to kickbacks. Local private practitioners would purchase an expensive piece of high-tech surgical equipment and rent it to a surgical center that would pay the physician owning the equipment a fee for each use.[218] Although the physicians were not paid for referrals, the rental arrangement allowed them to earn fees by referring patients for surgery that requires the equipment.

In practice, physicians, providers, and suppliers can mix and match their financial arrangements to suit their needs. Hospitals that have used kickbacks to generate referrals also bring other financial incentives into play, as is illustrated by the example discussed earlier of Russell Furth, the administrator at Pasadena General Hospital.[219] To bolster patient admissions, Furth paid physicians kickbacks. But he also used other means. He placed doctors who admitted more than 12 patients a month on an advisory committee that paid $1,000 a month for attending a one-hour breakfast or lunch meeting, subsidized the office rent of certain doctors, and was planning a joint venture with physicians for the purchase of a CT scanner.[220] When a physician who received rent subsidies asked to be put on the paid advisory committee, Furth told her this would be unfair, because she would be getting extra money for the same admission "activity" as other physicians.[221]

Certainly there are differences between the various financial arrangements discussed. But the common risk to patients and the ease with which one practice can metamorphose into another underlies them all. To protect patients from physicians' conflicts of interest requires policies that focus on the general problem, not simply the specific organizational form.

4

The Dangers of Incentives
to Increase Services
and the Ineffectiveness
of Current Responses

[W]here a high percent of Medicare recipients reside, there is a correspondingly high percent of physicians invested in laboratory ownership arrangements. The government in allowing such [practices]. . . might as well issue the physician owners their own money press. The physician controls the demand for the services, owns the supply of the services, and is guaranteed payment for the service by the government[1] (Jim Codo, a medical laboratory salesperson).

Proponents of the six activities discussed in Chapter 3 say that these serve some useful and legitimate functions. They also think that any negative side effects are negligible and can be dealt with by existing peer review and regulation. These claims are mistaken. Each of the financial arrangements discussed creates conflicts of interest that divide the physician's loyalty between patients and other parties. Each is also expendable or can be severely curtailed, with a net gain for patients, as well as for the practice of medicine.

This chapter explains why the conflicts of interest produced by these incentives are serious rather than negligible, why utilization and peer review mechanisms cannot offset their negative effects, and why most other existing institutions, laws, and policies are also insufficient.

The Dangers of Financial Incentives

Kickbacks

Kickbacks from hospitals encourage physicians to choose a hospital for patients based on their own remuneration rather than patients' interests. They prompt physicians to admit patients to hospitals when patients would be better cared for outside the hospital. They also discourage desirable market competition. In the absence of kickbacks, hospitals can compete for patients by delivering high-quality medical and nursing care or by providing amenities to patients. If physicians acted as loyal agents for patients, they would weigh these factors in choosing a hospital. But when hospitals pay them kickbacks, physicians may ignore these considerations, and hospitals have less incentive to improve their services.

Kickbacks paid by specialists, clinical laboratories, and medical suppliers to referring physicians also have perverse effects. They reward physicians for promoting a service, whether or not it is desirable. This encourages physicians to recommend the provider that pays them, or that pays them the most. Kickbacks undermine a doctor's ability to offer patients neutral advice about whether services are needed, which kinds are preferable, and who should provide them. Physicians who receive kickbacks use their position as patient adviser or surrogate purchaser to increase the market share of the kickback payer and take a cut of the resulting profit. No financial benefit accrues to patients. Once payers have assured a flow of purchasers through kickbacks, they have little reason to lower prices or improve quality. And physicians will be discouraged from looking for better alternatives.

Nevertheless, kickbacks do not *necessarily* require that physicians act contrary to their patients' interests. Physicians can selectively accept kickbacks and refer patients to kickback payers when it is in their patients' interest—and turn down kickbacks and refer patients elsewhere when it is not. Kickbacks can also counter other perverse behaviors—for example, physicians neglecting to refer patients to specialists when they should. This has led economist Mark Pauly to argue that general prohibitions on kickbacks are too broad.[2] Pauly points out that inappropriate physician referral has two sides: (1) incentives may cause physicians to refer when purely medical criteria suggest they should not and (2) in the absence of incentives, physicians may not refer when medical criteria suggest they should. Prohibitions against kickbacks address the first concern but aggravate the second.

Consider referral patterns from primary care physicians to specialists. Primary care physicians may undertake tasks performed with greater expertise by specialists. A general practitioner can perform a gynecological exam, but gynecologists, because of their training and specialization, will be able to diagnose problems with greater specificity and sensitivity than generalists. General practitioners have a financial incentive to perform services because they will be paid for the work, while they receive no payment for making referrals. Therefore, they may perform procedures or services even when it is in the interest of patients to be treated by specialists. Payments from specialists to general practitioners for referrals will counter incentives for general practitioners to treat patients who deserve specialized care.[3]

Pauly is correct in noting that incentives to provide services rather than to refer patients to specialists can prompt physicians to act contrary to patients' interests, just as incentives to refer can.[4] But the two situations are not analogous. The incentive for physicians to perform services is built into their dual role as advisers and expert practitioners paid for each service. Much of medical practice involves evaluating patients' needs, advising patients, and performing the service in close proximity. It is difficult, if not impossible, to eliminate this incentive without encountering significant negative effects. However, the incentive of physicians to refer to *particular* specialists, hospitals, or providers is not inherent in physicians' activity. It can be eliminated easily, with no, or only minor, negative consequences.

Despite the fact that kickbacks provide incentives that encourage appropriate referrals in some situations, they do not generally promote patients' interests: they encourage fewer appropriate referrals and more inappropriate ones. Pauly's argument in defense of kickbacks works only when physicians are able to perform the same service (or a credible alternative) as the provider to whom they could refer. And this includes only a small number of situations. More often, physicians refer patients for services that they cannot provide: specialized diagnostic and therapeutic services, nursing care, or the purchase of medical equipment and pharmaceutical products. In such situations, even without a kickback, physicians would have to refer to others rather than perform the service themselves. Furthermore, physicians will have an incentive to provide services, rather than refer, only if their practice lacks patients. Physicians with a full practice have no financial incentive to avoid making referrals.

In addition, for kickbacks to provide desirable effects, the correct price would have to be attached. Low payment will not yield appropriate referrals; if too high, it will encourage medically inappropriate referrals, in addition to appropriate ones. There may be no price that encourages only desirable referrals. In any event, one cannot rely on kickback payers to set their prices at optimum levels. They are, after all, paying kickbacks to promote their own interests, not those of patients.

Even though some kickbacks may benefit patients, there are reasons for prohibiting them all. It is not worth the cost of evaluating each transaction to determine whether or not it is socially desirable. Since kickbacks are usually kept secret, evaluations may not even be possible. A broad prohibition will serve patients better than a laissez-faire policy, since most kickbacks do not benefit patients.

Furthermore, kickbacks achieve a negative impact beyond their immediate effect. The practice of paying kickbacks explicitly calls forth self-interested behavior and encourages physicians to consider their own economic welfare above that of patients. Kickbacks in medicine chip away at the patient-centered ethos.

Physician Investment and Self-Referral

Some partnerships and closely held corporations seeking physicians as investors are merely devices to "lock in" referrals. They will not allow anyone to invest who cannot make referrals. They may also require physicians to use only *their* services.[5] Sometimes the effort to raise capital through physician ownership is a ruse. No significant capital is raised, or if it is, the cost is much greater than is possible through bank loans or other means. Many such financial arrangements are marketed to physicians in terms that openly advertise income from referrals. These arrangements border on kickback schemes.

Proponents of joint ventures maintain that not all physician ownership plans are shams and should not be treated as if they are. Physicians' Clinical Services Limited Partnership (PCS) of Exton, Pennsylvania, has been cited as one example of the kind of arrangement that should be encouraged—not prohibited.[6]

PCS was a limited partnership organized to provide clinical labora-tory testing for Pennsylvania, New Jersey, Maryland, Delaware, Virginia, and Washington, D.C. In contrast to many limited partnerships, health care providers and investors other than physicians were allowed to invest. In 1987 PCS planned to sell 1,200 limited partnerships, and unlike many ventures in which physicians invest, the sale would raise substan-tial capital: up to $12 million. The arrangements established by PCS had several other redeeming features. Each investor's ownership interest was small; a share purchased for $11,000 gave the owner only 1/1,200th of the limited partnership.[7] With such a small share, physician investors had only a small financial incentive to order tests. The effect of any individual physician's clinical decisions on the firm's revenue was also very small. Furthermore, investors made and risk an out-of-pocket investment, and their earnings were limited to a pro rata share of any profits earned by the firm. These factors ensured that PCS was a legiti-mate investment and its financial structure mitigated some of the worst effects of physicians' conflicts of interest.[8]

Nevertheless, even PCS offered perverse incentives for physicians to make referrals. PCS planned to have at least 75% and perhaps as much as 90% of its business issue from physicians and health care partners.[9] The sale of partnerships to others provided respectability, but the busi-ness still relied largely on physician owners to generate business. Even though each physician alone owned only a small percentage of the laboratory, and could not substantially affect profits through his or her clinical decisions alone, all physician investors had the same pecuniary interest in using the lab's services, which tends to lock in referrals and undermine the benefits of diluting ownership.[10]

In sum, the organizational and financial arrangements of facilities such as PCS provide a more diffuse incentive to prescribe services than many, if not most, investments by physicians in medical services. But such ventures still depend on their investors to send them most of their business. This distinguishes them from other investments. If a doctor's decision to generate business involved only his or her own welfare there would be no problem. But it does not. All physicians' self-referral to medical facilities in which they have an interest constitutes an avoidable conflict of interest that compromises loyalty.

Some proponents of physician self-referral argue that by holding a financial stake in a medical facility, doctors will be advocates for their patients and ensure that they receive top-notch care.[11] Public-spirited physician investors, so the argument goes, could exert pressure to provide high-quality care because they might refer their patients elsewhere if the facility did not respond. As an investor, the physician would be involved, come to know the personalities, and wield some clout.

This argument is plausible in theory, but the facts belie it. Most, if not all, physician investments are passive limited partnerships. Medical facilities can give such investors no control over the day-to-day operation or management of the facility without undermining their status as limited partners. Physician investors' ability to intervene is no greater than if they used the facility but had made no investment. Moreover, physicians can always refer patients to a facility's competitors, whether or not they invest. Medical facilities that seek physician referrals are just as apt to cater to the views of unaffiliated physicians who can send patients.

Far from making it easier to refer patients elsewhere, investing in a facility makes it harder. When physicians remove patients from facilities in which they have invested, they rob their own pockets.[12] Unaffiliated physicians have no such barriers: they can refer patients elsewhere at no personal cost to themselves.

Other proponents of physician investment claim that whatever limitations they may have, physician investors provide an important source of capital for new facilities—unavailable elsewhere—and that physician investment is necessary for creating many facilities, especially in rural areas. In fact, most medical facilities that seek physician investors draw much of their capital from general partners or from bank loans, not from the physician investors; indeed, capital is more cheaply obtained from bank loans than funds from limited partnerships, based on typical rates of return. If facilities were seeking just capital, they would not target physicians as investors. As for the need for investment in rural areas, this too belies the facts. Most physician-owned facilities are located in or near urban markets rather than in the countryside.[13]

Dispensing Drugs, Selling Medical Products, and Performing Ancillary Medical Services

Physicians who dispense drugs and medical products and perform medical tests have been generally tolerated. This may be due to uncritical acceptance of tradition. Dispensing drugs and performing medical tests have thrived for another reason: they seem to be no more of a problem than fee-for-service practice. After all, physicians have an incentive to recommend their own services. Why, then, should we be concerned with a doctor who has an incentive to recommend ancillary services that he or she also provides? Not because the incentive to recommend ancillary services is stronger, or the risks are greater; nor is there a conceptual distinction between these two kinds of activity. Rather, the answer has to do with what is practical. Other than eliminating fee-for-service practice, there is no easy way to eliminate its perverse incentives. Health insurers often build in controls, such as requiring patients to receive a second opinion for elective surgery, to counter the incentive. But a check is not possible for every recommendation physicians make. It is quite easy, however, to reduce the incentives to recommend pharmaceutical products or medical tests simply by having other parties provide these services.

The benefits of physicians dispensing drugs are minor when compared with the disadvantages. Dispensing drugs is not an activity for which physicians have special expertise. Pharmacists are trained to dispense drugs; they, and not doctors, should dispense them.[14] Pharmacists can screen errors that physicians may make and can answer the questions of patients. The division of medicine from pharmacies allows checks and balances that are destroyed when physicians dispense drugs. The same rationale argues against physicians dispensing eyeglasses, as well as other medical products and supplies, and performing medical tests.[15]

Free-market proponents have argued that consumers will be better served by physician dispensing because it would allow competition in the market, which lowers prices and provides more choice.[16] But proponents focus too much on price and ignore an important point. Pharmacists cannot control the volume of their own prescription sales, while physicians can—by a stroke of a pen. The main problem with physicians dispensing is that drugs may be prescribed when not appropriate. Increased volume of sales can offset any overall savings arising from lower prices.

And with over 50,000 pharmacies in the country, price competition already thrives in retail sales. Physician dispensing is unlikely to inject significant additional competition in the market for prescription drugs. Moreover, whatever choice, in theory, a patient may exercise when picking from among a greater number of sellers, physician dispensing may actually constrain choices. The doctor's office is a perfect setting for a captive sale. The path of least resistance is to purchase immediately, rather than shop around. This is even more true for patients whose drug costs are covered by health insurance.

Not surprisingly, existing evidence suggests that physicians do not generally sell pharmaceutical products at lower prices than pharmacies. More often, they charge more.[17] The same holds true for physicians who own pharmacies. A 1975 study of their prescribing habits found that they tended to prescribe their own drugs and to prescribe drugs more frequently; the cost to consumers was approximately one-third more than the cost to patients of a comparable group of physicians who did not own pharmacies.[18] Small wonder then that consumer groups such as the Consumer Federation of America have opposed physician dispensing.[19]

While it is sometimes more convenient to purchase drugs from a doctor's office, convenience is generally greater when drugs are dispensed through pharmacies. Pharmacies are usually open for longer hours than doctors' offices and are located closer to where patients reside or work, which makes refilling prescriptions easier. In some rural areas, when a physician's office is located far from a pharmacy, physician dispensing does provide an advantage to patients. But physician dispensing is growing most rapidly in urban areas, not in rural areas.[20]

Allowing physicians to dispense in the name of free consumer choice has another disadvantage. If physician dispensing were to become a widespread phenomenon, it would impair the ability of our pharmaceutical distribution system to function efficiently without creating an adequate substitute. Physicians who dispense are likely to skim the market and concentrate on a few of the most widely used or most profitable drugs. Reducing sales of these staple drugs by pharmacies would cause pharmacies to lose an important source of revenue and be left holding mainly a large number (typically 3,000) of infrequently used drugs, thus raising their average costs and decreasing their revenue. Fewer pharmacies could survive under such conditions. Eventually, the wider range of drugs could be purchased at fewer locations, and at a higher cost to consumers.

Hospital Purchase of Physicians' Medical Practices

When hospitals own a medical practice, physicians work for the hospital while serving patients. But this relationship differs from the corporate practice of medicine, where the employer seeks profit through the difference between the fees generated and the salaries paid and other office costs. When hospitals own a practice, they maintain an interest in the promotion by their employed physicians of the economic goals of a separate institution: the hospital. The hospital has aims that can conflict with those of the physician or patient: it needs a steady flow of patients. It is true that different organizational missions can complement each other. A well-respected practice can operate as the source of hospital admissions. A practice that generates a high volume of patients may allow physicians special access to hospital administrators, who will be willing to take account of their needs and their views on ways to make the hospital perform better for patients. Hospital ownership will not necessarily lead to bad medicine, and it can lead to positive changes.

But when hospitals own practices, physicians lose their independence, which they could otherwise use to promote patients' welfare. Normally, a physician can choose which hospital to send patients, but this choice diminishes and perhaps even disappears when a hospital owns his or her practice. Independent physicians can monitor the actions of hospitals and intervene when it is to the patient's benefit. They can assess the work performed for the patient, and they can privately or publicly criticize the hospital. While these options are still possible, in theory, when physicians are employees, the personal cost to physicians of exercising the options is likely to be much greater. The hospital can dismiss the physicians, lower their salaries, channel patients to other doctors, or make their work less pleasant. When a hospital owns a medical practice that refers patients, the institution has less incentive to compete for patients in other ways—by providing better-quality care, for instance.

Hospitals may exert pressure in three main ways on physicians whose practices they own. First, hospitals will want physicians to admit patients to their facility rather than to others, to admit as many patients as possible if they are not full, and to plan admissions in a manner that helps the hospital schedule.[21]

Second, hospitals are likely to put pressure on physicians to refer patients to other hospital-owned or -affiliated practices or ancillary facilities.

Third, hospitals are likely to pressure physicians to be frugal in using services and hospital time for Medicare and other patients. Third-party payers that reimburse hospitals at a set rate per admission, such as

Medicare, give hospitals incentives to reduce their costs. These incentives are usually tempered because physicians are paid separately, and attending physicians determine what kinds of services patients should receive and when they should be discharged. But when physicians are employed by hospitals, this check on underuse of services is lost because doctors have an interest in promoting the financial goals of their employer. They are likely to know and promote these goals even without pressure; but if not, the hospital can exert greater leverage over their decisions than if the physicians were independent. The physician's and patient's options diminish if physicians in private practice are captive employees of a particular hospital.

Payments from Hospitals to Recruit or Bond Physicians

Physician bonding programs, recruitment plans, and other financial ties with hospitals create problems similar to those caused by hospital ownership of private practice. When hospitals subsidize the practices of physicians, the hospitals do not enjoy the full extent of legal leverage over them that they have when physicians are their employees. But depending on the extent to which they subsidize practice, the amount of income physicians derive thereby, and the sensitivity of physicians to these subsidies, hospitals can still exercise considerable economic clout. Indeed, if the money is substantial enough, hospitals may have equal or superior leverage.

Once physicians have grown accustomed to subsidies, business support, and other perks of bonding programs, kicking the habit may be hard. To leave their turn-key office practice would require them to relocate and take on greater management responsibility, a major obstacle for some physicians. Moreover, physicians may derive income from hospital referral services or from participation in joint ventures with hospitals. While many practices are nominally independent, their survival or well-being may in fact be linked to the hospital through a web of economic ties that are as strong as actual employment.

If the hospital provides only minor financial support, the physician has greater independence. Income and benefit supplements may then function more like a quid pro quo for specified returns or a gift that induces favors. Physicians who do not reciprocate risk losing the hospital's largess in the future.

Gifts from Medical Suppliers

Scholars have identified two distinct gift traditions. In one, gifts express altruism: the donation of blood, body organs, or even money, without seeking anything in return.[22] In the other, gifts are a form of social exchange, bestowed in return for past favors, to induce others to do something in return, to remain in the receiver's good favor, or to indebt him or her to the donor.[23] What makes gifts from sellers of medical products and services to physicians troubling is their ambiguity: they may appear to be tokens of appreciation, with no ulterior motive, but are usually meant to extract favors.[24]

In daily life we often distinguish between gifts and kickbacks. Kickbacks are made in exchange for producing income; gifts do not require any returned favor. Kickbacks usually presuppose a specified return; receiving gifts can produce feelings of indebtedness and gratitude, which may yield unspecified reciprocation.[25]

But the line between gifts and kickbacks can blur. Pharmaceutical firms may link gifts to conduct it seeks, such as the hospital's adding their drug to the hospital formulary.[26] Firms can also monitor the behavior of physicians and tender gifts, depending on the pliant behavior of a physician. Here, firms make gifts in exchange for desired behavior, even though there is no explicit agreement. Gift relations can become routinized and turn into kickback arrangements. This, in part, is why the Medicare fraud and abuse statute defines kickbacks much more broadly and prohibits any payments or income that can induce referrals.[27]

Proponents of gifts argue that government should be careful in regulating these practices because they offer significant benefits.[28] Gifts, so the argument goes, are a necessary tool used by the pharmaceutical and medical supply industries to market their products. Allowing firms to promote their products through gifts gives them an opportunity to recoup their investment and thereby encourages firms to invest in product innovation. Moreover, gifts are an integral part of providing information about products to doctors, information that is transmitted more economically by the firms themselves than by other means. Restrict the use of gifts, proponents say, and you will also cut the flow of information that doctors now receive, discourage research, and slow the dissemination of new useful medical therapies, all to the detriment of patients.

In fact, gifts are neither necessary nor particularly useful. Patent laws already protect the investment of firms in research and development, and gifts are only one of many options that firms use to promote their products, not a necessary means. The use of gifts by medical suppliers has waxed and waned, and many firms selling medical care and other products market their products without using gifts. Moreover, although gifts may facilitate the dissemination of information to doctors, the information is biased.

A 1992 study published by the *Annals of Internal Medicine* found that pharmaceutical advertisements published in leading medical journals often contained inaccurate or misleading information and that 62% needed major revisions.[29] Experts reviewing the advertisements felt that, in 40% of them, information on efficacy was not balanced with facts on side effects or situations in which the drug should not be used. And nearly one-third of the expert reviewers believed that the graphs and tables used in advertisements misrepresented the conclusions of clinical studies cited. Reviewers disagreed with the advertisements' claim that their product was the drug of choice nearly one-third of the time. There is no reason to believe the expert reviewers were hostile to pharmaceutical firms. Quite the contrary. Over three-quarters of the reviewers had received some form of payment from pharmaceutical firms within the past two years. Fifty-eight percent had received payments greater than $5,000 and 18% received smaller payments.[30]

There is some value in medical suppliers dispensing information to physicians through seminars and other means despite the potential bias. However, such contacts will have greater value and less risk of distorting clinical judgment if firms do not offer gifts. Many physicians insist that they retain their objectivity despite receiving gifts. They resolve to evaluate critically the promotional efforts of donor firms and to make clinical decisions that are in their patients' interest. But as one physician asked, "If you were a patient with a medical problem for which there was more than one possible medication, would you be interested in what gifts your doctor had recently accepted from the manufacturer of one of the options?"[31]

Gifts can influence the judgment of physicians, though they may not be aware of it. They may favorably dispose physicians to the donor's products. They may make physicians willing to spend more time with sales representatives. And they can create an emotional bond between the physician and the donor firm, thereby leading physicians to regard the firm's interests and their own as related. All these factors can increase the tendency of physicians to use a firm's medical products, or to make decisions, unintentionally, that are not in the patient's best interests.

A study conducted by Dr. Jerry Avorn showed that advertising influences physicians' beliefs about pharmaceutical products. Avorn asked physicians to state the properties of certain drugs and their appropriate uses. The answers revealed many beliefs that did not correspond to published medical reports but did reflect the claims producers had made in advertisements.[32] Yet the physicians studied contended that they based their assessment of medical products only on scientific evaluations, literature, and experience. Avorn concluded that advertising affected physicians' subconscious perceptions. And if advertising can influence physicians' beliefs about medical matters, gifts may also compromise their judgment or loyalties.

Consider, for instance, the pharmaceutical industry's practice of sponsoring scientific symposia at resort locations. These are generally sponsored by a single firm and are focused on a product it sells or a medical problem for which its products may be used. The more sophisticated of these promotional symposia are well enough respected to receive continuing medical education credit. In fact, pharmaceutical companies now subsidize nearly all continuing medical education for physicians.[33] One would assume that if physicians could receive credit for a course, it would be objective. Many universities that help to organize continuing medical education programs have policies to enhance objectivity and limit the influence of sponsors.

Nevertheless, in two studies, Dr. Marjorie Bowman found a bias affecting how the drugs were discussed and the prescribing habits of physicians after completion of the course despite policies to ensure neutrality. One study of continuing medical education at the Georgetown University School of Medicine in 1986 examined the content of two courses on the same topic, sponsored by two firms making comparable calcium channel blocker drugs.[34] The research found that the instructors assessed the drug made by their sponsoring firm more favorably, even though both drugs were comparable in potency and price, and despite guidelines to prevent sponsor interference.[35] The more positive assessment was made in several ways. The sponsor's drug was mentioned more frequently than others, and the clinical effects of the sponsored drug were cast in a more positive light. References to non-sponsor drugs tended to be negative or equivocal. When instructors made direct comparisons between drugs, they usually claimed that the sponsor's drug was better.[36]

Dr. Bowman's second study in 1988, also organized at Georgetown, examined physician prescribing patterns in the wake of three continuing medical education courses sponsored by drug companies.[37] The courses dealt with a limited range of drugs for specified purposes; the drugs had similar properties, effects, and costs, and none was clearly superior. Two courses discussed comparable calcium channel blockers, and one course discussed comparable beta blockers. The study consisted of surveys taken before participants took the courses and six months afterward. Physicians were asked to report the frequency with which they used the drugs. Three firms were each the primary sponsors of different courses. Overall, after taking the course, physicians favored the drugs produced by their course sponsor. Taking the course increased the prescribing of many drugs, but physicians increased their use of the sponsor's drug the most. These biases occurred even though Georgetown subscribed to guidelines established by the university and the American Council on Continuing Medical Education. These included disclosure of sponsorship and affiliation of speakers. Drugs were referred to only by their generic names.

The influence may stem not only from "buying" a physician's loyalty. By giving physicians gifts, medical suppliers can increase their access to very busy people. Having more time to make their pitch may be all that sellers need to promote their products in ways that influence physicians. A study by Dr. Nicole Lurie and her colleagues suggests as much.[38] Dr. Lurie and her colleagues surveyed physicians in internal medicine at seven universities over a ten-year period. They examined the frequency of their contacts with pharmaceutical sales representatives, including brief meetings and lunches. They asked whether physicians had accepted gifts of medicine for personal or family use, accepted paid trips, received honoraria for lecturing, or received research support. They also asked about changes in doctors' clinical practice, and whether they had suggested that a new drug be added to a hospital formulary.

They found a strong association between frequent contact with sales representatives and reported changes in clinical practices. There was also a strong association between receiving honoraria or research support and recommending that new drugs be added to the hospital formulary. A large number of physicians reported contacts with sales representatives. Forty-five percent of the faculty surveyed said they had received research support. Twenty-five percent of the faculty said they had made practice changes at least once in the past year, based on a discussion with a sales representative. Twenty percent said they had recommended changes in their hospital's formulary. The patterns were similar but less pronounced for residents. Nearly one-third of residents said that they had changed medical practice at least once in the past year, based on a discussion with a sales representative. Four percent said they had recommended changes in the formulary.

This trend in medicine is not surprising. Although very few studies of the effects of gifts on marketing medical care have been published, medical firms apparently believe that the practice increases sales, since they spend large sums of money on gifts. Business journals have published reports on the use of gifts to market products in other fields. One study shows that giving consumers small gifts can alter their perceptions of a product.[39] Salespeople have long used gifts to increase sales.[40]

Different kinds of gifts may have different effects. Large gifts may act more like bribes or kickbacks. Small ones may serve as advertising or samples. Large gifts seem more suspicious than small gifts. They lead one to ask: "Why is the firm giving the gift, and what does it expect to get in return?" But small gifts can influence physicians as well, even if the monetary value of what is received is trivial. The notepad and pen or paperweight with the drug's name emblazoned on its side is a constant reminder of the product. Receiving such gifts may not act as a strong financial inducement to use the supplier's services, but it is an effective form of advertising. Moreover, no clear border divides gifts of value, which might compromise judgment, from gifts as advertisements. Thus, a case can be made for restricting even the smallest gifts.

Conventional wisdom holds that it is not necessary to prohibit these six practices, that it is possible to cope with these problems through utilization review, peer review, and other legal and regulatory mechanisms. What, in fact, has been the experience of these monitoring measures?

Countering Financial Incentives: Utilization and Peer Review

Over the years, the federal government, third-party payers, and business corporations have developed programs to review the clinical decisions of physicians.[41] These are intended to counter financial incentives to dispense services, particularly those arising out of fee-for-service practice.

Starting in the 1950s, insurers and large companies initiated private utilization review programs.[42] Government programs started with Physician Standard Review Organizations (PSROs) in 1972. They were replaced with Peer Review Organizations (PROs) in 1982.[43] Most private programs were designed to cut excess use of medical services. Peer review programs, such as PSROs and PROs, have a broader mandate: to improve the quality of medical care. Yet traditionally, they too, have focused on deterring unnecessary surgery and medical procedures.

Utilization review programs use three main techniques: (1) preauthorization review, (2) concurrent review, and (3) retrospective review. *Preauthorization review* programs require physicians to receive approval before admitting patients to hospitals for routine or elective surgery. Some programs offer or require patients to obtain a second opinion when their physician recommends a major medical procedure. Others set standard lengths for hospital stays for particular medical conditions. Physicians must receive program approval to deviate from protocols. *Concurrent review* programs monitor patients' medical charts while they are receiving hospital care. They can intervene if excess services are being provided or if alternative therapies are preferable. *Retrospective review* programs analyze hospital records after the patient has been treated. If the program finds that physicians or hospitals provided unnecessary, inappropriate, or overly costly services, they can deny payment.

PSROs created administrative controls. They monitored physicians' behavior and assessed the appropriateness of hospital care; they audited hospital admissions and length of stay; and they designed protocols for reviewing medical treatment. But PSROs produced dismal results. For hospitals and physicians enjoyed built-in incentives to increase the volume of their services. Eventually they were eliminated.[44] There was little impetus for hospitals to perform utilization review vigilantly. Moreover, providers were organized and represented concentrated interests, whereas regulators and reviewers were not.[45] Providers easily overrode regulatory restraints.

Much greater reductions in utilization occurred after 1983, when Medicare switched from cost-based hospital payment to prospective payment based on Diagnosis Related Groups (DRGs). The new system gave hospitals an interest in using resources frugally. PROs met with more success than PSROs, partly because of the new incentives for hospitals to limit expenditures for Medicare patients. PROs review hospital care and ambulatory surgery. They are intended to focus on quality of care (including both under- and overuse of services). But they are still designed to identify primarily incidents of overuse of medical services.[46]

Private utilization review programs are managed by insurers, employers, and HMOs that pay physicians and have an interest in ferreting out unnecessary medical services to limit their expenditures. Some studies have found that utilization review programs can cut hospital admissions by 12% and the number of days patients spend in hospitals by 8%.[47]

The effect of utilization review on patient health status is less certain. Ample evidence suggests that a great deal of unnecessary medical care continues in spite of these programs. But other critics point to errors leading to denial of services that are beneficial or even necessary. So, even though utilization and peer review may reduce some unnecessary services, they are not a panacea for controlling overuse of services, let alone conflicts of interest. And they are costly and burdensome.

Until now, utilization review programs have focused on medical care in hospitals.[48] They were not geared to outpatient services and so slighted overuse in physician dispensing of drugs and physician self-referral to clinical labs, diagnostic facilities, and free-standing surgical facilities. Overuse of these services abounds. A study by the Blue Cross/Blue Shield Association indicated that between 20 and 60% of clinical laboratory testing is unnecessary.[49] But a study evaluating the possibility of using utilization review to address this problem concluded that too many clinical services are performed for effective monitoring by utilization review techniques.[50] The cost of evaluating claims would be greater than any savings produced.

The main limitation of utilization and peer review programs is that they do not come to grips with the core problem—the incentive to overtreat. They leave self-serving incentives intact and try to compensate for them: a strategy that will always follow one step behind the problem. They *counter* financial incentives to overtreat with administrative controls which can catch some inappropriate services, particularly flagrant abuses. But utilization review cannot identify the full measure of over-treatment because medicine involves so much uncertainty and ambiguity. In the absence of clear clinical standards, reviewers have difficulty second guessing the clinical decisions of doctors.[51]

Another limitation of review programs is that they are not designed to identify whether referrals were made to the most appropriate clinician. So long as reviewers do not identify gross errors on the part of providers, they are incapable of determining whether an alternative provider would have given better care or whether the risk to patients would have been less. Review programs cannot ascertain whether physicians should have used their discretion to refer patients to other providers.

Nor can they uncover biases that flow from financial conflicts of interest. From the perspective of most health policy makers, bias in choosing a provider is a subtle issue, one with which government policy should not concern itself. But from the patient's perspective, the issue matters. Patients have a right to expect that their physicians will make referrals in their interest, not to further the financial interests of the physicians or third parties.[52] When more than one acceptable therapeutic choice is possible, the physician should take into account the patient's values and interests in making a choice.

Another drawback of utilization review programs is that they entail significant social costs. Utilization review programs that interfere with the details of clinical decisions cause physicians great frustration. They require administrative expenses, and physicians must spend considerable time complying with procedures. These programs often remove a measure of clinical autonomy from doctors and place them under the control of payers who watch their pocketbooks, sometimes at the expense of patients. In their quest to eliminate unnecessary services, they cut down some useful services as well.[53] It therefore makes sense to rely on other approaches—such as eliminating incentives to overtreat—to the extent possible.

Still, we will need utilization review and quality assurance programs, even if financial conflicts of interest are eliminated. Most physicians have developed styles of practice based on fee-for-service payment that rewards offering services. It would take time to change these practice patterns even if physicians are not paid on a fee-for-service basis. Moreover, other forces encourage overtreatment. Some originate from institutional providers and medical suppliers who will, no doubt, continue to promote their products and services. Another problem is the perception of many physicians that in case of uncertainty, providing treatment will reduce the risk of malpractice liability. Social and psychological factors enter as well. Professionals spend years training and generally like their work. They tend to view it as important and may overvalue the need for the services they perform.

Nevertheless, utilization and peer review programs will have an easier time   achieving their goals if they do not come into conflict with the six practices previously discussed that encourage overtreatment. A far more effective approach is to eliminate these practices or to address directly the financial conflicts of interest.

The Limitations of Current Law and Policy

Current law and policy do not address physicians' conflicts of interest as such. State boards control licenses and discipline physicians. Some state and federal policies address a few conflicts of interest, such as kickbacks and self-referral. In addition, the federal government and private organizations are beginning to develop policies on hospital recruitment payments and gifts. But authority is fractured and existing law is piecemeal, inconsistent, and generally inadequate. It also addresses only a small range of problems and often is not enforced. While these laws make doctors, hospitals, and other providers modify the manner in which they organize their financial affairs, they have not prevented providers, suppliers, and physicians from putting into effect a wide range of sophisticated and lucrative schemes fraught with conflicts of interest. The lack of an adequate legal framework to address these issues as a whole, rather than individually, ensures that conflicts of interest will be treated as discrete, fragmented issues, despite their common ground.

State Licensing

Virtually every state has used its authority to protect the public's health and to set up a medical licensing board that establishes competency standards, grants and revokes licenses, and disciplines physicians.[54] In theory, these boards could help control excessive use of services or other inappropriate medical practices or could regulate conflicts of interest. But due to limited resources, institutional obstacles, and restricted state mandates, medical licensing boards in fact perform much narrower functions.

Licensing boards establish minimal standards for medical competence, including medical school education, medical board exams, internships, and continuing medical education. In granting and revoking licenses, state boards consider an applicant's fitness to practice the profession.[55] And one criterion for refusing or revoking a license is "character unbecoming to a physician." Yet boards usually revoke a license or apply sanctions only in the cases of incompetent or impaired physicians, or when doctors have been convicted for criminal activity or have engaged in other egregious conduct. Typically, licenses are revoked for kickbacks, fraudulent medical records, false billing, sexual abuse of patients, or sale of a medical license to a nonphysician.[56]

State licensing boards do not currently formulate conflict-of-interest policy.[57] The Federation of State Medical Licensing Boards knows of no state licensing boards with either a code of conduct or guidelines relating to physicians' conflicts of interest, although officials on state licensing boards are themselves often subject to conflict-of-interest regulation.[58] But some states empower state boards to discipline physicians for certain specific conflicts (dispensing drugs, fee splitting and kickbacks, and self-referral).

Several other factors undermine the ability of state boards to discipline physicians and control the quality of medical care. Most boards lack funding. In many states, licensing fees subsidize general state revenues, rather than the other way around.[59] Boards possess only limited authority to investigate cases, conduct hearings, and discipline physicians. Many states do not expect or permit state boards to police the quality of care. Staffed primarily by physicians, the boards may serve to protect physicians, not the public. (For example, they usually require a very high standard of proof.) Doctors disciplined in one state can move to another and easily escape detection or discipline. Unsurprisingly, several reports (including those of Senate committees, scholars, the Health and Human Services Inspector General, the Public Citizen Health Research Group, and investigative reporters) have concluded that state boards do not discipline physicians as they should.[60]

Another problem stems from the division of functions between PROs and state licensing boards. PROs review the quality of care that physicians provide, and can deny payment for unnecessary service or recommend that a provider with a record of poor quality be barred from the Medicare program. However, PROs lack the authority to discipline physicians. State licensing boards, which have this power, may not be in the know; PROs rarely inform state licensing boards when physicians overuse services or provide poor-quality care.[61] Surveys in 1988 and 1990 indicated that about two-thirds of PROs had not referred cases to state boards in the last year. When PROs and other agencies did refer cases to licensing boards, more often than not they did not provide detailed information.[62]

A federal statute enacted in 1990 aims to remedy this situation.[63] It requires PROs, Medicare carriers, and state Medicaid agencies to inform state licensing boards whenever they take action against an errant physician.[64] But even with this information, it is doubtful that state licensing boards can counter the incentives to provide services. Their resources are too meager.

Regulation of Specific Conflicts of Interest

Some medical licensing boards do have authority to regulate three kinds of activity involving conflicts of interest: (1) fee splitting and kickbacks, (2) physician self-referral, and (3) dispensing pharmaceutical products. What can be said about this experience?

Fee Splitting and Kickbacks. Thirty-seven states prohibit physicians from paying or receiving kickbacks for patient referrals.[65] The breadth and effectiveness of the prohibitions vary. Some states prohibit kickbacks generally;[66] others target only kickbacks between physicians or between certain specialties.[67] Still others concern Medicaid patients exclusively[68] or referrals to clinical laboratories.[69] But states do not strictly enforce these laws. A survey conducted by the Department of Health and Human Services Inspector General's Office showed that the overwhelming majority of states lack the resources to monitor compliance with antikickback and related laws.[70]

Self-Referral to Physician-Owned Facilities. Twenty-three states restrict self-referral arrangements in some way, but these restrictions vary greatly.[71] Only ten states have any significant restrictions on physician self-referral (Florida, Illinois, Maryland, Michigan, Minnesota, Missouri, Montana, Nevada, New Jersey and New York).[72] Only three—Illinois, Michigan, and New Jersey—have relatively broad restrictions.[73] But all these state statues have carved out exceptions that reflect the effective lobbying of medical subspecialty groups. Other states have limited restrictions. For example, California does not issue pharmacy permits to physicians or to a partnership or a corporation in which a physician owns more than a 10% share, and Pennsylvania bars physicians from owning a controlling interest in a pharmacy.[74] Colorado physicians may not own more than 10% of some medical enterprises.[75] Washington State does not allow physician self-referral in ophthalmology services.[76] Connecticut, at one point, did not issue certificates of need to ambulatory surgery centers owned by physicians planning to refer their patients to the center.[77]

Eighteen states require physician investors to level with their patients if the doctors have invested in a facility to which the patients are referred.[78] But only eleven states require disclosure in writing.[79] Most do not specify the language, timing, or content of disclosure. Some states require disclosure only for certain medical specialties or in certain circumstances, such as when the referring physician holds a greater than minimum equity interest (5 or 10%) in the facility.[80]

No statistics on prosecutions under state laws restricting self-referral are readily available, but their effectiveness appears dubious. A study conducted by the Department of Health and Human Services Inspector General's Office, including 143 interviews with enforcement officials in 50 states, found that only two states could monitor compliance. The officials cited lack of staffing and resources, inadequate enforcement mechanisms, and vague statutes as insuperable challenges.[81]

Obstacles to Enforcing Self-Referral Laws: The Example of Michigan. When states have attempted to develop strict laws, physicians have sought to evade or overturn them. Michigan, which enacted a strict statute in 1978, is instructive. The Michigan statute prohibits physicians from "directing or requiring" patients to use medical facilities in which the physicians have a financial interest.[82] In 1979, two physicians filed a lawsuit challenging its constitutionality. A circuit court judge issued a preliminary injunction against enforcing the law. This remained in effect until 1982, when the court ruled that the law was constitutional.[83]

Physicians then attempted to reinterpret the language of the law to limit its effect. The Attorney General had previously issued an opinion stating that the law prohibited physicians from referring patients to clinical laboratories in which the physicians had a financial interest.[84] But in 1988, two other doctors sought a ruling from the state board of medicine to distinguish between "referring" and "directing or requiring." They contended that they could refer patients to a facility they owned so long as they posted a sign in their office stating their ownership and informing patients of the right to choose another facility. This, they argued, would not constitute directing the patients. In 1989 the board of medicine ruled that such referrals were prohibited, despite the written disclosure. The physicians then brought suit challenging the board's decision.[85] In an unusual ruling in May 1990, a circuit court judge ignored the main issue in the legal challenge and ruled that the board of medicine had not promulgated rules under the statute and therefore had failed to give physicians proper notice. The court held that the board of medicine had no authority to discipline the plaintiffs for referrals. Although the ruling technically applies only to the two plaintiffs, the Attorney General's office has brought to a halt all further legal actions for self-referral until a final resolution. The Attorney General's office appealed the decision. The appellate court overturned the lower court's decision in August 1992 and remanded the case for further hearings.[86] It may take another two to three years for the issue to be fully resolved.

Thus, due to legal challenges and outright resistance, the effects of the law are unclear. For lack of resources and court challenges, from its enactment in 1978 until December 1992, the Attorney General's office has initiated only four suits against doctors under the statute, three of which are in abeyance pending resolution of legal challenges to the regulation.[87] No data are available on the extent of compliance with the statute, although the history of legal challenges and the small number of enforcement suits suggest that it may be low. In any event, a 1989 study by the Health and Human Services Inspector General's Office found that physician-owned free-standing medical facilities in Michigan had a 20% higher rate of use of services than free-standing facilities overall.[88]

Physician Dispensing. Most states regulate physician dispensing in some way. The aim generally is not to prohibit or limit dispensing—only five states do that—but to control quality.[89] In recent years, when states have considered prohibiting physician dispensing altogether, the Federal Trade Commission has opposed such measures, claiming they would reduce competition.[90]

Existing state regulation of dispensing is much less restrictive for physicians than it is for pharmacists; three of the four states with the greatest number of practicing physicians enforce minimal regulations. Even so, a survey indicates that the laws are not well enforced for several reasons.[91] State licensing boards lack funds and power. Regulatory authority is diffuse, fragmented, and uncoordinated. Physician licensing boards have little authority to investigate complaints or inspect physicians' offices. Statutes that regulate dispensing may also be unclear or contradictory, further complicating enforcement.[92]

Traditionally, it is the states that regulate physician dispensing. Yet Congress has considered intervening. Bills severely restricting dispensing were introduced in 1964, 1970, 1987, and 1988, but they were never enacted.[93] The AMA opposed the legislation, arguing that physicians should have the right to dispense so long as they did not take advantage of patients, informed patients that they could purchase drugs elsewhere, and did not violate state laws.[94] The guidelines of the AMA's Council on Ethical and Judicial Affairs allow physicians to dispense drugs but discourage doing so on a regular basis.[95]

Federal Legislation and Regulation of Kickbacks and Self-Referral

The federal government, one of the largest payers of medical care, regulates physicians reimbursed under the Medicare, Medicaid, and other programs.[96] Medicare and Medicaid statutes include prohibitions against receiving or paying kickbacks and, in some narrowly specified cases, Medicare prohibits self-referral activities as well. The laws, while setting standards, leave many patients outside these programs unprotected and address only a few egregious conflicts of interest.[97] And the laws have not been well-enforced. To promote reform where politically feasible, legislators have added changes bit by bit, tacking on items to major legislation. As a result, some provisions have been passed and then repealed, others watered down in compromises to ensure enactment.

The oldest and broadest law is the Medicare and Medicaid fraud and abuse statute. The aim of the initial legislation was to deter fraud, misrepresentation, unnecessary use of medical services, and excessive program costs.[98] Enacted in 1972, the legislation initially prohibited soliciting, offering, or receiving kickbacks, bribes, or rebates. It was expanded by amendments in 1977, 1980, and 1987 to include paying or receiving both cash and in-kind remuneration to induce referral of Medicare and Medicaid patients or for ordering goods or services paid for under these programs. The statute now imposes both criminal and civil penalties for violators. Civil penalties allow the Secretary of Health and Human Services to exclude providers who violate the statute. Criminal penalties include fines and prison terms.[99]

Prior to the 1977 amendments, judicial decisions interpreted the statute literally and did not enlarge the traditional definition of kickbacks: payment of a percentage of income to a person or organization that has made the income possible. Moreover, courts initially considered whether or not payments in question caused Medicare or Medicaid to lose money or whether overt corruption existed.[100]

After the 1977 amendments, the statute was interpreted by courts to include payments intended to induce referrals, whether or not recipients provided services legitimately needed. According to such judicial decisions, the statute is violated if one of the purposes of payment was to induce referrals—even with additional, legitimate reasons for payment.[101] Under this standard, many existing practices that pose conflicts of interest risk prosecution.

Yet the government has prosecuted relatively few cases; most have involved the more classical and egregious kickbacks, or disguised kickbacks, and usually overuse of medical services. Difficulties in proving cases, lack of resources, and other priorities have limited the number and kinds of suits initiated by the government.[102] As a result, in the early and mid-1980s many lawyers advised clients that income earned from self-referral to physician-owned facilities was probably acceptable if earnings were based on a return from the investment, rather than on the number of patients referred, if the services are essential, and if certain other conditions were met.[103]

Lawyers have offered more conservative advice since then, especially since 1989, due to a stricter regulatory climate. In the summer of 1989 the Inspector General issued a fraud alert indicating that certain physician joint ventures were suspect. In the summer of 1992 the Office of Inspector General announced it was investigating two major home infusion companies—T² Medical and Caremark, Inc.—for possible criminal violations of the fraud and abuse law.[104] It also announced that they were conducting over 200 other investigations under the fraud and abuse statute. Furthermore, the Federal Bureau of Investigation has increased staffing for investigations of health fraud by 30% and now has approximately 150 agents assigned exclusively for health fraud.[105] The Department of Justice has also established a Health Care Fraud Unit. Now lawyers are more cautious and look to regulations defining safe harbors (discussed below) as an index of protected activities.

As for the hospital recruitment of doctors, there are signs that the law may soon limit the scope of permissible subsidies. In May 1992 the Department of Health and Human Services Inspector General issued a fraud alert warning that certain payments from hospitals to physicians used in recruitment may violate the Medicare fraud and abuse statute.

The alert cited as suspect payments hospital income guarantees, payments for consulting services in excess of market value, discounted office space, below-market-rate loans, free billing, nursing services, reimbursement for continuing education, and travel to conferences. In the summer of 1992, in *Polk County Memorial Hospital v. Peters*, a Texas court ruled that a hospital could not recover funds it had advanced to a doctor under a recruitment contract when the doctor failed to use it as his primary hospital. The court held that the contract violated public policy and was unenforceable because the contract made payments which induced referrals, thereby violating the Medicare fraud and abuse statute.[106] In December 1992 the FBI initiated an investigation when Kennestone Hospital at Windy Hill, Georgia, reportedly offered $1.2 million in income guarantees, rent subsidies, medical equipment, and public relations services to Dr. George J. Kanes, one of its top admitters.[107] The IRS is also reviewing hospital recruitment practices and is expected to issue a General Council Memorandum or other guidelines soon.

Still, recent developments suggest that the tension between the broad reach of the law and the more narrow examples of prosecution will probably persist in the future.

In the fall of 1991, in *Inspector General v. the Hanlester Network*, the Department of Health and Human Services Appeals Board interpreted the fraud and abuse statute to preclude payments of partnership income to physician investors in certain situations. In *Hanlester*, three joint ventures were created with physicians as limited partners to channel business to SmithKline which served as manager of the labs. The appeals board ruled that distributions of profits to limited partners violate the law if they are intended to influence the judgment of physician investors in making referrals.[108] The board noted that even though physician investors were paid only a pro rata share of the profits, most referrals came from limited partners and so tended to increase their income. It was therefore irrelevant that the profits each self-referring physician earned were not "mathematically proportional to his referrals."[109] On remand, the administrative law judge held that the payments and management contracts violated the statute and excluded participating labs from Medicare and Medicaid. Earlier, SmithKline had settled its suit with the Department of Health and Human Services for $1.5 million.

While the legal standard set forth in *Hanlester* is very strict, the facts of the case suggest that Health and Human Services targets only egregious cases of self-referral for prosecution and courts may be unwilling to impose penalties unless they find such facts. The Hanlester labs made payments to limited partners based on the expected rather than actual earnings, a situation more akin to traditional kickbacks. The expected earnings paid were always greater than the actual receipts—presumably they were advances—but it is unclear whether SmithKline ever balanced the accounts. When promoting investment, employees for the Hanlester Network told doctors that the number of shares sold to any individual would be based on expected volume of referrals and that physician investors who did not refer business would be pressured to increase referrals or sell back their shares. Some employees of the Hanlester Network were compensated, in part, based on a percentage of the revenue generated by referrals from doctors who bought shares from them. And although the Department of Health and Human Services imposed penalties on the clinical labs, the doctors taking the kickbacks were never prosecuted which sends a mixed signal to physicians about the risks they face.[110]

Other trends also suggest a limited scope for the Medicare and Medicaid fraud and abuse statute. In the summer of 1991, the Department of Health and Human Services Inspector General issued "safe harbor" regulations defining payment practices deemed not to violate the fraud and abuse statute and therefore safe from prosecution.[111] These were originally proposed in response to concern over the wide scope of the statute and aimed to *protect* activities even though they would be illegal if the statute was strictly interpreted. Practices outside these safe harbors are not necessarily illegal, but they are not protected.

Many activities that are illegal under a strict reading of the fraud and abuse statute and not protected by safe harbors still are unlikely to be prosecuted. (The trade press noted as much after the draft safe-harbor regulations were released.[112]) The safe harbors include protection for many activities, including physician investment in companies whose stock is publicly traded, physician investment in private medical facilities to which doctors refer patients, physician income from equipment lease arrangements, rental of space, industry discounting practices, hospital referral services, sale of physician practices, hospital waiver of patient insurance co-payments, warranties, and personal service contracts. Although the safe harbors are narrowly drawn, nearly all exclude from prosecution some practices that place physicians in situations prone to conflicts of interest.

The provisions for physicians' self-referral illustrates the latitude that still exists. To fall within this safe harbor, physicians and businesses must follow several rules.[113] Individuals in a position to make referrals must purchase the investment on terms available to all investors; the income earned by investors must be proportional to the capital they invest; the business cannot loan funds or guarantee loans to individuals to finance their investment; and the business cannot market its services as part of a cross-referral program on terms that distinguish between investors and other individuals.

Investments in businesses with net tangible unprotected assets over $50 million must be made through securities that are registered with the Securities and Exchange Commission. Physicians and others who invest in smaller businesses must meet three additional requirements. All physicians and others who do business in any manner with such an entity or benefit from the entity can collectively own no more than 40% of the facility or can generate no more than 40% of its revenue in any twelve-month period. The business facility cannot require that physicians make referrals, generate other business, or be in a position to make referrals in order to retain ownership. The terms upon which investments are offered cannot vary with the previous or expected volume of referrals.

Businesses that create joint ventures with physicians and meet these restrictions will avoid the most offensive kinds of kickback schemes— the crude payoffs that end up being tried, such as the Balasco and Furth cases. But these restrictions do not generally prevent self-referral or physician investment that pose conflicts of interest. When probed, the restrictions do not even appear to be particularly strict. Consider, for example, the 40% revenue rule. Many facilities that would fail or be marginal performers in a competitive market get a boost if they can secure nearly half of their income from physician investors. Although this requirement reduces the income that would accrue from self-referral, it does not eliminate incentives to establish businesses that are financially driven by physician self-referral and does not prevent physicians from entering situations prone to conflicts of interest.

Other requirements for safe-harbor protection are neither particularly onerous nor by their nature effective.[114] For example, requiring that the earnings of investors be proportional to the income invested merely clarifies standard investment practices. As for the prohibition on *requiring* that physician investors be in a position to refer patients, physician-owned facilities do not need to require referrals because financial incentives induce them. Every physician investor recognizes the incentive to make referrals. The effect of each referral on income is usually stated (or implied) in prospectuses, which explain potential earnings and business risks, that are sent to all potential investors. Most prospectuses disclose a business plan, the volume of referrals expected from investors, and projected returns based on various assumptions and volumes of referrals.

Furthermore, business practices that violate other safe-harbor standards, but are hard to detect, get around the prohibition on requiring referrals. Most private-placement memoranda formally allow anyone to invest; but the subscription agreements usually allow the management or general partners to sell shares to whomever they wish and require potential investors to submit information that would indicate whether or not they are a good potential source of referrals. The general partners can therefore sign up physicians who are in a good position to refer, and who are likely to do so, without an explicit requirement. For prosecutors to identify such improper practice would require an in-depth, time-consuming investigation, an unlikely prospect unless other factors signaled clear abuse.

In November 1992 the Inspector General's Office announced that it would soon propose new safe harbors for ten new activities including hospital recruitment of physicians.[115] An unofficial draft of a safe harbor for physician recruitment, leaked the year before, indicated the standards the Inspector General might propose.[116] The draft safe-harbor allows hospitals to subsidize the private practices of physicians who relocate near a hospital for up to three years. No upper limit caps the amount of income the hospital can guarantee.[117]

The proposed hospital recruitment safe harbor does not permit all existing physician recruitment practices, particularly those that explicitly require admissions. But it does protect the more conventional recruitment payments. Although such payments do not require referrals, it is clear that most will have that effect. Hospitals make the payments to generate referrals, and physicians subsidized by a hospital will tend to admit patients there frequently, even if they are not bound by contract. Why else would a hospital want to incur such a financial burden?

The small number of prosecutions to date under the Medicare and Medicaid fraud and abuse statute, combined with evidence of frequent and extensive activity that contravenes the statute, suggests that it is not being effectively enforced, but there are indications that this neglect may change in the future. Stricter enforcement of the statute and more narrowly drawn safe harbor regulations may reduce abusive and scandalous practices. But it would still allow doctors to engage in a wide range of conflicts of interest without offering any significant social benefit in recompense.

New Legislation on Self-Referral

The first federal provision on this subject dealt with home health care services in 1982. Regulations barred physicians who own more than 5% of a home health agency from designating that agency for treatment of Medicare patients or from treating such patients.[118] They imposed the same prohibitions on physicians who were paid as officers or directors of the home health agency or who were paid more than $25,000 (or 5%) of the agency's assets in any year. The statute prohibited (with limited exceptions) home health care providers from supplying services to Medicare patients if the referring physicians retained an ownership interest in the provider or received compensation from the provider.

In the last five years, Representative Pete Stark (D.-Cal) has sponsored several other measures to restrict physician self-referral, some in narrowly defined fields, some for the Medicare program generally. They have met with only partial success. To help build momentum, Representative Stark has sought reports on the limitations of the Medicare and Medicaid fraud and abuse statute and the effects of physician ownership from several agencies, including the Health and Human Services Inspector General's Office and the Government Accounting Office. In 1989, the Inspector General, who is charged with enforcing the Medicare fraud and abuse statute, wrote that the statute "will never be effective in deterring business practices where the ultimate objective may be the same [as kickbacks] but where the payments are masked as 'dividends,' 'rent,' or 'consulting fees.'"[119] Bolstered by these reports, Representative Stark has pursued new legislation to eliminate physician self-referral in Medicare.

Representative Stark added another provision to the Catastrophic Coverage Act of 1988, which was to take effect in 1990. The statute would have expanded Medicare coverage for home use of intravenous therapies and restricted physician self-referrals by any physician who prescribes or establishes a plan for the therapy.[120] The provision would have eliminated or limited many arrangements such as the T^2 Home Health Care arrangements discussed in Chapter 3. However, the Catastrophic Coverage Act was repealed in December 1989, annulling this provision.

Another legislative foray by Stark attempted to eliminate virtually all physician self-referral within the Medicare program.[121] The original bill would have prevented physicians from referring their Medicare patients to *nearly all* medical facilities in which they had an ownership interest or from receiving any compensation from facilities to which they referred patients.[122] The intent was to restrict physicians from referring to institutions in which they or their families were investors or to which they had financial ties. The medical profession was divided over the bill. The AMA opposed the legislation, as did many other medical societies and health providers.[123] Other groups, however, were in favor, such as the American College of Radiology, the American College of Surgeons (ACS), the American College of Nuclear Medicine, and the American Clinical Laboratory Association.

To pass legislation in 1989 required a compromise. The law, which went into effect in 1992, only prohibits physicians from referring Medicare patients to entities furnishing clinical laboratory services in which the physician or a member of the physician's immediate family has an ownership interest or compensation arrangement.[124] And even the scaled-down legislation contains numerous exceptions. Physicians may self-refer to the following: clinical labs whose stock is publicly traded, with assets of over $100 million; labs operated by a physician within his or her own office, or within a narrowly defined group practice in which the physician is a member; labs in rural areas; any hospitals in Puerto Rico; hospitals in which the physician owns shares of the whole hospital (rather than part) and is on the medical staff; and HMOs.

The ban on compensation arrangements does not include payments from hospitals to physicians who are employed there or who provide administrative services. Nor does it include payments by hospitals used to recruit physicians or payments for leasing office space.[125] The exceptions open up all sorts of conflicts of interest. Medical suppliers and providers can still forge financial links that bond physicians to an organization and give them an incentive to refer in general, even if not for clinical lab services. But the legislation includes significant sanctions for noncompliance, such as denial of Medicare payment for service, civil penalties of up to $15,000 per service, and exclusion from Medicare.[126] It also requires all entities with referring physician investors to file reports with the Department of Health and Human Services so that they can monitor the practice.[127]

Future self-referral legislation is on the agenda. President George Bush's health reform program, proposed in 1992, would have prohibited self-referral under Medicare in radiology, radiation therapy, durable medical equipment, home health care, physical therapy, and rehabilitation services, a proposal similar to the original legislation proposed by Representative Stark.[128]

Federal Tax Policy and Nonprofit Hospitals

Federal tax law also affects physicians' conflicts of interest, albeit indirectly. The Internal Revenue Code (IRC) exempts nonprofit hospitals and other charitable institutions from paying taxes. To qualify for exemption under Section 501(c)(3) of the IRC, the revenue earned must be used for charitable purposes, and no income can inure to the benefit of private individuals.[129] The policy's aim is to prevent institutions from exploiting their charitable status for private gain. Charitable institutions can pay reasonable compensation to employees and others for needed goods or services. But any benefits to individuals must be incidental and necessary to achieve the public purpose. Unusually large salaries, bonuses or dividends, or rent subsidies may constitute gifts that violate Section 501(c)(3).

Traditionally, the IRS has tolerated common hospital payments to physicians.[130] However, as early as 1986, the IRS warned that hospital income guarantees and other perks used to recruit physicians may violate the ban on private inurement, depending on the details of the transaction.[131]

Recently, the IRS began to coordinate its policy on this issue with the Inspector General of the Department of Health and Human Services. In the fall of 1991 the IRS took its first step by issuing a General Counsel Memorandum.[132] It reviewed three cases in which hospitals created joint ventures with their staff physicians. In each, the joint venture entity purchased the revenue stream of certain hospital outpatient facilities; thus participating physicians had a proprietary interest in the net profits of part of the hospital and would earn income based on hospital revenues. The IRS concluded that such ventures gave physicians payments indistinguishable from dividends—payments that are not necessary for, or incidental to, the hospital's achieving its charitable goals and therefore improper. Although General Counsel Memoranda are not official policy, they do indicate the IRS's considered position. Hospitals that sell revenue streams in the future risk losing their tax-free status.

Now hospitals are in a double bind. They are reluctant to claim that recruitment and bonding payments are made in exchange for patient referrals because this violates the Medicare fraud and abuse statute and some state laws. However, if payments are not for patient referrals, then what is their purpose? Unless explained, the IRS may consider them payments to insiders, in violation of their prohibition on private benefit or inurement. Hospitals must show that payments promote their public purpose and that any private gain is only incidental.

If the IRS expands its policy along the lines set forth in the General Counsel Memorandum, nonprofit hospitals are likely to limit their payments to physicians in order to comply; the risk of losing their tax-exempt status is a strong deterrent. Even an unsuccessful IRS challenge to a hospital's tax-exempt status would complicate fund-raising through tax-exempt bonds. Thus, IRS policy, although seeking to promote other objectives, could limit practices that now create significant conflicts of interest.

Relying on the IRS to police conflicts of interest, however, has its limitations. For one thing, it affects mainly non-profit hospitals. Also, the IRS is unlikely to cavalierly strip charitable hospitals of their tax-exempt status because of their importance and their wide public support. Policies that match the practices of private hospitals may be tolerated on the grounds that they are necessary to compete. And future IRS policy is uncertain.

Antitrust Law

Federal antitrust statutes prohibit many business practices that restrict market competition.[133] These laws have the potential to restrict medical care practices that create conflicts of interest if they are anticompetitive.[134] They also limit the power of professional associations, such as the AMA and ACS, to develop ethical codes prohibiting self-referral, fee splitting, and other conflicts of interest if these provisions also limit market competition.[135]

Unless a practice can be used only to limit competition—such as price fixing—in which case it is considered per se illegal, courts must examine the impact of the practice on each market, balancing effects that limit competition with those that increase it. Only if the practice significantly restricts competition or if the actor exercised market power will courts find a violation of antitrust law.

Some judicial decisions have indicated that tying sales of one medical service to those of another may be anticompetitive and subject to antitrust liability.[136] But to challenge successfully on antitrust grounds practices such as tie-ins, financial incentives for referrals, or self-referral, plaintiffs must show that the parties engaging in these practices exercised market power.[137]

So far, antitrust law has not been a significant force in addressing physicians' conflicts of interest. This is due in part to the difference in frameworks and aims of antitrust law and conflict-of-interest law. Some commercial practices that promote market competition can produce physicians' conflicts of interest. But antitrust laws only restrict conflicts of interest that significantly restrict competition.

An attempt was made to amend antitrust laws to address one kind of physician self-referral. In the 1960s, Senator Philip Hart (D.-Mich.), chairman of a Senate subcommittee on antitrust and monopoly, held hearings on physician ownership of pharmacies and pharmaceutical repackaging firms.[138] He proposed legislation that would prohibit such physician ownership on the grounds that it restricted competition.[139] But the legislation was not enacted. And the Federal Trade Commission (FTC), whose job it is to promote competition, has actually promoted physician self-referral. In 1988 the FTC opposed proposed Medicare and Medicaid safe-harbor regulations limiting physician self-referral arrangements, arguing that these practices promote market competition.[140]

However, the FTC may help use antitrust law to restrict such practices in the future. In January 1992, the director of the FTC's Bureau of Competition indicated that it was considering prosecuting certain physicians who referred patients to ancillary facilities in which they had invested and breaking up such joint ventures.[141] The FTC staff now believes that in certain markets, specialists who invest in ancillary facilities might be able to use referrals to channel patients to their facility, thereby cornering the market for a specialized service, creating market power, and lessening competition.

Policies on Gifts

Doctors working for the Veterans Administration and other branches of the federal government are subject to laws (regulating all federal employees) that prohibit accepting gifts from individuals or firms that may benefit from decisions made by government employees. (Similar restrictions may cover physicians employed by state or municipal governments.) In effect, such physicians are restricted from accepting gifts from most medical suppliers and manufacturers, because physicians can help these groups by prescribing products or placing products on the Veterans Administration formulary. There is no evidence that such restrictions hamper these doctors from acquiring useful information about new medical products.

Physicians in private practice are not subject to any federal or state laws on accepting gifts. But the Food and Drug Administration is now considering guidelines on the promotion of pharmaceutical products and the sponsorship of scientific and education programs that could limit certain gift-giving practices.[142] This development follows several congressional hearings.

In 1974, the Senate Subcommittee on Health of the Committee on Labor and Public Welfare held hearings on promotion in the pharmaceutical industry. They focused public attention on the extensive use of gifts for marketing medical products.[143] In response, the organized medical profession and the pharmaceutical industry proposed self-regulation. Drug manufacturers reduced such practices for two years, but there was no lasting effect.[144] In 1977, Senator Ted Kennedy introduced a bill that would have regulated pharmaceutical promotion and prohib-ited the tendering of gifts if the purpose was to influence prescribing, but the legislation was not enacted.[145]

In December 1990, the Senate Committee on Labor and Human Resources again held hearings on promotional practices in the pharmaceutical industry.[146] In anticipation of the hearings (planned for over two years), the pharmaceutical industry and the organized medical profession developed new code provisions for gifts.

The AMA had not addressed gifts in its code early on. However, in 1959 the AMA revised its principles of medical ethics to deem unethical any inducements for referrals including *gifts*. But the restrictions against gifts were dropped when it revised its principles the following year. From then until 1990 the medical profession has passively accepted the practice of industry giving gifts to physicians, viewing it as harmless.

The AMA announced a new policy on gifts in an ethical opinion and report adopted the week before the 1990 Senate hearings.[147] The opinion prohibits doctors from accepting substantial gifts or cash with strings attached. But modest meals, pens and other tokens, and hospitality at conference social events were deemed acceptable if they primarily benefited patients or had educational value (such as textbooks). Further, the AMA allowed physicians and medical schools to accept funds for conferences and medical education, as well as the costs of travel and lodging, so long as these were channeled through the conference sponsor rather than reimbursed directly to individuals.[148]

The AMA opinion is notable because it would restrict many existing practices outright, rather than merely recommend that physicians follow their consciences. Still, the policy has limitations. First, it confuses the benefit of the patient with the benefit of the physician. The AMA sanctions some gifts, but the form of the gift should not change what it potentially represents. Gifts of textbooks are less offensive than luxury goods, vacations, or cash. But textbooks serve as income subsidies to physicians, not to patients.

Educational and luxury gifts alike may influence physicians to change their behavior. If the gift of a textbook induces physicians to prescribe a drug when it is not needed, or when another is preferable, the gift does not primarily benefit the patient. Firms that switch from cash to textbooks to comply with AMA policy will serve the same marketing aims as before. It is also likely that more respectable gifts will have a similar influence, or perhaps an even greater influence, cloaking the medical supplier with an aura of benevolence. Firms that truly wish to benefit patients can do so by eliminating gifts and reducing the cost of their products or by providing products gratis to needy patients. Gifts that only presumably benefit patients find their way into doctors' pockets and may well raise the price of drugs to patients. Internal company decisions revealed at the hearings by former employees suggest that companies are *not* motivated to provide gifts for the benefit of patients.[149]

Another drawback is that AMA policy does not place an upper limit on the value of gifts physicians can receive from any one source over several transactions. And even educational gifts can run high: a sales representative who visits a physician on a regular basis could finance hundreds or thousands of dollars of a physician's practice expense.

A third problem is that the AMA's interpretation of the guidelines opens up new loopholes.[150] For example, the AMA allows physicians to accept charitable contributions of up to $100 in their name for attending a dinner in which a firm promotes its products. Physicians will thereby receive a tax deduction that can reduce their federal income tax liability. The interpretations also allow physicians to receive medical supplies, such as Gram stain test kits, stethoscopes, and other diagnostic equipment because, the AMA claims, these benefit primarily the patient. But such gifts subsidize the private practice of physicians, and patients receive no direct benefit. And the AMA allows physicians to be paid for conference attendance and travel as long as the funds are disbursed through a medical school. It is hard to see what difference this pass-through of funds will make if the recipient knows the sponsor.

A fourth problem is enforcement. As seen in Chapter 2, the medical profession has long been unable to enforce ethical guidelines. Perhaps enforcement will be more successful in the future since the AMA has taken stronger official stands on gifts. So far, though, evidence suggests that the AMA's gift guidelines are not being scrupulously followed. A 1992 survey of physicians by the Department of Health and Human Services Inspector General found that pharmaceutical firms offered gifts—defined as inappropriate by AMA and Pharmaceutical Manufacturers Association guidelines—at least once to 27% of physicians overall and to 36% of physicians who wrote over 50 prescriptions a week.[151]

A 1992 investigative report featured in the *American Medical News*, (which is published by the American Medical Association), revealed that at the annual dermatological meeting "the scene [was] no different" from what was described in an 1989 article critical of gift giving at dermatology meetings. "Physicians and their spouses loaded up on cosmetic samples and other giveaways, stuffing them into suitcase-sized canvas bags with a drug company logo on the side."[152] The article documented widespread violation of the AMA and Pharmaceutical Manufacturer Association (PMA) guidelines, including, among other things, sumptuous entertainment, sweepstakes, and trick-or-treat giveaways. A subsequent *American Medical News* article reported on "rumblings in the ranks" about the guidelines. While noting that pharmaceutical firms had cut back on some practices, it quoted physicians who said they would accept payment of expenses to attend meetings, a violation of the guidelines. Other physicians reported that they had sent letters criticizing the guidelines to all members of their medical society.

Other medical associations have developed policy statements on the relations of physicians and pharmaceutical companies. Their purported aim is to prevent gifts and other financial ties with pharmaceutical firms from compromising physicians' judgments and prescribing habits. These policies are typically voluntary and do not offer an easily identified or workable standard. Some groups even state that their guidelines cannot be enforced. For example, the Infectious Diseases Society of America "recognizes its inability to legislate the morals of its members."[153] The American Surgical Association says that its position "does not connote any direct restriction."[154]

The 1990 position paper of the American College of Physicians (ACP) illustrates the problems with such policies.[155] The ACP accepts the propriety of gifts and honoraria and directs policy toward "excessive or inappropriate rewards." It is concerned first with public confidence in the profession and only secondarily with the possibility that physicians' judgment may be compromised. It urges professional societies to develop guidelines to "discourage excessive" industry-sponsored gifts and offers a policy of its own: gifts, hospitality, and subsidies should not be accepted if doing so might influence or appear to influence physicians' objectivity. But physicians are supposed to make this judgment individually. To help them decide whether financial arrangements are acceptable, the ACP proposes that doctors ask themselves whether they would be willing to disclose these financial arrangements publicly. But it is not necessary for physicians to disclose this information to patients, the ACP, colleagues, or the public. Physicians are merely counseled to imagine their reaction (and the reactions of others) in deciding what is appropriate. They never have to test it.

5

Incentives to Decrease Services in HMOs and Hospitals

Traditional ethical notions must be modified because doctors can no longer say the "patient comes first," for they must also consider the hospital, the group practice, and the publicly approved reimbursement scheme[1] (Troyen Brennan).

Withholding Services and Conflicts of Interest

Many policies that give physicians incentives to withhold services originate from private institutions and government agencies as responses to the distortions of fee-for-service medical practice.[2] A simple syllogism has governed policy: giving physicians incentives to perform services produces undesirable effects. Ergo, eliminate these problems by giving physicians incentives to refrain from performing services. Only one thing was overlooked: rewarding physicians for using resources frugally does not eliminate financial conflicts of interest. It creates new conflicts with different effects.

Attempts to limit services are often born of good intentions: to eliminate waste and to limit expenditure on medical care, thereby making it more affordable. We need to limit medical care expenditures because we have goals other than health, and we do have budget constraints. But when we need medical care, we generally don't want our limited personal income to keep us from attaining it. Most people do not want to pay for medical care out of pocket. Likewise, providers would prefer to avoid depending on out-of-pocket payments. So we spread the responsibility and financial risk through private insurance and government programs. This third-party involvement weakens incentives for individuals to monitor the costs of medical care and for providers to use or recommend services in a frugal way.[3]

Insurers and government programs now bear most of the direct financial burden of health care. As health care expenditures rise, they must raise premiums or taxes to pay the costs. And here we face limits. As costs rise, more employees and employers reduce their insurance coverage or do not purchase or provide insurance. And if taxes rise too much, the public will exert pressure on government.

These trends have prompted insurance companies and third-party payers to cap the outlays to HMOs and hospitals. Medicare now pays acute care hospitals a set fee per inpatient patient, depending on the diagnosis.[4] Sometimes Medicare pays HMOs through a similar fixed-payment system. In such arrangements the entity bears a portion of the financial risk.

HMOs and hospitals often pass the buck. They force physicians to carry some of the financial risk for recommending tests, performing medical procedures, and making referrals. Proponents say these incentives will persuade physicians to cut out wasteful tests and procedures, so everyone will benefit, even patients.[5] But the incentives discourage use of resources in general, resources that can also benefit patients.[6] Paying physicians to act as cost-control agents for third parties pits the interests of physicians against those of patients. It motivates physicians to consider their own financial interests in balancing the concerns of the payers and patients. And it compromises the ability of physicians to offer patients disinterested professional advice.[7]

One way to avoid perverse consequences is to pay physicians a salary. This form of payment insulates them from direct financial incentives to provide more or fewer services; it removes a major distorting influence in making clinical decisions. Paying a salary eliminates the conflicts of interest in fee-for-service practice without creating the reverse conflict.[8]

However, employed physicians encounter both *indirect* and *nonmonetary* incentives to promote the interests of their employers. Employers can block salary increases or promotions. They can even dismiss physicians who perform too many medical procedures. No physician's salary is more secure than his or her employer's financial solvency, so salaried physicians have a reason to generate income for their employers.

Who is employing the physician can affect the physician's behavior. If the employer is a hospital or other provider, salary may encourage patient admissions. If the employer is a large group practice, peer pressure may encourage referrals. And when government agencies or other third-party payers employ physicians, they may discourage providing services.

Still, there are important practical differences between indirect or nonmonetary incentives arising from salaried employment and direct financial incentives. Indirect and nonmonetary incentives are ubiquitous. They often exert less effect than direct financial incentives. It would be difficult to identify them all or gauge their seriousness, and it would therefore be exceedingly difficult, if not impossible, to control them—or even to develop a policy in response.

Moreover, the social significance of direct financial inducements is different from indirect ones. When we pay a physician to provide more or fewer services, we call forth self-interested behavior. We legitimize such motivations and actions and explicitly reward them. But physicians making clinical decisions ought to consider the interests of their patients and to comply with appropriate standards of medical practice, not consult their own financial well-being.

Although physicians, like other people, are motivated by earning money, we should not encourage personal financial gain as a criterion for particular clinical choices. A combination of motives, drives, and desires prompts everyone to act as they do. It would be imprudent to try to suppress them in order to promote desirable conduct. We need not worry about the complex range of motives of physicians, or all the indirect incentives that influence them. But at least we can try to avoid encouraging self-interested action when it creates conflicts of interest.[9]

Yet HMOs and hospitals now do precisely that. To see how this occurs, consider some of the incentive plans that HMOs and hospitals now use.

HMOs and Financial Incentives

HMOs provide comprehensive medical care to subscribers, using a closed panel of physicians. Members pay a fixed monthly premium and only nominal fees for services rendered (copayments).[10] HMOs perform two distinct functions: they insure subscribers by guaranteeing comprehensive medical care, and they deliver these services. Medical providers that charge for each service have an incentive to perform many services. HMOs do not. They incur costs by performing services but do not increase their revenue. They have an incentive to minimize services. Federal law and policy have promoted HMOs to increase public access to reasonably priced medical care; to reduce excessive, inappropriate ordering of medical services; and to reduce unnecessary federal spending.[11]

The first HMOs, now called *staff model HMOs*, owned medical care facilities and employed a group of physicians on salary. But changes in health care markets spawned several variations. For example, *group model* HMOs contract with an organization that employs the physicians. *Network model* HMOs contract with two or more physician groups. *Independent Practice Association* (IPA) HMOs contract with a separate organization, which in turn contracts with physicians who have their own practices, offices, and non-HMO patients. Usually their primary care physicians are paid either on a discounted fee-for-service basis or on a per-capita basis, with a set fee for each member for which the physician is responsible. The later is called a capitation payment.[12]

The Preferred Provider Organization (PPO) is a hybrid between IPA HMOs and traditional indemnity insurance plans that reimburse beneficiaries up to a set level for medical expenses they incur. Subscribers can receive medical care from a closed panel of physicians, as in an IPA-style HMO with only nominal copayments. They can also receive treatment from any other physician they choose, as in indemnity insurance, if they make a significant copayment (usually about 20 to 30% of the fee). Insurance coverage kicks in only after the patient has paid a deductible.[13]

HMOs and PPOs are managed-care providers. They attempt to control standards of practice and referrals to specialists and to hospitals. The term *managed care* refers to HMOs, PPOs, and increasingly, to most indemnity plans with management structures that control practice standards and referrals.[14] Managed-care providers attempt to organize systematically the use of medical care and the manner in which it is delivered in order to achieve explicit objectives. The objectives can range from reducing expenditures and the use of services to expanding the range of services provided or improving patients' quality of life. Managing care requires restricting patients' choice of providers and medical options and physicians' clinical autonomy. Both the physician and the patient are managed.

The management is usually done by physicians, nurses, and trained administrative staff. It involves the use of medical protocols to assess clinical decisions, individual case managers to coordinate medical care in complex and expensive cases, the use of retrospective reviews of utilization of services, and a host of other devices. The crucial factor is that choices traditionally made exclusively within the patient-physician relationship are explicitly controlled by organizational and institutional arrangements.

Staff model HMOs are a classic example of managed-care providers because such HMOs can effectively exercise control over all physicians they employ in a single location. The advent of utilization review, which allows insurers to monitor the behavior of physicians, now makes it possible to manage care in other ways as well. Here we focus on HMOs. However, physicians working for other managed-care providers often face similar conflicts of interest.

Over time, physicians have developed practice styles based on fee-for-service incentives that encourage high utilization of medical services.[15] These practice styles are now deeply ingrained; many people believe they persist even when physicians are paid by salary. To counter them and reduce inappropriate use of medical services, HMO managers use several administrative techniques. They make primary care physicians gatekeepers who coordinate medical treatment and approve referrals to specialists. They monitor physicians' clinical decisions, determine their appropriateness, and deny payment for unnecessary medical care. And doctors often need to receive administrative authorization before admitting patients to hospitals.

HMOs and Physician Risk Sharing

Most HMOs also use payment incentives to tie the interests of physicians to the financial goals of the organization. They frequently make physicians—particularly primary care physicians—bear part of the financial risk for providing services, so that their incomes decrease as the cost of treating patients rises.[16] HMOs and physicians carry two kinds of risk for the cost of medical care: one for the clinical decisions physicians make, another for the health status of their patients. They can reduce their exposure by reducing the amount of services provided or by choosing relatively healthy patients (who are less expensive to treat). Such incentives encourage physicians to ask themselves "How much will this cost me?" before providing or recommending medical services. As a result, physicians may recommend too little medical care.

Physicians can bear financial risk in an almost unlimited number of ways. But all risk-sharing plans rely on common approaches. One way is to compensate physicians on a per capita basis (*capitation*). In this system, doctors' incomes are fixed by the number of patients they have; providing additional services to these patients reduces the doctor's time and resources.

Frequently HMOs use both bonuses and financial penalties for physicians paid by salary, or fee-for-service. Many HMOs withhold part of the basic payment to primary care physicians and make them forfeit the payment if HMO costs exceed targets. HMOs also often pay a bonus to physicians who refer frugally. With either the carrot or stick approach physicians can increase their income by making clinical decisions that reduce services and lower the costs for the HMO. Sometimes the HMO considers only the use of services and referrals of physicians individually. At other times, HMOs base their bonus payments on the performance of a group of physicians or on the HMO's profitability.[17]

HMOs often link risk-sharing payment and penalties to the primary care physician's role as a gatekeeper. Gatekeepers are supposed to coordinate medical care to eliminate unnecessary services and properly channel appropriate ones. They determine what specialty care patients receive, and some HMOs will not pay for or provide services without their approval. Many HMOs make primary care physicians responsible for part of the costs of specialty care, laboratory tests, and hospital care. This gives them an incentive to reduce their referrals. Without such incentives, primary care physicians, paid by salary or capitation, have an indirect incentive to substitute treatment by specialists for work they could perform themselves.

Risk sharing is the norm in HMOs.[18] A 1987 study by the Group Health Association of America, an HMO trade association, found that 85% of HMOs use financial incentives for physicians. Approximately two-thirds withheld part of physicians' fees, salary, or capitation payments—usually not more than 20 to 30% of the base pay—and returned all or part of the funds withheld later, depending on the amount and cost of referrals.[19]

A study of HMOs in Medicare's risk-contracting program found that 29% shared both profits and loss with physicians; 21% shared only profits; and 20% shared only losses.[20] Most studies estimate that between 13 and 18% of HMOs distribute funds based on individual physician performance. But one study found that at least 60% of HMOs used individual physician performance, at least in part, to determine the level of incentive payments. In recent years the industry trend has been to reduce the amount of risk individual doctors bear.[21]

Elements of Risk Sharing

Five features of risk-sharing plans limit the financial risk and resulting incentives: (1) the risk pool size, (2) whether physicians risk loss or stand to profit, (3) the services for which physicians bear risk, (4) the extent of risk sharing and whether there is any cap on potential profit and loss, and (5) how profits or losses are distributed among physicians.

Risk Pool Size. HMOs can force physicians to bear risk for their use of medical referrals alone or pool the risk with those of other physicians in their department, health center, or some other unit. The greater the number of physicians in a risk pool, the smaller each one's pro rata share. The larger the group, the less financial risk physicians bear for their own decisions.

Some HMOs spread financial risk based on a combination of individual and collective risk pools. For example, they may create two risk pools: one collective and one for each physician. A surplus in the collective risk pool will be distributed, but only to physicians who have a surplus in their individual risk pools.

Profit and/or Loss Sharing. HMOs can share both loss and profit. A typical arrangement is to set a base payment (either salary, capitation, or fee-for-service) and to hold a portion of this payment (typically about 20%) in an escrow account. The funds set aside are released to physicians at the end of the year only if the individual physician or the physicians as a group did not provide more than the projected number of services. If physicians used more services than expected, the HMO draws on the withheld funds to cover the increased costs. The greater the amount by which services performed exceed the target, the greater the proportion of the withheld funds the HMO uses to cover its costs. HMOs use similar strategies for sharing profits. They often provide bonuses when the volume of physicians' clinical tests and referrals falls below a target. HMOs frequently use both of these carrot-and-stick approaches simultaneously.

Risk Sharing for Different Services. HMOs can make physicians bear risk for the cost of several different types of services: primary care, diagnostic tests, specialty care, drugs, hospitalization, and nursing facilities. Some HMOs give physicians the option of assuming risk for certain services.[22] HMOs usually place physicians at risk for the cost of some services but not others. They can also establish one kind of risk sharing for one service and a different kind for another. The more services for which a primary care physician is responsible, the more risk borne and the stronger the incentive to reduce services.

Limiting Risk and Profit. Usually HMOs limit the risk borne by physicians, establishing a threshold for loss and placing caps on the profits that can be earned. Stop-loss and profit-cap provisions help temper the effect of incentives. The aim is to prevent the cost of caring for seriously ill patients from placing undue financial pressure on physicians, and to prevent physicians' desire for personal gain from unduly tempting them to reduce medical services. Typically, HMOs limit the risk of loss or profit to 20% of the base income, but policies vary. One approach is to set a cap on loss for each patient. Another caps each doctor's financial loss for his entire pool of patients. A third varies each physician's upper limit on financial risk for different kinds of services, setting one limit for referral services, another limit for hospital services, and so forth.

Distribution of Profit and Loss. HMOs can distribute the profit or loss to physicians in several ways. Most risk-sharing plans concern primary care physicians. However, specialists can share in the savings or deficits.[23] Risk-sharing plans can distribute the profit or loss based on individual or group performance or a combination of both. Distributions may also reflect the number of patients, the physician's seniority in the HMO, or stock ownership. Profits are distributed quarterly or yearly, or upon retirement, as part of a deferred compensation plan.

The more frequently HMOs evaluate and reward physicians, the fewer clinical decisions and patients are involved. And this links financial reward closely to individual clinical choices. In addition, when physicians receive payments soon after taking specific actions, there is a clear link between performance and reward. The more directly rewards are linked to action, the stronger the inducement.[24]

Some Risk-Sharing Plans

As an example of an HMO risk-sharing plan, consider United Health-care in Seattle, Washington, operated by the Safeco Insurance Company.[25] United Healthcare paid each primary care physician a set monthly fee for each patient to compensate them for providing or arranging all medical care. At the end of the year, the doctor shared any remaining funds with Safeco and was partially responsible for any deficit. But risk sharing was limited. Depending on the size of the physician's practice, the risk of loss was capped at between 5 and 10% of reimbursed charges. Profit sharing was limited to between 10 and 50% of reimbursed charges. In addition, to prevent distortions due to a few patients needing unusually expensive medical care, each physician's risk was limited to $5,000 per patient per year. Physicians paid on a fee-for-service basis (i.e., specialists) had a separate incentive plan. If United Healthcare ran a deficit, payment could be lowered to 85% of the ordinary fee. With a surplus, payments would be adjusted upward to 105% of ordinary charges. In 1979, slightly over half of the physicians realized year-end surpluses. The average was $413; the highest surplus was $5,000. The average deficit was $169 and the highest $1,833. Despite these financial incentives, the HMO was unsuccessful and eventually went out of business.

Another such plan was Bluechoice, owned by Blue Cross/Blue Shield of Missouri.[26] Bluechoice made primary care physicians gatekeepers, responsible for coordinating all specialty care. It paid primary care physicians by capitation, and offered financial penalties and rewards to encourage them to reduce the amount of services they provide. Bluechoice withheld 20% of each physician's capitation payment and placed it in a pooled risk fund (PRF). The PRF was used to fund a portion of catastrophic patient care (i.e., care costing over $50,000). It was also used to fund unanticipated costs of hospital and specialists' services. Unused funds are returned to contributing physicians.

Bluechoice created a specialty comprehensive referral fund (CRF) for each physician's office. This fund was used to pay for the cost of each office's services provided by hospitals, specialists, and laboratories. The funds placed in the CRF were based on the anticipated usage of these services by each physician's patient group calculated using the patient's age, gender, and other factors. If a physician exhausted his or her CRF, then the 20% withheld from that physician's office, set aside in the PRF, was used to cover the costs. If the sum was exhausted, remaining PRF funds, contributed by other physicians, were used. If a surplus existed in the CRF at the end of the year, the primary care physicians split the surplus with Bluechoice, up to a maximum bonus of $50 per patient per year.[27] Depending on the HMO's finances and the clinical decisions made by physicians, Bluechoice paid primary care internists between $55,334 and $185,426.[28] The clinical decisions made by physicians on the scope and amount of services and referrals provided to their patients could increase their net income more than threefold.

The Physician's Perspective

In effect, doctors paid under risk-sharing arrangements participate in a kind of joint venture with HMOs. By keeping costs down for the HMO, doctors promote their own financial well-being. Dr. Robert Berenson, an internist, explained the effect well: "Long accustomed to providing too much . . . medical care, physicians now have powerful incentives to withhold [it]."[29] This is because risk sharing offers doctors no economic incentive to be aggressive in providing services and will even reduce their income as they increase the number of tests and procedures they order. Doctors make daily clinical decisions that can reduce the medical risk to patients but increase the costs of HMOs. Under risk-sharing arrangements they may be reluctant to do so. From the doctors' perspective, they are paying for part of every consultation, test, ancillary service, or hospital care a patient receives. Their share may be small, but the incentive can change perceptions.

Berenson recounts the change in attitude he underwent in caring for an elderly woman with a rare form of cancer when he was paid under risk-sharing arrangements. She represented an economic loss, and he "ended up resenting the seemingly unending medical needs of the patient and the continuing demands... [of] her distraught family."[30] The problem was not the patient's requests or performing the work. But under the risk-sharing system, very sick patients devastated his accounts. Risk sharing makes "patients who come in often for care from me . . . or who want a referral for specialty care begin to look like abusers."[31]

Many doctors adjust to these new financial rules. But others don't. Dr. Devra Marcus, a Washington internist, left her HMO practice just after joining. Her first two patients were diabetic, and she referred them to an ophthalmologist to check for retinal changes because diabetes can lead to blindness if not treated. Following these referrals, a colleague told her that her use of specialists would reduce her referral fund and could reduce her salary. "I pulled out. I didn't want to think about whether I would be losing money if I ordered an ophthalmologic consultation. I wanted to think about what was best for the patients."[32] Something is perverse in a payment system when it makes well-intentioned physicians look at sick patients they treat as a drain on their income.

Gauging the Effect of Financial Incentives

There is little hard data concerning the effects of financial incentives on physicians' clinical decisions. One study found no relation between distribution of risk-sharing bonuses and physicians' referral decisions. But paying physicians by capitation led to lower rates of hospitalization, and placing physicians at financial risk was associated with lower rates of outpatient visits.[33] HMO managers generally believe that the withholding of funds and bonuses affects doctors' clinical decisions. A 1989 survey of managing directors of 643 HMOs found that nearly four-fifths believed that withholding between 5 and 30% of payment would affect the volume of tests ordered and elective hospitalization, and nearly one-half believed that bonuses of between 5 and 15% would also affect clinical choices. Over one-third expressed concern about withholding payments of between 15 and 30%. But managers in general believed that the incentive payments used by *other* HMOs were more worrisome than the incentives they used.[34]

As we shall see in more detail later, several patients have sued HMOs, claiming that risk-sharing incentives led physicians to withhold necessary services to their detriment. And many anecdotes suggest cause for concern. In an article on HMOs "earning more for doing less," the Associated Press reported the example of Dr. Denise Hart, a nephrologist. She recalls a patient who had kidney failure and spent the night in a hospital without receiving dialysis or seeing a nephrologist because the HMO primary care physician denied authorization despite the emergency room physician's informing him of the urgency. During the night, the patient suffered from cardiac arrest and had to spend a week on a respirator.[35]

The *Chicago Tribune* reported the case of Daniel Bohnen, who was accidentally shot in the face with shot gun pellets. Shortly before he was scheduled for emergency surgery to repair his right eye, the HMO business office called and insisted that a consultant confirm the need for surgery. The surgeon warned the HMO that a delay would endanger Daniel's vision, but the HMO insisted on the second opinion, in the consultant's words, "to save money." The result: Daniel lost vision in one eye, and the HMO later paid Daniel's parents $1.2 million to settle a malpractice suit they brought.[36]

Presumably, HMO doctors serving as consultants, reviewers, and gatekeepers will place the patient's interest first, but the payment mechanism can define loyalties. Dr. J. Kristin Olson-Garewal, former medical director of University Family Care, an HMO in Tucson, Arizona, told of her role in convincing doctors to substitute less costly medications. Asked if this might conflict with her obligations as a physician she replied, "When I became the medical director, I represented the payment entity."[37]

In the absence of definitive data on the impact of risk-sharing incentive payments, we must draw inferences from what we know about the likely effects of incentives. In general, plans with strong financial incentives for reducing services are more likely to compromise physicians' loyalty to patients than plans with weak incentives. Incentives are strong in several circumstances: when physicians bear risk individually or in a small risk pool, when they are at risk for expensive services, when stop-risk protection starts at a high level, when HMOs link penalties and bonuses directly to individual clinical decisions, and when physicians risk losing or gaining a large percentage of their baseline income.

While it is relatively easy to isolate factors that affect the financial risk of physicians, it is hard to determine the dollar value to a physician of any incentive arrangement. Dollar value depends on several factors noted earlier: the size of the risk pool, the extent of risk sharing and stop loss, the services for which physicians bear risk, how the profit or loss is distributed, and whether there is profit and/or loss sharing.

Another reason why dollar value resists definition is that risk-sharing incentives do not reward physicians each time they forego a service or referral. Indeed, it is impossible to identify all the possible services physicians avoid. Nor do risk-sharing plans penalize physicians for each service they use. Rather, they pay out benefits or impose penalties only if doctors perform more than a specified number of medical procedures or make more than a specified number of referrals.

Even under incentive plans in which physicians bear risk individually, physicians cannot know whether or not they will be penalized until after there is a tallying of all their referrals, their patients hospitalized, their orders for tests, and so forth.

Even when a physician's utilization of services exceeds a threshold that triggers the financial incentive, the cost to the physician of a decision depends on the total volume of utilization. The same clinical decision has different financial implications depending on the choices the physician makes for all patients before and afterward. When risk-sharing plans spread risk among a group of physicians, it is very difficult, if not impossible, for physicians to predict the cost to them of performing a service. Together, these factors make it hard to determine precisely how strong an incentive there is for physicians to withhold a particular service.

Still other factors—for example, the level of fees, salary, or capitation rate paid by an HMO—can affect how physicians will respond to risk sharing. If the base level is low, physicians may be more sensitive to financial incentives than if the base level is high and allows them to earn a comfortable income without profit sharing or despite any financial penalties.[38] Some physicians also work exclusively for an HMO, while others do so only part-time and earn income from an outside practice. The more a physician relies on an outside practice for income, the smaller the bonus or penalty he or she will receive from the HMO and the less sensitive the physician will be to HMO financial incentives.

Despite the complexities of determining the effects of particular clinical choices under risk-sharing plans, physicians know that it is generally in their financial interest to limit the number of procedures, tests, and referrals. And even when the risk borne by individual physicians is small, incentives may create group pressure to use resources frugally, with ripple effects that spread beyond those caused by the financial incentive alone.[39] Most HMOs inform physicians when they deviate from the norm and use services heavily. The message is reinforced, explicitly and implicitly, on a regular basis. Physicians are also aware of the total amount of income they can gain or lose. One suspects that doctors contracting with or employed by an HMO will, with time, develop an intuitive sense of what style of medical practice best serves their interest. Their practice style will reflect the incentives offered by the HMOs.

Although economic theory suggests that strong incentives to reduce services place patients at greater risk than weak incentives, the effect of small incentives may outweigh their size, especially when applied to every clinical decision physicians make. Even small rewards can shift perceptions and attitudes. Payment also has symbolic value. It can bond physicians to payers, producing commitments disproportionate to the sums of money involved.

Hospitals and Financial Incentives

Until recently, hospitals had strong incentives to increase the number of services they provided and to disregard costs, since they were paid based on their cost of providing services. Medicare was particularly generous. In reimbursing hospitals for their costs, which included overhead and capital, Medicare fueled expansion and high utilization of services and technology.

But that situation has changed. Since 1983, Medicare has paid hospitals a set fee per patient, based on the doctor's diagnosis of the patient's illness using 486 Diagnosis Related Groups (DRG). The DRG payment is based on the average cost of treating the patients in each group of diagnoses.[40] Medicare makes an exception for unusually high-cost patients, paying one-half of the cost beyond the DRG payment. But in general, hospitals are at risk for the full costs of medical care. If their costs are, on average, higher than their revenues, the hospital will run a deficit. If, on average, hospitals keep their costs lower than revenues, they will profit. These changes reverse previous incentives and tilt it in the hospitals' interest to use resources frugally. Medicaid and most private insurers have not yet adopted similar fixed payment systems. But they now monitor hospital charges closely and refuse to pay for services they believe are inappropriate or could be just as well delivered at lower cost outside the hospital.

The economic interests of hospitals and physicians are often at odds with each other.[41] Most physicians are still paid for each service and have an incentive to increase services. Physicians are not financially responsible for hospital costs, although they contribute to them by using hospital facilities and making routine clinical decisions, such as ordering tests and deciding when to discharge patients. In response, hospitals now encourage physicians to take account of the hospitals' financial interests in practicing medicine. Hospitals often inform physicians of treatment costs, especially when physicians make clinical decisions that cost the hospital more than the average amount.[42] When they do, studies show doctors order fewer and less costly diagnostic tests.[43] Hospitals monitor physicians and use persuasion to encourage frugality.

Hospitals have also devised programs that encourage physicians to reduce the services they provide. These include physician investment and self-referral in joint ventures, hospital purchases of physicians' practices, and physician recruitment and bonding programs. Variations of these practices include plans that make direct incentive payments to physicians, joint ventures with hospital staffs, physician ownership of hospitals through limited partnership and evaluation of the doctor's economic performance, a process called *economic credentialing*.[44]

One of the most criticized hospital incentive plans is one devised for doctors by the Paracelsus Healthcare Corporation at its Hollywood Community Hospital in 1985. What made the Paracelsus cost containment strategy different from others is that any resulting hospital profit was shared with the physicians. The hospital shared with physicians the difference between hospital charges, based on costs, and the Medicare DRG payment. The greater the hospital profit per patient, the larger the physician incentive premium. Payments to physicians were based on a sliding scale. They would range from 10% to 20% of the difference between the hospital's retail charges and the Medicare DRG payment.[45] In short, doctors gained income if they provided less treatment, discharged patients earlier, or simply used resources more efficiently.

Initially, the California State Board of Medical Quality Assurance reviewed the program and found it to be legal. But the AMA and other critics charged that the Paracelsus plan provided too strong an incentive to withhold appropriate medical care, and it was discontinued after government investigations.[46] Congress later enacted legislation that prohibited hospitals receiving Medicare funds from making payments that gave physicians an incentive to reduce medical care for an individual patient.[47]

A number of other hospitals have become interested in incentive plans. Central DuPage Hospital in Infield, Illinois, made plans to develop a deferred compensation plan using incentives for reducing care. The hospital planned to pay physicians additional compensation based on their performance and several other criteria, including average length of patient stay and use of ancillary services for each patient. Each physician's "efficiency" performance would be compared to the revenues generated by treating patients. Physicians using fewer resources than average, or discharging patients earlier than average, would receive credit. The compensation was to be invested by the hospital and paid upon each physician's retirement; however, it was never put into effect.

Under another physician incentive plan—the so-called Medical Staff Hospital (MeSH) joint venture—the hospital would make incentive payments to physicians. As proposed, the medical staff would form a joint venture with the hospital. The hospital would make incentive payments to physicians if the cost of treating Medicare patients were less than a certain percentage of costs.[48] The incentive for reducing services would be spread across the medical staff, presumably diluting the incentive for each physician individually.

Hospitals and medical staff often undertake joint ventures. Such ventures have certain common features. They "harmonize the economic interest of hospitals and physicians," according to Robert Rosenfield, a lawyer who specializes in these issues.[49] Hospitals use these ventures to acquire or "capture" the loyalty of local physicians who control admissions and utilization of medical services.[50] One wonders how patients will fare if their interests conflict with those of physicians and hospitals once the latter two are "harmonized."

Hospitals also try to influence physicians by hiring medical staff organizations as part of a utilization review program. The organization reviews records to determine the appropriateness of admissions and treatment and to teach physicians how to reduce unnecessary use of resources. Sometimes hospitals pay physicians on the basis of their cost savings, thus giving physicians an incentive to reduce their use of resources.[51]

Another tactic is for privately owned hospitals to syndicate themselves and sell shares to local physicians.[52] Physician investment takes several forms. Frequently, a hospital corporation will retain a majority share in the facility and sell off the remainder as limited partnerships to local physicians. In other cases, hospital employees own shares through employee stock ownership plans.[53] Physician owners have an incentive to admit patients to the hospital but also to reduce the services they provide to Medicare patients because their payment is fixed in advance.

Still another emerging trend is for hospitals to deny or revoke admitting privileges of physicians, based on the expense to hospitals of their clinical decisions.[54] Though an indirect measure, the power to cut off the means to a livelihood is a serious economic threat. In the past, hospital by-laws only authorized the administration to grant and revoke medical staff privileges on the basis of clinical competence and the quality of medical care. Now many hospitals are evaluating physicians in financial terms. Some lawyers recommend that hospitals revise their by-laws and their credentialing process to give them the power to deny, limit, or revoke privileges to physicians whose clinical decisions result in hospitals losing money or earning little money under Medicare's prospective payment system.[55] The lawyers suggest that hospitals develop economic profiles of physicians by compiling information about patients' average length of stay. Hospitals could conceivably terminate physicians who deviate from an acceptable standard.[56]

An American Hospital Association (AHA) study indicates that a negligible number of hospitals—only 1%—have by-laws that require physicians applying for admitting privileges to submit information on the cost effectiveness of the medical care they provide. Slightly more hospitals use financial profiles based on cost of treatment in renewing physicians' privileges. But some commentators believe these programs are destined to grow significantly in the future. The programs typically look at patients' length of stay, the volume of medical tests the physician ordered, and the use of other resources that affect hospitals' costs. Despite the label *cost-effective*, the programs generally do not examine the clinical impact of resource decisions. In effect, they evaluate physicians for behavior that reduces costs, with little attention to benefits.

Hospitals also provide incentives for physicians to use resources frugally through their bonding program, as described in Chapters 3 and 4. Bonding programs include recruitment incentives, income guarantees, rent subsidies, advertising, patient referral programs, and in-kind services. They seek loyalty from physicians with admitting privileges. Although bonding programs do not specifically reward physicians for reducing medical services, they indebt physicians to hospitals for income and thereby encourage them to promote the hospitals' goals. Bonding programs have traditionally been used to induce patient admissions. But this situation is changing. In some cases, such as patient referral programs, hospitals already explicitly exclude so called high-cost physicians.[57] With the increasing emphasis on containing hospital costs, physicians indebted to hospitals are apt to provide fewer services to Medicare patients and to discharge them earlier.

6

The Dangers of Incentives to Decrease Services and the Ineffectiveness of Current Responses

It is one thing to entrust your life and health at times of crisis to a physician who is committed to the practical ethics that involves a quest for excellence and who may err on the side of doing too much. It is quite another to entrust your life and health at times of crisis to a physician whose diagnostic and therapeutic intervention are limited by the new regulatory constraints or incentives of competitive efficiency that "place the provider at economic risk"[1] (Alan Stone).

A physician having a financial interest in decreasing utilization of premium dollars would have the appearance, if not the reality, of being a self-serving denial-of-care agent for the benefit of the "buyer" of care seeking "cost control" to the "healthcare industry"[2] (Robert Geist).

The Dangers of Financial Incentives

Both Health Maintenance Organizations (HMOs) and hospitals have developed strong long-term organizational and financial ties with physicians that enable them to influence their clinical decisions. As we have seen, they often use financial incentives to manage physicians' behavior and cut costs. Many incentives can promote patients' welfare or at least have no detrimental effect. But there are HMO risk-sharing and hospital incentive plans that encourage physicians to reduce the number of services they provide. They compromise physicians' loyalty to patients and reduce their independent judgment. These problems are not minor. They are growing more serious, and regulatory measures are not yet coping with them adequately.

The Corrosive Effects of Risk-Sharing Incentives

Society makes a statement about the role of physicians when it provides incentives for them to help government or health care organizations reduce their costs. This is especially so if there are no equivalent financial incentives for physicians to improve quality of care. By using financial incentives to change the clinical practice of physicians, society calls forth self-interested behavior. In asking physicians to consider their own interest in deciding how to act, we alter the attitude we want physicians ideally to have. For if physicians act intuitively to promote their patients' interests, we will worry less that they will behave inappropriately. But if their motivation is primarily self-interest, we will want their behavior to be monitored more carefully.

Incentives also undermine other practices, such as informed consent. Law and ethics now require physicians to inform patients of the risks, benefits, and any alternatives of proposed treatment or nontreatment. To fulfill this role, physicians must provide patients with disinterested assessment and advice. Rewarding physicians for reducing services, however, tends to compromise their ability to give disinterested advice. It is likely to shape their views of what kinds of activities are desirable.[3] Even if most individual doctors rise above the lure of incentives and provide good advice, patients will still have reasons to doubt their neutrality. This suspicion alone weakens the informed consent process, for it requires communication, cooperation, and trust between patient and physician. If patients doubt the neutrality of their doctors, that process is impaired.

Physicians, like others, will always have private interests that may influence their judgment. But we can encourage institutions to temper self-interest, channel it in socially desirable ways, and counter it.

The Problem with Hospital Incentives to Physicians

Hospitalized patients rely on physicians to act on their behalf more than other patients do. Usually weak or severely ill, they lack the autonomy of those living outside of hospitals. Ordinarily, they cannot switch physicians in midtreatment. When hospitals pay physicians to promote the hospital's financial goals, this compromises physicians' loyalty to vulnerable patients.

Hospitals enjoy an advantage over patients in competing for the loyalty of physicians. Patients consult doctors when they have a medical problem—just once in a while. Physicians have many patients, and each patient can augment a doctor's income by only a small amount compared to the total earned. The economic influence each patient exerts over a physician is usually small. And so, physicians have to divide their loyalty, or at least their time, between patients.

But the relation between hospitals and physicians is entirely different. Most physicians have frequent, ongoing, and long-term relations with just a few hospitals.[4] Hospitals depend on physicians to admit patients, and many physicians, in turn, need hospital privileges to earn their livelihood. Physicians' clinical decisions affect hospital costs, hospital referrals, and other economic ties, which can, in turn, benefit physicians.

Hospitals and physicians increasingly depend on each other for employment and income and rely on each other's cooperation. Despite tensions that can emerge between hospitals and doctors, their relationship is one of economic symbiosis. Each party must work with, watch, court, and cater to the other. It is essential to both parties to promote good long-term relations with the other. Even though physicians are expected to be loyal to patients, hospitals have far greater leverage over physicians' decisions than do patients and far greater economic clout.

These factors skew the relationship between hospitals, physicians, and patients in favor of common interests between hospitals and physician. As a result, hospitals and physicians often do not fully respect the rights of patients. The hospital has even been called a "human rights wasteland."[5] Hospital incentive plans did not create this structural imbalance between hospitals, physicians, and patients, but they are not neutral. They undermine physician loyalty to patients even further.

Are Physician Incentives Effective or Necessary?

Many HMO managers fear that without economic incentives for reducing the use of services, nothing will ensure that physicians use resources prudently.[6] They say that other approaches, such as administrative monitoring and penalties for overuse, are less effective.[7] They also discount the possibility that these incentives will encourage physicians to provide too few services. Peer review and quality assurance programs, they argue, identify and deter underservice.[8]

Such reasoning is suspect and prompts questions. If incentives to provide services cause physicians to use too many resources and to perform unnecessary procedures, would not incentives to reduce services result in too few services? If financial incentives encourage physicians to reduce their services, how can we be sure physicians will reduce only unnecessary or wasteful services? Why should incentives have negative effects in one respect and not the other?

Moreover, if peer review and quality assurance review programs can adequately control underservice, why can they not adequately control overuse? If administrative reviews of physicians' practices effectively identify and limit one kind of practice, then they should prove effective in the other. And if they are ineffective in one setting, why should we not suspect their efficacy in the other?

No substantial evidence supports the claim that incentive plans are necessary to control use of services. The first HMOs did not use financial incentives to reduce the volume of services, and they significantly reduced hospitalization—with no discernible harm to patients.[9] Incentive plans did not even exist a few years ago. Other more suitable methods for controlling unnecessary use of services exist; new ones can be developed.

Proponents of risk sharing acknowledge that *strong* incentives can produce negative effects, and would prohibit them. However, there is no natural or easily identifiable threshold level for determining when incentives become too strong. Moreover, there are great obstacles to regulating risk-sharing and incentive plans based on the amount of risk borne. The danger of particular arrangements depends on the probability and extent of risk. Both are influenced by many factors—not their broad structural features. So many different variations of risk-sharing plans exist that it would be impractical to evaluate each one, to distinguish the acceptable from the unacceptable, and harder still to monitor and regulate them—a quagmire of unknown dimensions.

Proponents argue also that the negative effects of incentives can be mitigated by spreading the total risk among a pool of physicians and limiting the risk assumed by any individual.[10] These measures could reduce the size of the incentive and prevent its undue influence. Here, too, proponents of risk sharing want to have it both ways. They argue that if incentives are weak, no harm will be done. But even if weak, incentives will—they say—produce desirable changes in physician behavior. However, if incentives are strong enough to produce desirable changes, they could produce *undesirable* changes.[11]

Financial Incentives That Help Patients

Not all physician incentives are undesirable. Incentives rewarding behavior that promotes patients' interests should be encouraged. So should incentives that promote other desirable goals and do not compromise loyalty to patients. For example, HMOs and hospitals can use financial incentives to encourage physicians to provide high-quality care, devote extra hours of service, perform particularly hard or unpleasant work, produce high patient satisfaction, undertake research or publications, develop their skill and competence, or assume essential administrative duties.

HMOs and hospitals might also use incentives to encourage physicians to practice efficiently, that is, use the fewest resources needed to achieve a result. Many HMOs and hospitals claim they do just that. Their incentives, however, are usually designed only to reduce expenditures, which does not necessarily make a practice more efficient—it may reduce the benefits. Incentives to reduce the volume of services do not target waste. They discourage all services, not just inappropriate ones. To encourage efficient physician practices, HMOs should offer incentives directed to particular practices.

Effective incentive plans could build on existing peer review programs. Hospitals employ Peer Review Oranizations (PROs) to review patients' charts and evaluate the appropriateness of medical care. Often, third-party payers will deny payment for inappropriate medical procedures. HMOs use quality assurance programs to identify inappropriate underuse of medical care. Hospitals and HMOs could hire evaluators to review patients' charts and identify both inappropriate provision and denial of services. HMOs and third-party payers could then pay physicians bonuses if they made no, or very few, errors and impose penalties for overuse and underuse of services. Such incentives would discourage both skimping and waste, would reward physicians for providing good medical care, and would not undermine fidelity to patients. Reviewers could be independent experts unaffiliated with the hospital or HMO; the identity of the physicians evaluated should be kept confidential.

At least two Independent Practice Association (IPA) HMOs, U.S. Healthcare and Av-Med, have developed physician payment plans that include incentives both for reducing utilization and for promoting some measure of quality in care.[12] The plans attempt to counter incentives for quality care with incentives for reducing services and are therefore preferable to incentives for reducing services alone. But neither program balances both incentives equally.

U.S. Healthcare has used several variations on its quality incentive formula. Initially it paid primary care physicians by capitation. The payment plan included two main components: incentives for reducing services and incentives for so-called quality measures. The lower the volume of services each physician performed, the higher the capitation rate and the more frequently it was paid. The capitation rate was also adjusted upward or downward based on quality of care. Quality was measured by a review of medical records, results of patient satisfaction surveys, transfer rates out of physicians' offices, and what the IPA called an assessment of physicians' "managed-care philosophy."

U.S. Healthcare reviewed medical records to determine whether physicians immunized infants, measured the blood pressure of high-risk individuals, and screened for high cholesterol. The patient survey asked about physician availability, waiting time, patient satisfaction with office personnel, and whether the physician appeared concerned with patient welfare. Physicians received high or low scores in managed-care philosophy, depending on whether they used preventive care programs, participated in quality-assurance advisory or membership committees, and helped patients receive high-quality care.

This program was headed in the right direction, but incentives were still skewed.[13] Physicians were not penalized for reducing services inappropriately, except for a few specified services included in the quality measures. There were too few of these measures, so inappropriate reduction of services was still rewarded. Incentives to reduce services overshadowed incentives to increase them. U.S. Healthcare's quality incentives encouraged only low-cost services, such as immunization or testing for cholesterol level and blood pressure in high-risk groups. No direct financial incentive spurred the use of valuable but costly services. Moreover, many of the incentives for quality focused on patient satisfaction and participation in quality-review administrative work, which do not involve rewards for physicians providing services. Such incentives do not counteract conflicts of interest that discourage referrals to specialists and hospitals. They simply add incentives to provide patients with different low-cost services and keep them satisfied.

Measures of patient satisfaction and transfer rates out of a practice provide some useful information to HMOs and can indicate quality problems. But they are also marketing tactics. They do not touch the most crucial aspects of medical care, and they do not encourage the provision of services most likely to be reduced by physician risk sharing. They do encourage physicians to play a role that sociologist Erving Goffman calls "cooling out the mark" (i.e., acting to reduce the client's anger and frustration).[14] Physicians may please patients by reducing office waiting time and adopting a friendly, caring manner. They can help to prevent patients from choosing another provider due to frustrations with the HMO, perhaps because of reduced services. Incentives to keep patients satisfied are generally desirable.[15] But when used in conjunction with incentives to reduce services, they may help cover up, rather than eliminate, inappropriate reductions in medical care.

In 1992, U.S. Healthcare adopted a more complex compensation formula.[16] Multiple factors affect the payment doctors will receive, including quality measures. Still, each doctor's capitation rate can be adjusted upward by 5% if his or her patient's use of hospitals, specialists, and emergency rooms is low and downward by 2.5% if utilization exceeds targets. As with the previous formula, quality measures provide some check on utilization. But there are still stronger incentives to use services frugally.

Incentives for Physicians to Allocate Scarce Resources

Using markets and administrative mechanisms, society limits the resources used for medical care. Budget constraints impinge on social goals. Increasingly, spending more on medicine requires spending less on other desirable social goods, and—beyond a certain point—further spending for medicine produces diminishing returns. Physicians are strategically situated to help society control medical expenditures because their clinical choices affect the allocation of resources. But resource allocation is at odds with physicians' traditional obligation: to act in the interests of their patients.

Physicians can play three distinct roles: (1) they can act as ideal fiduciaries, promoting their patients' interests without regard to those of other parties;[17] (2) they can act as neutral resource allocators, distributing resources to maximize social benefit or promote some principle of fairness; and (3) they can promote their own financial interests or those of third parties, such as HMOs or hospitals. Medical ethics adjures physicians to act as their patients' agents. But the world of practice is not compartmentalized, and most physicians perform all three conflicting roles at different times.

As ideal fiduciaries, physicians have to promote the interests of their immediate patients even if the same resources could produce more good for still other patients. But physicians who treat a group of patients in triage or under severe budget constraints usually focus treatment on a few because very ill patients will die regardless of treatment, and patients with minor problems will survive and heal even if treatment is delayed or foregone. Doctors treat first those patients who would die without medical intervention. In triage, physicians' obligations to promote the best interests of each patient conflict with their obligation to care for all patients. Here, doctors must balance the interests of one patient against those of others.

Some countries control medical spending by imposing regional or hospital budgets that place physicians in a position similar to triage. Some Canadian provinces, for example, assign hospitals a budget for all patient care. To stay within the budget, hospitals set their own priorities on allocating funds. In this system, doctors have to consider the good of patients collectively. This arrangement also prevails in Britain, where doctors have to make difficult decisions on how to use resources because the National Health Service has a limited budget.[18] Physicians working in staff model HMOs occupy a similar position. With limited resources, they must make difficult choices in caring for their patients. Too many resources donated to one kind of care or patient will leave less available to others or even threaten the solvency of the HMO.

Physicians caring for a group of patients under budgetary constraints cannot act as ideal fiduciaries; they are expected to adjudicate the allocation of resources. Even though this creates risks for patients, it also provides benefits. In theory, clinical choices and allocative choices are distinct; in practice, they merge. If physicians don't act as allocators, others will. This will constrain clinical choices and interfere with physician discretion. But since medicine constantly involves uncertainty, tradeoffs, and conflicting goals, the art of doctoring requires discretion and subtlety of judgment.

To illustrate the risk to patients, consider a range of ways to pay physicians and the resource allocation roles they perform along a continuum from 1 to 6 (Table 6-1). At one end (1), the physician is a nearly perfect agent for a single patient, acting solely on his or her behalf. At the other (6), the physician is an agent whose clinical decisions are highly self-interested. Between these extremes are several intermediate positions.

Physicians can work for several patients (2). Here, the interests of one patient may conflict with another's, putting a doctor in the middle. For example, if a physician treating two patients must decide which one to admit to the one bed remaining in the intensive care unit, he or she is forced to choose between them, and the medical prognosis alone may not dictate an answer.

Further along the continuum (3), the physician serves as an agent for patients and for society. When a doctor treats many patients subject to a budget, then society is, in effect, asking the doctor to allocate resources. The physician must decide which medical care should be a priority and which must come second.

Next on the scale (4) is the salaried physician, paid by a hospital or a private firm to offer medical care to its patients or employees, or remunerated by an insurance company to offer care to insured parties. In each instance, the physician is subject to pressure to limit medical interventions in order to protect the resources of the payer and has conflicts of interest.

In (5), the payer hires the physician to provide medical services and offers incentives to reduce the use of resources. The physician is actually rewarded for limiting services.

At the end of the continuum (6), the physician is paid a set fee per patient to provide all the medical care that is necessary and bears full risk for the cost. Here, each time they make a clinical decision, physicians must balance their own interests against those of patients.

Some people say that if it is acceptable for physicians to help allocate resources, then encouraging them to do so with financial incentives is also acceptable. But the risks to patients are less onerous when physicians do not have a personal stake in the choices they make.

Table 6-1. Physician Payment Continuum

1	2	3	4	5	6
Salary paid to care for one patient.	Salary paid to care for many patients.	Salary paid by government. Physician administers budget for a group of patients.	Salary paid by providers or payers. Physician provides medical services to patients.	Physician paid by providers or payers with financial incentives to reduce expenditures.	Physician paid a set fee per patient and bears the full risk of providing medical services.

To the extent that physicians allocate scarce medical resources to promote their appropriate, efficient, and just use, they perform this role better when they do not have financial incentives to reduce services. This helps ensure that physicians are neutral and do not make rationing decisions for their own private gain. Physicians practicing under budget constraints can act as disinterested judges of conflicting claims and promote the welfare of individual patients to the extent possible when the welfare of other patients is considered.[19] The situation is different, though, when HMOs pay physicians to limit the use of resources. Physicians in that case are encouraged to use their own well-being as a criterion in making difficult medical allocation choices.[20] This tips the scales against patients. Doctors are then more likely to limit medical care to increase their income.[21] If society or HMOs need to limit resources, why not do so by using explicit, publicly agreed-upon criteria based on some sense of fairness, patient need, or social priority rather than rely on decisions of individual physicians skewed by considerations of personal gain?

Countering Financial Incentives:
Peer Review and Quality Assurance

Federal law requires that hospitals receiving Medicare funds use PROs to ensure quality of care. Similarly, federally qualified HMOs must have quality assurance programs. In addition, many hospitals, HMOs, and third-party payers have their own peer review and quality assurance programs. All aim to identify and eliminate practices that cause poor quality of care, including underservice. Proponents of physician incentives think that such review mechanisms can assure the quality of medical care and counteract any adverse effects of financial incentives.[22] Peer review and quality assurance programs are relatively new and rapidly changing, so it may be premature to criticize them.[23] But experiences with two kinds of regulatory controls—Physician Standard Review Organizations (PSROs), the precursor of PROs, and certificate-of-need laws—indicate that the prospects are not encouraging.[24]

Created by the federal government in the 1970s, PSROs were intended to reduce excessive use of medical services by monitoring and reviewing physicians' clinical decisions. They assessed the appropriateness of hospital care received by Medicare and Medicaid beneficiaries. Federal and state certificate-of-need laws regulated the expansion of hospitals and other medical facilities. State agencies, prompted by federal law and funding, established a regulatory apparatus to control hospital growth.

As we saw in Chapter 4, both programs, which countered financial incentives to provide services and expand facilities, produced disappointing results.[25] More recent utilization review programs have had more success; they are operated by insurers, employers, and HMOs that control physician reimbursement. As such, they have an incentive to ferret out unnecessary medical services. However, quality assurance programs are less likely to prevent underuse of medical services. Insurers, employers, and hospitals with a high percentage of Medicare patients lack a direct financial incentive to eliminate underservice.[26] Providers and insurers will probably concentrate on activities that more directly affect their short-run profits.

The Limitations of Professional Review Organizations and Quality Assurance Programs

Quality assurance technology remains undeveloped. Its methods, derived from tools intended to control excessive use, are still evolving.[27]

The underuse of medical service takes several forms. They include insufficient medical care, tardy treatment, and inappropriate treatment settings.[28] As yet, no single method can measure the various dimensions of underuse. Some analysts even doubt that a single measure can be found.[29] The Institute of Medicine (IOM) has concluded that existing technology limits what PROs can accomplish.[30]

Underuse is often more difficult to detect than overuse. Overuse leaves a record of medical intervention that can be evaluated. With underuse, there is often no record—or an inadequate one. If a primary care physician does not record symptoms suggesting the need for medical tests, referrals, or treatment, reviewers will be unable to identify errors of judgment. Likewise, when doctors do not order clinical tests or do not consult specialists, there is less evidence of inadequate care.

The problems are magnified because Medicare and PROs pay close attention to controlling utilization and costs, a focus that can conflict with ensuring quality of care.[31] For example, Medicare carriers and intermediaries usually monitor physicians with atypical billing practices, which are not a good indicator of medical quality problems. With few exceptions, PROs cannot review patients' complaints of underuse but can investigate complaints of overuse.[32] Yet a report commissioned by the IOM suggests that there is more underuse of medical care among the elderly than overuse.[33] Some PROs have even expressed concern about service underuse that they are unable to track.[34]

PROs concentrate almost exclusively on hospital care, thereby excluding quality-of-care issues arising outside of hospitals. In HMO risk-sharing contracts, PROs do examine some outpatient cases, but these are only a small percentage of their cases. PROs also focus on individual cases of hospital care, rarely evaluating general hospital practices.

Reviewers are often not neutral parties. Many private sector programs are financed by, and cater to, the interests of employers or insurers. They emphasize reducing costs over increasing quality. Many HMOs (especially IPA HMOs) employ their own physicians to conduct peer review, but such physicians obviously have an interest in bolstering their HMO's financial performance. This is especially true of HMOs that reward physicians for reducing utilization of services.

Medicare employs an independent contractor called the *SuperPRO*, and an internal management system called *PROMPTS-2*, to review the performance of PROs.[35] Both examine how well PROs evaluate cases. But neither SuperPRO nor PROMPTS-2 evaluates whether PROs correctly identify which cases to review for quality problems.[36] A 1988 Government Accounting Office (GAO) study of Medicare's quality assurance programs reports that PROs use methods of dubious validity and that their data may not be accurate.[37] No independent evaluation has yet determined how effectively PROs identify quality problems or whether they improve practitioner performance. Nor, contrary to hopes, have PROs demonstrated any impact on the quality of care.[38]

Several organizational problems suggest that PROs do not adequately monitor quality or protect patients from underservice. Medicare does not coordinate the activities of fiscal intermediaries, insurance carriers, and PROs. Each has developed independent standards and review practices; there is no agreed-upon method to report quality problems to PROs or other government agencies.[39] The GAO reports that PROs lack institutional mechanisms to improve the performance of providers when they identify poor quality.[40] The IOM found that PRO intervention for serious problems are largely ineffective.

As early as 1987, a Senate report found that some HMOs, contracting with Medicare under its risk-contracting program, provided poor quality of care and did not implement quality assurance programs. The report also found that the Health Care Financing Administration and other government agencies did not adequately monitor HMOs for underservice and other quality problems.[41]

A recent study of quality assurance commissioned by the IOM confirms that HMOs have problems.[42] Many lack adequate management information systems and claims processing procedures to track data, and the data they use often lack integrity. The medical director in charge of utilization review programs may have little influence on the HMO decisions that affect quality. Many HMOs also fail to give adequate feedback to physicians on their performance. In general, HMOs accord low priority to quality assurance, because it has little direct impact on their financial performance.[43] They often fail to implement effectively their quality assurance plans.[44] It is prudent to be wary of descriptions of how quality assurance plans are supposed to work when such descriptions are not verified.[45]

The Limitations of Current Law

In 1973 and 1982 federal statutes and regulations gave qualified HMOs the option of sharing risk with physicians as part of their required program to control costs and utilization of services.[46] Medicare, in particular, has a *risk-contract* program for HMOs that allows them to allot part of their financial risk to affiliated doctors. The risk-contract program takes its name from the way the HMOs, not physicians, are paid. Medicare pays participating HMOs 95% of the adjusted average per capita costs to the Medicare program of beneficiaries in the HMO region. Since HMOs generally have lower costs than average, this provides them an incentive to participate in the program. Nonparticipating HMOs that have Medicare patients are paid on a fee-for-service basis. Several states also explicitly allow HMOs to establish risk-sharing arrangements.[47]

In general, federal and state policies have initially tolerated, and even encouraged, risk-sharing arrangements with doctors, although some states are considering legislation that would require HMOs to disclose these incentives.[48] However, in 1986 Congress enacted legislation prohibiting HMOs that participate in the Medicare risk-contract program from using financial incentives to induce physicians to limit services.[49] The legislation was also applicable to other managed-care providers similar to HMOs called *competitive medical plans.*[50]

HMOs and insurers with managed-care plans opposed these provisions and succeeded three times in getting Congress to defer the date for putting them into effect. In 1990 the HMO and managed-care industry was able to convince key legislators that physician risk sharing posed only minor hazards to patients, especially if risk-sharing plans adopted certain protective measures. Congress rescinded the prohibition on incentives to reduce services, except for one egregious kind described below. Congress also required the Secretary of Health and Human Services to regulate physician risk sharing to reduce dangers to patients.[51]

The law now prevents HMOs participating in the Medicare risk-contract program (or managed-care providers in a similar *cost program*) from issuing specific incentive payments to physicians as inducements to reduce medical care to individual patients. It prohibits incentive arrangements analogous to those made by the Paracelsus Hospital for reducing services to individuals by splitting the Diagnosis Related Group (DRG) payment with physicians (described in Chapter 5). Even the most ardent proponents of incentives and HMO risk sharing now concede that this incentive is too strong, too direct, and too immediate to be used safely.

Whatever other considerations may have been involved, these concessions by the HMO and managed-care industry constituted good tactical moves to preserve risk sharing. No HMOs have used these directly targeted incentive payments. HMOs and the managed-care industry have shunned the use of one payment, offered to one physician, to reduce care to one patient. The law thus prohibits an abuse, albeit one that has never occurred.

The new law allows any risk sharing by primary care physicians or physician groups for their own services. However, it requires the Department of Health and Human Services to regulate providers that make primary care physicians bear "substantial" financial risk for the cost of hospital care, services of specialists, and other services. In the past, the department has expressed the view that physician risk sharing is not a problem. That attitude was maintained, in December 1992, when the Department of Health and Human Services proposed regulations.[52]

These regulations would limit the amount of risk that an HMO or other managed care organization can make physicians bear for the cost of services they recommend but that are provided by other parties. If the organization makes incentive payments to doctors no more than once a year, it would be barred from making doctors responsible for over 30%

of the cost of referral services. If the incentive payments are tendered more frequently, organizations would not be allowed to make doctors responsible for more than 20% of the cost of the referral services.

The rule would also require some organizations participating in these programs to conduct yearly surveys to learn whether members were satisfied with the care they received and whether they believed they had been denied care. However, only organizations that place doctors at risk for more than 25% of their compensation, if paid annually, or 15% of their compensation, if paid more frequently, would have to make such surveys.

The proposed regulations would do little to protect patients from most existing risk sharing arrangements. Indeed, Erling Hansen, general counsel for the Group Health Association of America, a HMO trade group, says that "these rules are not intended to modify industry practice or physician behavior."[53]

Furthermore, the statute and regulations are not comprehensive in scope. They apply only to HMOs and managed-care providers participating in a few Medicare and Medicaid programs. The programs cover 5% of Medi-care beneficiaries and 3% of managed-care members nationwide. Approximately 1.3 million people are enrolled in plans that are subject to such federal regulation.[54] Moreover, most patients are enrolled in HMOs that do not ask physicians to bear the risk of other providers and are not subject to the regulations.

Federal policy on hospital incentive payments to physicians is also only partial. In response to the Paracelsus incentive plan discussed earlier, Congress prohibited hospitals receiving Medicare funds from splitting Medicare DRG payments with physicians or from rewarding individual physicians for withholding medical care from individual patients.[55]

However, no restrictions exist for hospital plans, either current or in the offing, that provide other incentives to reduce services. For example, hospital corporations can still bring in physicians as limited partners and physician investors have incentives to reduce services for Medicare patients because the hospital receives a fixed fee.

The percentage of the population that is elderly and covered by the Medicare program is growing. Therefore, incentives for physicians to reduce hospital services will become more significant over time. Many private insurers are already setting limits on fees they pay hospitals; the trend is likely to continue.

Common Law Suits as Remedies

Although some plaintiffs have brought lawsuits involving physicians' conflicts of interest, courts have not yet developed a body of law addressing these problems. Several private lawsuits for civil damages have challenged HMO risk-sharing arrangements. So far, most of these suits have been settled out of court, and so they provide no legal precedent. Others are still being litigated or have failed. Attempts to challenge risk-sharing arrangements illustrate two points: first, judge-made law lacks a framework designed to regulate physicians' conflicts of interest; second, aggrieved HMO members face sizable obstacles when challenging risk sharing arrangements under existing laws.

One of the more interesting lawsuits illustrating these trends is *Teti v. U.S. Healthcare*, which was brought on behalf of all enrollees in U.S. Healthcare, a national HMO (see Chapter 5). The suit challenged U.S. Healthcare's policy of requiring its physicians to share part of the financial risk of referrals to specialists and hospitals. The plaintiffs claimed that this practice provided physicians with financial incentives that "compromised the[ir] independent medical judgment . . ., thereby resulting in a substantial diminution in the quality and comprehensiveness of health care services available."[56] They declared that U.S. Healthcare had breached its contract and did not provide the comprehensive services promised. They also argued that U.S. Healthcare did not disclose these incentive arrangements to prospective members, and that this constituted fraud and violated state consumer protection and unfair trade practice laws, as well as the Racketeer Influence and Corrupt Organizations Act of 1970 (RICO).

Current law lacks a conflict-of-interest standard for physicians. The U.S. Healthcare plaintiffs could not challenge the legality of physician risk sharing directly because the federal HMO statute explicitly allows such arrangements, as do some state statutes. Nor could they directly challenge the legality of physicians receiving incentive payments. No statutes, regulations, or court decisions discuss the legal relations between physicians and patients using a conflict-of-interest framework. To the extent that the law addresses physicians' conflicts of interest at all, it considers them as problems in isolation. A further obstacle is that HMO members contract with the HMO, not with physicians. This may preclude them legally from raising objections to payments of doctors by HMOs.

The plaintiffs, therefore, used an indirect approach. They claimed that the public enrolled in U.S. Healthcare based on incomplete, misleading, and false information; had prospective members been informed of the risk-sharing incentives, they would not have joined. Such claims might have convinced the judge to rule in favor of Teti but would not set a precedent that forced HMOs to eliminate risk sharing. If courts require HMOs to disclose details of risk-sharing plans to prospective members, some HMOs might discontinue such practices. But more will probably reveal the information in ways that discount the risk, thereby calming members.

U.S. Healthcare has recently changed its physician compensation package.[57] Incentives to reduce services still exist but now appear more palatable because other incentives spur quality of care. Disclosure of incentives may enlighten members as to the limits of their physicians' loyalty, but it will not protect them from abuses. If risk sharing in HMOs remains pervasive, patients will have few options.

The plaintiff's lawyers in *Teti* relied on fraud, consumer protection, and RICO legislation that was not directed specifically to the problems of patients but is part of contemporary commercial law. The court found their claims insufficient to allow the case to proceed to trial.[58] The attorneys might have relied on legal principles governing fiduciary relations in other settings, or they could have drawn analogies to similar conflict-of-interest problems in other areas of law. They might even have asserted new claims or rights. Judges can create new remedies when existing ones are inadequate. The strategy of the *Teti* lawyers reflected the law's conservatism. Lawyers trying to advance their clients' interests usually assert well-tested claims; these have a greater chance of success.

Recent Malpractice Lawsuits

In the late 1970s and early 1980s, lawsuits against HMOs alleging bad faith denials of promised benefits proliferated.[59] In 1987, however, the Supreme Court eliminated this option for individuals covered by group insurance. In *Pilot Life Insurance Company v. Dedeaux*, it ruled that the Employment Retirement Insurance Security Act (ERISA) preempted state consumer laws and common law remedies—including bad faith breach-of-contract claims—against health insurers and HMOs.[60] Since then, aggrieved HMO members have used other strategies. Now they claim that HMOs are liable on three grounds: that physicians are their agents; that HMOs failed to supervise physicians; and that HMO policies caused physicians to commit malpractice.[61]

In a pathbreaking case, *Wickline v. State of California*, the court ruled that when third-party payers deny medical treatment inappropriately, they are responsible for consequential harm done to patients.[62] Imposing liability on HMOs for negligence caused by risk-sharing plans would merely extend the holding in *Wickline*. Several patients have already pursued this approach and sued HMOs, claiming that their risk-sharing plans promoted malpractice by inducing physicians to withhold appropriate medical care.

In one of the first reported malpractice lawsuits against HMOs for using risk sharing plans, Mr. Pulvers sued the Kaiser Health Plan, one of the oldest HMOs.[63] Pulvers claimed he had been led to believe that he would receive the best quality of care and treatment possible, but in fact the treatment he received for Bowen's disease was negligent because Kaiser rewarded physicians for providing less expensive medical care. Before the suit was resolved, Pulvers died, and his claims—along with additional claims for breach of warranty, fraud, and wrongful death—were pursued by his wife and children.

The outcome of the case is confusing and has not served as a useful precedent. A jury rejected Pulver's claim for malpractice but found Kaiser and its doctors liable for wrongful death and breach of warranty. The trial judge upheld the plaintiffs on their claims for breach of warranty but ordered a new trial to resolve the claims of wrongful death and fraud. Kaiser appealed the trial verdict; the appeals court rejected the claims of fraud, noting that HMO incentive plans are specifically authorized under the Health Maintenance Organization Act of 1973.[64] The appeals court found no evidence that Kaiser doctors had acted negligently, withheld required medical care, or deviated from accepted standards of professional conduct.

Two more recent cases illustrate typical malpractice situations but do not offer much legal guidance because they were settled out of court. In *Bush v. Dake*, Sharon Bush sued Group Health Services of Michigan, Inc., an HMO, claiming that its risk-sharing plan encouraged affiliated physicians to be negligent in providing medical care.[65] Ms. Bush said that her physician, Dr. Paul M. Dake, didn't take a routine Pap smear because Group Health Services made him bear the financial risk of paying for tests and referrals. This led to late detection of her cervical and uterine cancer.[66]

Sharon Bush had consulted Dr. Dake about vaginal bleeding and mucous discharge in August 1985. Dr. Dake prescribed medications for infection. But in January 1986 the symptoms persisted, so Bush requested a referral to a gynecologist. When Ms. Bush was examined by Dr. Frederick W. Foltz, who took a Pap smear, the test was negative; but the doctor recommended a follow-up visit if the bleeding persisted. Although it did persist, Dr. Dake refused to make another referral to a gynecologist or take a Pap smear. In May 1986, Ms. Bush went to an emergency room, where a physician took a biopsy and diagnosed cervical cancer.

Ms. Bush claimed that the HMO's financial risk-sharing plan was illegal because it violated public policy. The court, noting that both federal and state statutes regulating HMOs mention risk-sharing arrangements as an option, ruled that risk sharing is not contrary to public policy.[67] But the court concluded in ruling on pretrial motions that the risk-sharing plan could have contributed to the doctor's negligence, in which case the HMO would have been legally responsible. Before trial, however, the parties reached an out-of-court settlement.

In *Sweede v. CIGNA*, Kelly Sweede sued her physicians and CIGNA Healthplan, a Delaware IPA HMO, claiming that CIGNA's risk-sharing arrangements had prompted her primary care physician, Dr. Thomas A. Neef, to withhold appropriate medical care.[68] She alleged that Dr. Neef did not authorize a biopsy despite the urging of her gynecologist—and despite her symptoms of breast cancer. Had he authorized a biopsy when it was first recommended, Ms. Sweede claimed, he would have detected her breast cancer early enough to stop its spread. It was not until a year after she had first told him of a lump in her breast, and only when clinical signs emerged of advanced-stage cancer, that he authorized a biopsy. Ms. Sweede said that Dr. Neef refused the referral earlier because the risk-sharing plan penalized him for making referrals; CIGNA, she added, was negligent in supervising and training physicians. She maintained that CIGNA engaged in deceptive trade practices, consumer fraud, and deceit, and breached contract and fiduciary obligations to subscribers by purposely not informing patients of these incentives and their consequences.

The court decided to try CIGNA and the physicians separately. At the trial against her physicians, the court prohibited Ms. Sweede from introducing evidence about CIGNA's financial incentive plan, saying that the evidence would be prejudicial and not highly relevant.[69] The trial ended in a hung jury. Before the retrial of Ms. Sweede's doctors or the CIGNA trial, the parties reached an out-of-court settlement. A short time later, Ms. Sweede died.

In the initial stages, CIGNA attempted to have the lawsuit dismissed claiming it was not responsible for the medical decisions of physicians. Several reasons were given: that CIGNA paid the IPA, not the physicians, and in fact had no direct contact with physicians; that the medical director who oversaw the quality assurance and utilization review programs worked for the IPA, not CIGNA; and that the medical director never prevented Dr. Neef from making any referrals for Ms. Sweede, so that CIGNA itself could not be held responsible for his denial of the biopsy.[70]

Ms. Sweede argued that CIGNA, directly or indirectly, through its physician payment plans and its utilization review program, exercised control over physicians. She also said that CIGNA paid the physicians directly rather than the IPA, notwithstanding an agreement that states otherwise, and that the medical director had worked for CIGNA. CIGNA's contract with the IPA also specified that doctors must "agree to the risk-sharing arrangement required by the IPA," thus assuring that the IPA would use a risk-sharing plan and physicians would have an incentive to promote CIGNA's interests.[71] In addition, Sweede said, CIGNA, directly or through its IPA, required physicians to receive authorization for referrals and for hospital admissions and discharges; and through its advertisements, CIGNA led the public to believe that physicians were working for, and were supervised by, them. Even if not, CIGNA should still be held responsible for its acts, Sweede argued, because CIGNA induced subscribers to rely on the physicians as CIGNA's agents.

Like other HMOs, CIGNA finances and organizes its plan in order to influence physicians' behavior. Yet CIGNA structures the plan to shield itself from any legal responsibility for the consequences of risk sharing. It is organized so that as much work as possible is implemented by other parties. This allowed CIGNA to claim that Ms. Sweede failed to show any causal connection between risk sharing and her physician's decision to disallow a biopsy, and that, in any event, CIGNA does not control individual physicians' conduct.

In *Boyd v. Albert Einstein Medical Center*, Mr. Wayne K. Boyd sued HMO-PA on behalf of his deceased wife, claiming that the HMO's risk-sharing arrangement had led to her death.[72] Boyd said that because of the risk-sharing plan, when his wife's physician suspected she was having a heart attack, he required her to leave a hospital emergency room and be evaluated at his office—to save money. Had his wife been tested and treated in the hospital, Boyd said, she would not have died that afternoon.

Boyd added that HMO-PA misleads members about its policies by distributing brochures promising comprehensive health care benefits of the highest quality while failing to mention that physicians received incentives to limit their services. The court decided that Boyd had a basis for suing the HMO and a trial was scheduled to decide whether Mrs. Boyd's physician was negligent in providing her medical care and, if so, whether the HMO was responsible.[73]

Before the trial, however, another lawsuit against HMO-PA involving similar claims came before the appellate court. In *McClellan and Shotel v. HMO-PA*, Marilyn McClellan alleged that her primary care physician, Dr. Joseph A. Hempsey, removed from her back a mole that had undergone changes in size and color and failed to obtain a biopsy or histological exam that would have revealed she had cancer.[74] McClellan claimed that as a result her cancer was not detected or treated in a timely manner. Her suit against HMO-PA claimed, among other things, that they were responsible for the doctor's negligence because their system of paying doctors made it "against the primary care physicians' personal or pecuniary interest to give proper medical advice and make appropriate referral." HMO-PA attempted to have the case dismissed claiming it lacked any legal basis. The appellate court has allowed the lawsuit to proceed but did rule that it was up to the legislature, not the courts to decide whether HMO risk-sharing incentives for doctors violated public policy.[75]

In May of 1992, shortly after the *McClellan* decision, the *Boyd* case went to trial. But the parties settled the suit midway through trial and all records of the case were placed under court seal at the request of the parties.[76]

As these five cases indicate, the law remains unsettled. Malpractice lawsuits based on HMO risk-sharing arrangements are likely to increase in the years ahead. Physicians frequently criticize the way our legal system resolves malpractice issues, protesting its negative effects on medical practice. Nevertheless, some physicians have opposed legislation and regulation as ways of dealing with conflicts of interest, arguing that it is more appropriate to rely on medical malpractice as a deterrent and to punish those who violate patients' trust, rather than impose regulations on all physicians. Whatever the merits of legislative and regulatory approaches to conflicts of interest, malpractice law offers only a partial remedy for the harms of HMO incentive payments.

Malpractice in Perspective

If courts hold HMOs responsible for their own malpractice and that of their affiliated doctors, HMOs will have an incentive to monitor medical practice more closely in order to reduce liability. To the extent that this occurs, malpractice law will deter negligent practices. But HMOs seeking to avoid the cost of liability can take other, less costly actions, too. To shift the risk, HMOs can change their contracts with their members and physicians. Some HMOs already require members to arbitrate malpractice claims to avoid litigation and lower the amount of awards. More HMOs are likely to require such concessions from members in the future and might also use contracts to limit the amount of money received by injured members. In addition, HMOs may try to force their physicians to bear the cost. HMO contracts can require physicians to reimburse HMOs in the event that courts hold the HMO liable for the physicians' actions.[77] HMOs can also change their legal relationship with physicians, thereby preventing courts from holding the HMO responsible. Already lawyers are holding seminars instructing HMOs how to shift legal responsibility to doctors.[78] The measures will reduce the risk to HMOs— without reducing malpractice.

Recent studies indicate that only a small percentage of patients with legitimate malpractice claims are aware of the malpractice or bother to sue.[79] One study indicates that as few as 2% of patients harmed by malpractice file malpractice claims.[80] Many significant harms never result in a lawsuit because the expense of trying a case makes it uneconomical. Lawyers are usually paid for malpractice cases with a contingency fee. They recover between one-third and one-half of any judicial award or settlement. But since they are paid only if they receive a favorable result, they are cautious in bringing claims. Since the cost of going to trial is high, lawyers are reluctant to pursue cases in which the amount of money they can recover will be small in comparison to the expense of litigation.

The cost to HMOs of malpractice awards does not reflect the true cost of injuries. Even if it did, the real cost might not be high enough to justify a change of practice by HMOs, especially if risk sharing saves them large sums of money. Therefore, although malpractice suits can deter negligent conduct, their effect is smaller than one might suppose.

Moreover, society may soon cut back on tort liability for physicians.[81] A movement is afoot to use no-fault alternatives to compensate patients who are injured when undergoing medical treatment. Such reforms, modeled on automobile no-fault and worker's compensation statutes, would reduce the instances in which patients could sue physicians and limit the amount patients could recover if injured. To the extent that tort liability deters negligent conduct, the reforms would reduce the deterrent.

Nor will malpractice liability alone comprise an adequate remedy for injuries caused or even compensate all patients harmed. Malpractice pays money for lost income and medical expenses, as well as for pain, suffering, and injury. But money alone cannot heal people, restore lost life, or make up for suffering. From the perspective of most patients, it would be better to prevent improper medical care than to allow it and then provide compensation. Malpractice suits are worth pursuing only in cases of very serious harm. Yet incentive payments can lead physicians to provide poor-quality medical care that falls short of injuries for which the legal system provides compensation. Malpractice suits will not help these patients.

Such suits may encourage HMOs to limit the financial pressures placed by HMOs on physicians, encourage them to scrap risk-sharing plans, and impel them to pay for some injuries to patients. Fear of liability may also promote caution by doctors and make them err on the side of ordering more diagnostic tests and services, even if it is not in their direct financial interest to do so. But the deterrent effect will be only partial. Malpractice suits, therefore, attack only part of the problem of incentives to withhold services. It cannot be relied upon exclusively.

PART III

Inferences for Policy

7

Fiduciary Law
and the Professions:
Regulation of Civil Servants,
Business Professionals, and Lawyers

The fiduciary relationship between professional and client involves certain restrictions on the professional man's method of charging. It requires that the practitioner shall be financially disinterested in the advice he gives, or at least, that the possibility of conflict between duty and self-interest shall be reduced to a minimum[1] (M. C. Alexander and P. A. Wilson).

Fiduciary Principles and the Professions

Business, Government, and Law as Models for Medicine

Many professionals have conflicts of interest. Some resemble those physicians encounter; others differ. In many cases, society has developed policies to deal with the conflicts of interest among professionals. These problems and policies parallel a range of comparable options that now face physicians. Of particular interest are policies for federal employees, business professionals, and lawyers.

In the federal government, public service—rather than profit making—is the rule. The ethos of government resembles that of many doctors and medical organizations. However, its overriding ethical concern is with financial conflicts. Comprehensive statutes deal specifically and exclusively with conflicts of interest. These statutes apply to public servants including professionals employed by government, such as lawyers and physicians. It is possible, even likely, that government may some day extend similar standards to physicians and other recipients of federal funds.[2]

Business is at the opposite end of the spectrum from government. To the extent that comparisons to government service, with its nonprofit orientation, are inappropriate for doctors, analogies to business may be revealing. In recent years, medicine has become more businesslike; the trend is likely to continue. National policy encourages competition and financial incentives in the organization and delivery of medical services. Business responds to profit making, competition, and markets. Yet society has often intervened to protect vulnerable parties and demand high standards of conduct for certain financial professionals. Surprisingly, physicians are not even held to standards that exist for many business professionals.

Many observers contrast the ethic and role of physicians with that of the rugged competitor in business. As medicine becomes more businesslike, the physician is caught between an ethos of professionalism and an ethos of entrepreneurialism. However, the experience of business professionals shows that this tension is not unique to medicine. Many financial professionals enter into conflicts of interest resulting from professional advising, referral, and self-dealing—as do physicians. There have been public and private policies to address these problems in business for a long time.

Government and business have developed conflict-of-interest policies, but these activities differ from medicine: neither is considered a *classic* profession.[3] The legal profession—with its specialized knowledge, internalized norms, and self-regulation—is classic. The profession of law also is often compared to the profession of medicine.[4] Physicians of late have often called themselves *patients' advocates*. Lawyers' roles as advocates help define many of their conflicts of interest, and the adversary system of justice also helps to enforce standards of conduct for lawyers. This experience has implications for physicians as advocates.

A particularly prominent issue in medicine is the extent to which physicians can or should maintain professional autonomy and self-regulation. In law, standards developed by the profession for judging conflicts of interest are based on long-standing legal principles that apply to other groups as well. These standards are interpreted by judges and enforced by courts, thereby providing significant control to groups outside the bar. These features, too, make the experience of lawyers with conflict-of-interest regulation worth examining.

Although the law regulating each of these professionals is diverse, there is a common element: all are governed by what the law calls *fiduciary* principles. And the characteristics that define relationships between patients and physicians are similar in important ways to fiduciary relations.[5]

Fiduciary Relationships

Fiduciaries—people with legal obligations to serve others—are held to the highest standard of conduct known in law. They include trustees, agents, and various professionals. We may speak of the relationship between trustee and beneficiary, principal and agent, public official and the public, lawyer (or broker) and client. In all such relations, the party serving the other is the fiduciary. But no single word refers to the people on whose behalf the fiduciary acts. Therefore, I have coined the term *fiducie* to refer to the other party in fiduciary relationships.[6]

The concept of conflict of interest originates in fiduciary law. We speak of conflicts of interest when a person's activities or commitments compromise some fiduciary-like obligations. Examples illustrate fiduciary relationships and how law has shaped fiduciary obligations. They also situate problems of the patient-physician relationship in a broader context. To the extent that the roles of physicians and their ethical obligations to patients resemble the roles and obligations of other professionals, we can compare their respective conflicts of interest and the strategies society uses to address them.

Fiduciary obligations originated in trusts.[7] Trusts are a legal device to convey or control property. Through a trust, one party transfers property—often a gift—to a second for the exclusive benefit of a third.[8] The recipient of legal title to the property is the trustee. The person benefiting from the property is the beneficiary. Trusts divide ownership between legal title and beneficial enjoyment.[9] This distinction underlies the trustees' role of acting on behalf of the beneficiary.

Trustees have a legal duty to administer the trust solely in the interests of beneficiaries and in accordance with the terms of the trust.[10]

In exercising their authority, trustees may not consider the interests of third parties or themselves, or even of the person who appointed the trustee or established the trust. And trustees may not receive any incidental benefits or payment in connection with their work, except for previously agreed-upon, *reasonable* compensation for rendering services.[11] Trustees may not compete with the trust. Trustees cannot enter into personal financial transactions with a trust except in limited circumstances.[12] In these situations, full disclosure must take precedence, and the beneficiary must give knowing and intelligent consent.[13]

In enforcing the obligations of trustees, the main concern of courts is to deter trustees from entering into conflicts of interest. It is unnecessary for courts to demonstrate the presence of clear or present harm to beneficiaries or unjust enrichment of trustees in order to invoke preventive measures that limit the freedom of trustees.[14] Further, courts can declare void any transactions between the trust and the trustee acting in his or her personal capacity if the transaction is not fair, even if there was full disclosure.[15] Courts may also declare any benefits received by a trustee to be held in a constructive trust for the beneficiary.[16] If a trustee enters into a transaction that violates fiduciary obligations of loyalty, the beneficiary can object after the fact, the transaction will be legally void, and the beneficiary can receive restitution. The beneficiary can assert his or her rights even if the trustee acted in good faith, the price paid was fair, and the beneficiary was unharmed.[17] If a trustee is disloyal, courts have the power to remove the trustee or prevent the trustee from receiving compensation for work performed.[18]

Law has often treated delegated powers as a kind of property subjecting responsible parties to fiduciary obligations. A prime example is the agent.[19] An agent is a person who agrees to act for, represent, and be subject to the control of another party, a principal, for the principal's benefit.[20] Such agreements create a fiduciary relationship.[21] With limited exceptions, an agent's "duty is to give single-minded attention to the principal's affairs and to subordinate personal interests, except with the principal's consent."[22] Agents may not act for their own benefit, or help other parties to compete with their principal,[23] or disclose a principal's confidential information.[24]

Agents must not take unfair advantage of their position or use for their personal benefit information or opportunities acquired as a result of their position of trust.[25] Payments from third parties are suspect and may indicate a violation of loyalty. If an agent violates any of these obligations, the principal can disavow any agreement the agent has made, thereby shifting responsibility to the agent for fulfilling obligations. Agents who breach their duty of undivided loyalty may be liable even if there is little possibility of harm to the principal.[26] Principals can always terminate an agency relationship if the agent misbehaves; often, they can do so without cause.

The law has applied fiduciary principles developed for trustees and agents to government service and financial and legal professionals. Government officials hold office as a public trust for the benefit of those served.[27] The public delegates power to officials, but in return, officials must serve the public. Federal and state statutes hold government officials accountable as fiduciaries.[28] Justice Benjamin Cardozo once remarked that fiduciary standards are "stricter than the morals of the marketplace."[29] But it is more accurate to contrast standards of conduct for fiduciaries with those of the unregulated market-place. Fiduciary principles are part of the rules within which much of business functions. The law holds many business professionals, such as corporate officers, financial advisers, and broker-dealers, to fiduciary standards. Lawyers act as agents, representatives, advisers, and advocates for clients in courts and in business transactions. We expect lawyers to act in their clients' interests and to exercise independent judgment on their behalf. The law holds them accountable as fiduciaries.[30]

Common features characterize tasks performed by fiduciaries. They control the property or affairs of fiducies, or represent or advise them.[31] The work fiduciaries perform requires them to exercise independent judgment and discretion. Sometimes fiduciaries possess specialized knowledge. On other occasions, fiducies are not able to act on their own behalf or want to delegate the work.

Fiducies are vulnerable because they cannot monitor fiduciaries effectively or efficiently. So society imposes legal obligations on fiduciaries to ensure that they act as expected. Courts, legislatures, and government agencies supervise fiduciaries and define impermissible conduct. They fashion specific rules for individual problems and circumstances.

Although details vary, the law expects fiduciaries to be loyal to fiducies, to be scrupulously honest with them, and to act solely for their benefit.[32] Fiduciaries are not allowed to promote the interests of third parties or themselves, although they may receive reasonable compensation for their services. Fiduciaries cannot place themselves in a position where their obligations conflict openly with their personal interests or other commitments.

Who Are Fiduciaries?

Of course, many relationships require one person to trust or depend on another. Not all are fiduciary relationships. Who decides, and on what basis?

Courts and legislatures, not the individual parties in a relationship, ultimately determine who is a fiduciary. Parties can invoke court supervision by engaging in relations that are traditionally subject to fiduciary law. But individuals cannot simply remove themselves from fiduciary obligations.[33] Using their authority to *do justice*, courts can refuse to enforce contracts that eliminate fiduciary obligations. Courts can also apply fiduciary principles to novel transactions and relationships.[34] No simple criteria fully explain how courts decide which relationships they will recognize as fiduciary.[35] Courts make the decisions as they resolve individual disputes.[36]

Over time, courts have developed legal principles in several distinct areas of law, applied these principles to new situations that appeared analogous, and borrowed rules used in one situation for others. In addition, state and federal legislatures have enacted legislation that imposes fiduciary obligations on certain professionals. The result is a diverse set of rules held together by some broad common principles.

Although physicians sometimes call themselves fiduciaries, fiduciary law has been applied to physicians only for very limited purposes.[37] These include requiring that physicians not abandon patients, keep information they learn confidential, and obtain patients' informed consent to treatment.[38] Nevertheless, the roles played by physicians resemble those of professionals considered fiduciaries. They advise patients and act on their behalf. The medical ethos of acting in patients' interests embodies the fiduciary ideal. The patient-physician relationship, though unique, poses the same accountability problem as fiduciary relations.

Conflicts of Interest of Public Officials

Government service has not always been considered a public trust.[39] As late as the seventeenth century, public offices were sold in Britain.[40] In the seventeenth century, leading political theorists viewed monarchs as ruling by divine right with sovereign immunity.[41] As the power of Parliament grew, so did the idea of government as a representative institution. In 1690, John Locke espoused a theory of government that combined two powerful ideas from private affairs: the notions of a trust and of contract.[42] Locke argued that government was a social contract by the public that authorized government to act on its behalf. Public officials, he stated, held power as in a trust, to be used for the benefit of the public. The use of power for other means violated its terms and was illegitimate. This theory was the basis for the Anglo-American idea of government as a public trust.[43]

A central problem of modern democracies is reconciling governmental power with public accountability. Elections allow the public to recall public servants who do not represent their views, and presidents or judges who abuse trust can be impeached. But it is more difficult to hold appointed officials and civil servants accountable. There are many more of these than elected officials or judges, and their work usually involves details that are not easily understood by laypeople or seen by the public. Just as physicians are supposed to serve patients, public officials are supposed to act in the interests of the public. And, just as it is difficult for patients to scrutinize the details of what physicians do, it is hard for the public to review the details of public officials' work. If left unchecked, corruption may become a standard feature of government.[44] One way in which we hold public officials accountable is through conflict-of-interest laws, which prohibit public officials from being improperly influenced by private interests or divided loyalties. Conflict-of-interest rules also help maintain public confidence in government by helping to ensure the appearance of neutrality.

Initially, laws governing the conduct of federal government employees were developed in response to flagrant abuses, particularly bribes and kickbacks.[45] These laws were comparable to the state and federal laws regulating physicians, discussed in Chapters 2 and 4, which single out such obvious abuses as fee splitting. And, just as state and federal laws regulating physician fee splitting, dispensing, and ownership of medical facilities form a maze of rules varying with the jurisdiction, the laws governing the conduct of federal employees formed a patchwork of provisions lacking an articulated or systematic framework. Therefore, in 1962, 1978, 1989, and 1992, Congress enacted reforms to clarify and extend the law governing federal employees to a degree that has not yet occurred for laws governing physicians' conduct.[46] Federal law goes beyond penalizing misconduct: it prohibits public officials from engaging in activities that compromise their loyalty. Some of the newer provisions prohibit officials from engaging in behavior that may, but does not necessarily, give rise to abuse. They seek to avoid even the *appearance* of conflict of interest.

Federal law promotes institutions that reduce the risk that public officials will act in their own interests, or those of others, rather than in the interests of the public.[47] It established an Office of Governmental Ethics (OGE) to oversee the implementation of the executive branch ethics program. The office interprets conflict-of-interest statutes, promulgates regulations, monitors agency ethics programs, reviews presidential appointees' financial disclosure statements for compliance with regulations, and renders advice.

Federal government employees are subject to a number of conflict-of-interest constraints.[48] The most prominent include (1) prohibitions on government officials' participation in decision making that can affect their private economic interests; (2) restrictions on public officials' receipt of outside compensation and gifts that could affect their loyalty; (3) restrictions on public officials and former government officials helping private parties in dealing with the government; (4) prohibitions of officials' misuse of position in such ways as using government time, equipment, and the like for private purposes or using confidential information acquired in their official capacity for private gain; (5) rules requiring public officials to disclose their financial interests; and (6) provisions for the appointment of an independent counsel to investigate and prosecute wrongdoing by middle and high-level government officials.[49] Let us consider some of these in more detail.

Neutral Decision Making

To preserve the neutrality of executive branch officials, statutes prohibit any participation in decision making that could affect the decision makers' personal economic interests. When officials in the executive branch have acquired or pursued financial interests that could affect their independent judgment, they are disqualified from "participat[ing] personally and substantially" in governmental decision making on those matters.

The prohibitions are triggered by the financial interests of the employee, or by the employee's knowledge of the financial interests of his or her spouse, child, partners, prospective employers, or other people or organizations with which the employee has maintained strong affiliations.[50] The employee's superior can exempt the employee, in limited circumstances, but all exemption applications and decisions must be in writing.[51]

Officials who have to take action that may affect their private financial interests must recuse themselves, divest themselves of the interests, or place them in a blind trust. There is also the possibility of obtaining a waiver from certain conflict-of-interest rules in special circumstances. These provisions allow officials to keep investments in a manner that will not affect choices they make in their official capacities.

Outside Compensation and Gifts

Federal statutes and regulations bar public officials from receiving payments from private parties for performing their government services.[52] The aim is to prevent government employees from growing dependent on outside interests, as might occur if a corporation were to supplement the salary of a former employee. A regulation for executive branch employees prohibits them from receiving gifts worth more than $20 offered because of their official position. Such gifts are restricted from anyone who has or seeks business relations with the employee's agency, or who engages in activity regulated by the agency, or who has an interest that may be substantially affected by public officials performing their duties, or who seeks official action by the agency. With limited exceptions, present rules of the executive branch prohibit any gift from these same sources.[53] Also, Senate and House employees may not accept gifts worth more than $250 from any individual in a single year (except from family members), and any gifts worth $250 must be disclosed in writing.[54] High-level officials in all branches of the federal government may not earn more than 15% of an executive level II salary from outside employment, and the source of their outside income is restricted.[55]

For example, all officers and employees of the federal government, including members of Congress, may not accept honoraria.[56] They also must not earn outside income from certain professional activities, such as work that requires them to act as a fiduciary.

Work for Other Parties

A number of restrictions apply to the activities of former executive branch employees, and some newly enacted restrictions apply to members of Congress and their highest-paid staff.[57] These prohibit former employees from representing private parties before government agencies for which the employee worked, on matters in which they participated or that were part of their official responsibilities. They also are designed to provide a cooling-off period for the highest-level officials so that they do not trade on their positions in their former agency or Congress on any matter for at least one year. In addition, some restrictions prohibit not only representation but behind-the-scenes aid and advice in certain types of matters when those activities are engaged in on behalf of foreign governments or political parties or when certain confidential information about a trade or treaty negotiation would be used.[58] Penalties for violations of these restrictions range from civil fines up to $50,000 per count to felony penalties up to five years in jail and/or a $250,000 fine per count.[59]

Profit from Confidential Information

Public officials may not use inside or confidential information for personal gain.[60] In performing government service, employees often have access to information before the public does: for example, government statistics on agriculture harvests or trade balances could be used to speculate on the stock or commodities market. They may also acquire information that is not publicly disclosed.

Public Disclosure of Financial Interests

The Ethics in Government Act requires public disclosure of financial interests of middle- and high-level federal personnel and of nominees and candidates for office in the executive branch, the Congress, and the judiciary.[61] The disclosure includes the amount, type, and source of income and, in certain cases, those of spouses and dependent children. The statute specifies who must file disclosure statements, what must be disclosed, and the timing and filing procedures. The rules vary with the status of the official and the kind of income involved. In general, officials must disclose assets held for the production of income and sources of income including dividends, rents, interest, capital gains, gifts, and certain in-kind payments, such as entertainment, food, lodging, and transportation.[62] Employees must also disclose personal liabilities and debts, investment interests, real estate holdings, and securities transactions, plus significant affiliations with business, nonprofit institutions, labor organizations, and other institutions.[63] Public employees must also reveal arrangements for future employment, leaves of absence from government service, and continuing payment from past employers. Sources of income from qualified blind trusts are exempt.[64] There are also fines for failure to file reports or for filing false reports.

Invoking Justice Louis Brandeis' metaphor of sunshine being the best disinfectant, public interest groups promoted legislation in the 1970s to require public disclosure of government officials' financial interests. Disclosure advocates had two main objectives. First, it may be far easier to identify and prove violation of this standard than violation of the underlying conflict-of-interest rules. Second, reform groups did not trust the government to police itself. Public disclosure was intended to oversee the regulators as much as regulated officials.

The Government Accounting Office (GAO) found that in the past many officials did not file confidential financial statements, as required, with government review bodies. Even when government officials filed disclosure forms, the regulators often did not identify clear conflicts of interests. The advocacy group, Common Cause, attributed these deficiencies to secrecy. It believed that public disclosure would allow citizen watchdog groups, the press, and political adversaries to monitor the process and broadcast the dubious conduct of officials.[65] Publicity and the threat of a scandal would deter misbehavior. As a last resort, a scandal would arouse the electorate, which can vote delinquent officials out of office.

Appointment of Independent Counsel

After the Watergate scandal, Congress believed that because close political loyalties can create personal conflicts of interest, the Attorney General and high-level officials in the Department of Justice are sometimes unlikely to investigate and prosecute high-level executive branch officials for misconduct. Congress therefore established a procedure for funding and court appointment of independent counsel in such cases.[66] The special counsel provision has been used several times, most recently for the Iran-Contra scandal.

Limitations of the Policy

Governmental conflict-of-interest rules are not without their critics— those who believe the rules are ineffective and others who think they work too well. The former point to examples of misconduct by government officials as evidence that the conflict-of-interest rules are not working and note that institutions do not always function in practice as laws assume they should. The concern of the latter is that the rules will require many prospective government employees (particularly high-level appointees) to forego business opportunities, a cost they may not be willing to incur, thus deterring some of the most talented people from serving, and if so, society would be the net loser.[67] The 1962 legislation included provisions to address these problems. But no careful study has been conducted on the effects of conflict-of-interest rules on recruitment. Other critics aver that conflict-of-interest legislation reflects a desire for purity and seeks an unattainable ideal: the elimination of conflicts of interest. They argue against imposing restraints on action prior to misconduct.[68] Still others criticize the ban on earning honoraria as too strict, even unconstitutional. They say it makes sense only to ban earning outside income that is related to the work employees perform in their governmental employment.[69]

Implications for Physicians

Government conflict-of-interest laws aim to keep decision makers loyal by disallowing financial ties that may create private bias. The risk of economic bias is often greater for physicians than for public officials; physicians make decisions about the need for particular services and procedures from which they earn income. The tension is inherent in fee-for-service practice and exacerbated by the six financial arrangements described in Chapters 3 and 4.

Ideally, physicians making clinical choices should be indifferent to the effect on their own income: they should consider only what is good medical practice, given existing constraints. It is probably impossible for doctors to be completely detached from the effects of decisions on their own welfare. But it is possible to limit many financial arrangements that give physicians a vested interest in providing a particular kind or volume of service.

Although specific rules for government employees are not transferable to private medical practice, the idea motivating the law regarding public servants is relevant to physicians when viewed more broadly. As noted in Chapters 3 and 4, physicians in private practice often have ongoing financial arrangements with providers and suppliers that encourage them to increase services. Many receive gifts from pharmaceutical companies and other suppliers as well, or dispense medical products they prescribe, or refer patients to medical facilities in which they invest. Others are financially indebted to providers and suppliers through income supplements of various sorts. Many such outside sources of income that can bias decisions are restricted for government employees and could also be limited in private medical practice.[70]

Some problems may alert us to emerging practices that pose conflicts of interest for doctors. For example, the idea of a special counsel for investigation and prosecution appears to be a procedure unrelated to physicians' conflicts of interests, but it has some relevance. The case of alleged research fraud in 1985, at the Whitehead Institute in Boston Massachusetts is an example.

A research associate charged research fraud by Dr. Thereza Imanishi-Kari. Dr. David Baltimore, the institute's director, and Nobel laureate, was a co-author of the article in question. He defended his colleague and charged interference by congressional investigators. The institute used federal research funds to lobby Congress to cease its inquiry and denounced the investigation as a witch hunt. Yet after outside investigators found evidence of irregularities, Baltimore ceased defending his colleague and apologized for his own actions.[71] The example of an outside independent investigator to review charges of fraud or conflicts of interest in research or clinical cases may be an appropriate model in such circumstances. It also underscores an important point: individual doctors, like other professionals, are not always in a position to decide whether a conflict of interest biases their judgment.

A second example is the rule that prohibits government employees from using confidential information for their own benefit. No law directed to physicians includes such a prohibition. A recent case illustrating this gap in the law involved a psychiatrist, Dr. Robert H. Willis, who used information received from one of his patients during therapy to purchase stock. The patient was the wife of Sanford Weill, former CEO of Shearson Loeb Rhodes, who was attempting to become chief executive of BankAmerica. Dr. Willis pleaded guilty to violating securities law by trading using insider information. The court found that Dr. Willis violated fiduciary duties to his patient by his actions.[72]

Although securities law covered doctors in the case of Dr. Willis, doctors have other opportunities to profit from confidential information, and these are now becoming accepted practices. With increasing frequency, doctors sell information from patients' files to marketing firms, pharmaceutical firms, and third parties, which in turn sell it to insurers and others.[73] These files are a treasure trove for an industry that seek to sell drugs and other products to doctors, market to patients directly, and sell the information to other buyers. Some firms—such as Physician Computer Network, Inc. (PCN)—create arrangements that allow them to telephone into the doctor's computer and have access to patients' files, including medications prescribed and treatments recommended. PCN has signed up over 1,600 doctors by leasing them state-of-the-art computers and software at one-third of the commercial price and they plan to have over 15,000 doctors on line within four years.

PCN and other firms pledge that they will not record the name of the patient, but the potential for abuse exists. Health insurance firms can exclude patients with illnesses; confidential information about patients' illnesses can be released to others as well. Whether or not patients are harmed by the disclosure, information that ought to be held for their benefit is being sold by doctors for profit, and no income or other benefit accrues to patients; the records are sold without their consent. Such practices have no place in the doctor-patient relationship and should be prohibited.

Conflicts of Interest in Business

Conflict-of-interest policies exist in many areas of business.[74] For our purposes, the approaches are aptly illustrated with a few examples drawn from the law of corporations, pensions, and securities.

In each of these areas, business professionals control the use of other people's money. Corporate officers and directors have obligations to the corporation and shareholders, pension fund managers to pension beneficiaries, financial advisers, brokers, and money managers to investors in the securities market.

Corporation Law [75]

A well-known feature of the modern publicly held corporation is the separation of management from ownership. Shareholders have invested in the corporation and are entitled to part of the proceeds. Corporate officers presumably act for shareholders. Shareholders vote for corporate directors, who in turn can hire and dismiss corporate officers, including the chief executive officer. That's the theory.

But in fact, directors generally play a passive role in management, leaving corporate officers to administer day-to-day affairs and business strategy. One of the central problems in the modern corporation is holding management accountable to the corporation while allowing it sufficient discretion to perform its work. Corporate officers are supposed to work for all shareholders, not just one particular class or themselves.[76] This precludes their competing with the corporation for profitable opportunities, making corporate decisions considering the interests of other business entities, and using confidential information gained in their work to profit personally at the expense of the corporation. A comparable problem in medicine is ensuring that physicians act in the interests of their patients while enjoying the clinical freedom they need to do their work.

Just as physicians can make clinical decisions that affect their own remuneration, corporate officers can influence corporate decisions that may affect their own compensation or that of family and friends. This is seen most clearly in self-dealing. Corporate self-dealing has three main components: (1) a transaction between the corporation and another party; (2) interests on the part of corporate insiders in promoting the welfare of the party with which the corporation is dealing; and (3) influence or power exerted by corporate insiders over corporate decisions.

For example, corporate officers are well-situated to sell property that they own personally to the corporation in which they play an official role. They also are strategically placed to purchase corporate assets at bargain prices for their private use. In a private capacity, people are expected to act in their own interests. But as corporate officers, they must act for the corporation's benefit. Corporate officers who perform both roles simultaneously have conflicts of interest.

The legal rules governing corporate self-dealing have been relaxed over time. In the past, self-dealing was usually prohibited or presumed to be improper unless special evidence was presented. More recently, states have allowed self-dealing with few restrictions. But in many states, courts can still void such transactions if (1) the interested party does not disclose the conflict of interest and relevant facts;[77] (2) the transaction is not ratified, either by a majority of disinterested directors or by a majority of shareholders in good faith; or (3) the court determines that, despite disclosure and ratification, the transaction is unfair to the corporation.[78]

Some people have applauded the relaxation of restrictions on self-dealing, contending that—with proper disclosure—shareholders or a disinterested board of directors can appraise the fairness of a transaction by relying on the market price. However, leading corporate law scholars have criticized the current liberal attitude toward self-dealing.

Robert Clark, author of a treatise on corporate law, and now dean of the Harvard Law School, argues that it is generally better to prohibit self-dealing transactions but allow a narrow class of exemptions, subject to the approval of a regulatory agency, such as the Securities and Exchange Commission (SEC).[79] Self-dealing always presents some risk to a corporation, he says, but provides no benefits not usually available through transactions in which no self-dealing occurs; and shareholders are unlikely to serve as good judges of a deal's fairness. Evaluation will often require expertise and information that they lack; therefore, it is unwise to depend on their ratification as protection. It is also imprudent, Clark suggests, to allow self-dealing subject to court review because of the high social cost of reviewing a large number of transactions. Even if most self-dealing is fair, a rule that prohibits self-dealing, subject to administrative review for limited exceptions, will better protect corporate shareholders and be less costly to society than any alternative.

Physician self-referral is the medical equivalent of corporate self-dealing. When physicians refer patients to medical facilities in which they have a financial stake, they may use their position as a patient's adviser to benefit their private economic interests. But, unlike corporate self-dealing, which is usually reviewed by a group of independent professionals, and is at least subject to public scrutiny by shareholders, directors, and the courts, medical transactions are usually shrouded in secrecy. The patient may be informed, but not other independent professionals who might advise the patient.[80] Utilization review and quality assurance programs do review physicians' decisions, but utilization review programs promote the interests of their payers, which are not necessarily the same as the patient's interest. And their efficacy is questionable.

Whatever merit there may be in the argument that disclosure is not effective in protecting shareholders from corporate self-dealing holds all the more true in the case of physician self-referral because patients are more vulnerable than the shareholders. Patients usually do not decide voluntarily to bear the medical risk; they are personally and emotionally involved. Frequently they have to make quick decisions, and the lack of expertise and information impairs their judgment.[81]

Corporate self-dealing may also be more acceptable than physician self-referral because there are adequate remedies for misconduct.

Shareholders can be compensated financially for lost income. Since their money is at stake, shareholders also have a strong incentive to identify misconduct. Injured patients, on the other hand, cannot be adequately compensated by money: damage awards are a poor reward for injury, illness, pain, or death. And insured patients have little incentive today to monitor medical expenses because third parties pay most of the bills.

Pension Fund Managers

To obtain federal tax benefits, firms with pension plans must invest funds exclusively for the benefit of the employees. In the past, the firm for which an employee worked controlled pension plans, directly or indirectly. It was often to the firm's advantage to use the funds to purchase its own securities, or to promote the firm's interests or the interests of third parties. Pensions were promised, but their funding was not required. Pension fund managers, like doctors, could and did act contrary to the interests of the party they were supposed to serve.

In 1974 Congress enacted the Employee Retirement Income Security Act (ERISA) regulating private pension plans.[82] ERISA requires employers to fund pensions, holds managers of pension funds to fiduciary standards,[83] and establishes civil and criminal liability for violation of such standards.[84]

ERISA prohibits self-dealing, with only a few narrow exemptions.[85] Fund managers may not invest more than 10% of the funds in the firm for which the covered employees work. (There is an exception for employee stock option plans [ESOPs], which allow funds to be invested primarily in the employer's business: this allows employees to participate in profit sharing. However, firms offer ESOPs much less frequently than traditional pension plans.) Pension plan fiduciaries may not deal with plan assets for their own account, or be involved in any transaction involving the pension plan on behalf of a party with interests adverse to those of beneficiaries. Plan fiduciaries may not be paid by any party dealing with the plan in transactions involving its assets. ERISA also generally outlaws any financial transaction (such as a sale, loan, lease, or transfer) to or from a fiduciary or other designated persons for the plan, that is, persons providing services, an employee organization, or an employer covered by the plan.

To enforce limits on self-dealing and other fiduciary standards, ERISA grants the Secretary of Labor broad powers to investigate the records of pension plans and to promulgate regulations.[86] Pension administrators must file periodic reports with the Secretary of Labor, plan beneficiaries, and the public.[87] ERISA also sets standards under which pension plans must operate: who is eligible to participate, under what terms, rules for vesting of benefits, and minimum funding.[88]

ERISA takes a stricter approach to self-dealing than corporate law. It offers another model for addressing physician self-referral. Corporate law adopts a relatively lenient approach because adequate remedies exist for misconduct after the fact; disinterested professionals can often evaluate risk, and fiduciaries can be removed. Also, corporate business is intentionally entrepreneurial. ERISA, on the other hand, relies more on preventive measures because Congress wanted less risk for pensions even if this meant lower returns on fund investments. In medicine, health and life are often at stake, and monetary damages (and other remedies after the fact) are likely to be woefully inadequate. Society might therefore prefer a risk-averse approach to physician self-referral using broad prohibitions to self-dealing and regulatory oversight, as in ERISA.

Federal Securities Law

One way corporations obtain capital is by selling shares to investors. Securities are purchased and sold through broker-dealers. Investment advisers help individuals and firms to evaluate securities, and advise investors on how to design a diversified portfolio that suits their needs. Investment managers oversee clients' investments. These and other specialists help to operate the securities market.[89]

Although selling financial products, investment management, and advising clearly differ from the practice of medicine, financial professionals face analogous conflicts of interest. In both settings, professionals can increase their income by recommending services they provide.

Issuers, underwriters, broker-dealers, and investment advisers are expected to provide reliable information about securities. Yet they may be tempted to make misleading statements or to refrain from disclosing relevant information to increase their income.

Securities law requires issuers and underwriters to reveal even more extensive information than doctors must offer patients under informed consent law. Presumably full disclosure of pertinent information will help to protect investors. But disclosure is only one tool.

The securities industry also supervises the conduct of professionals and prohibits certain activities that pose risks.

Public oversight in the securities industry has two main aims: (1) to create conditions that enhance stable, efficient, and fair markets and (2) to set policies that protect investors and other parties who entrust their funds to fiduciaries. Federal statutes empower an independent federal agency, the Securities and Exchange Commission (SEC), to supervise the market, develop rules as needed to manage the industry, grant and revoke licenses of broker-dealers, conduct investigations, and impose sanctions for violations of rules.[90] The SEC also monitors industry self-regulatory organizations. Statutes allow private civil lawsuits against parties engaging in prohibited conduct injurious to those whom the securities laws protect.[91]

Disclosure

To protect purchasers, the Securities Act of 1933 and the Securities and Exchange Act of 1934 require full and accurate disclosure of material information.[92] Before making any public offerings or sales of securities, issuers must file a registration statement with the SEC. Since the SEC can delay their issuance, issuers nearly always correct any deficiencies noted by the SEC staff.[93] Buyers must receive a prospectus that provides much of the information in the registration statement.[94] The issuers, underwriters, and others are criminally and civilly liable for information and omissions that make the statement misleading. If prospectuses do not meet these standards, the SEC may suspend trade of the security and purchasers may sue to recover any loss.[95] Liable parties include every underwriter, every seller, and any person who signed the prospectus, was a director or partner of the issuer, or any professional (such as accountants, engineers, or appraisers) who approved the statement.[96]

Securities regulations also contain a catchall provision to prevent misrepresentation and fraud in trading. Rule 10-b(5) prohibits the making of untrue statements or the omission of facts that make a statement misleading. Violators may be liable under criminal and civil law. Any purchaser or seller harmed as a result of misleading statements may sue privately to recover damages.

Investment advisers must disclose conflicts of interest and other material facts.[97] Advisers are prohibited from *scalping*, that is, purchasing a large volume of a security just before recommending its purchase and profiting as a result from the rise in price without telling their customers.[98] When broker-dealers act as principals in relation to clients they have previously served as agents, they must disclose conflicts of interest, the best available market price, and other information.[99]

But disclosure and client consent will not cure all conflicts, especially when an adviser exercises influence over the client.[100] Broker-dealers, advisers, and money managers must deal fairly with their clients.[101] Payments for referrals and other arrangements that compromise an adviser's loyalty are always suspect and often considered fraudulent.

Regulation

Multiple functions with conflicting roles often create conflicts of interest for financial professionals. For example, broker-dealers act as agents and buy and sell securities on behalf of their customers, receiving a commission for their work. They may also act for their own account, buying securities from and selling them to customers, earning profits based on the difference in price. In addition, they often advise clients on purchasing securities. Combining these roles creates avenues for profit at the expense of their clients: for example, advising customers to buy from their own account even when it is not in their customers' interest. Because broker-dealers sometimes act as a client's agent, clients are apt to rely on them even when they perform a different role.

Many such conflicts of interest could be eliminated by limiting individuals or firms to only one function. This would be a costly solution, since having brokers or firms perform multiple functions produces economies of scale that can benefit purchasers. Securities law takes another approach. It allows specialists to perform multiple functions but subjects them to close supervision.[102] To the extent that the law tolerates conflicts of interest, it compensates by removing some of the discretion of financial professionals.

Society faces a similar choice with physicians who perform conflicting roles when they advise patients to purchase medical products they sell or when they engage in self-referral. We can either prevent such conflicts of interest by requiring physicians to refrain from self-referral and other activities, or we can allow conflicting roles but regulate physicians' conduct closely to reduce the possibility of abuse.

Securities laws supervise broker-dealers to ensure that they fulfill their fiduciary obligations. They hold liable those who "churn" their customers' accounts (i.e., trade excessively in order to earn commissions).[103] Broker-dealers who abuse their clients' trust to rake in unreasonable profits are liable for fraud; their registration may be revoked.[104] The SEC can sanction and customers can sue broker-dealers who recommend the purchase of a security but do not have a sound basis for their recommendation.[105]

Other rules limit the activities of broker-dealers. They may not charge more than the usual commission for transactions in which they act as dealers and already have the other party as a client. Statutes also regulate the financial structure and practices of broker-dealers, and impose standards for insurance and for segregating and safe keeping of clients' funds.

Implications for Physicians

Often financial professionals are self-employed, like physicians in private practice. Other times they are employed by large firms but, like physicians employed by HMOs, compensated in part based on the volume of services they provide. Doctors are now being partly pushed, partly lured, into arrangements that offer financial incentives based on the volume of services provided or the business generated. Some doctors hope that such market-like approaches will bring relief from government restrictions. Yet the securities industry shows that market competition and financial incentives, far from being incompatible with government regulation, require it. The securities industry epitomizes market competition, but it is also highly regulated to promote competition and ensure that professionals fulfill their fiduciary obligations.

The securities industry uses substantive regulation and supervised disclosure as tools to mitigate conflicts of interest. Unlike the medical profession, which relies on voluntary disclosure, the securities market has mandatory disclosure. The SEC specifies its timing and content in detail and monitors the information. Moreover, disclosure may be less helpful for patients than for investors. In the securities industry, information promotes an efficient market. Patients are quite different from investors and are unlikely to be able to use information in a similar way, especially because in medicine there exists no equivalent of the independent adviser who helps small investors make sense of financial information disclosed.

Conflicts of Interest of Lawyers

The role lawyers play as advocates in an adversarial system of justice
defines their obligations to clients and shapes the way courts and the
profession address their conflicts of interest. In litigation and negotiation,
one party's gain is often another's loss. Lawyers are expected to represent their clients zealously because lawyers for an opposing party
advocate their clients' interests.[106] Anything that compromises lawyers'
loyalty or judgment undermines their role and places clients at risk.

Lawyers' and doctors' roles differ, and so do many of their conflicts.
Nevertheless, comparisons are revealing. The medical profession has
only recently addressed conflicts-of-interest explicitly; it emphasizes
disclosure, and relies largely on voluntary compliance. The legal
profession has had explicit conflict-of-interest policies for nearly a
century. In addition to disclosure, it relies on prohibitions. There are
strong incentives for self-policing, a system of sanctions for noncompliance, and court supervision of lawyers' conduct.

Conflicts of interest were a central concern in American legal codes
of ethics as long ago as 1908, when the American Bar Association's (ABA)
Canons of Professional Responsibility were promulgated.[107] The *Canons*
were succeeded by the *Code of Professional Responsibility* in 1969 and by
the *Model Rules of Professional Conduct* in 1983.[108] Virtually every jurisdiction has adopted either the *Model Rules* or the *Code of Professional
Responsibility* as rules of court, and draws on them and judicial decisions
in regulating lawyers.

The conduct of lawyers is regulated by a disciplinary system
involving bar associations, state regulation, and courts. ABA codes are
used by bar associations in drafting ethics opinions and in disciplinary
proceedings. Courts have power to regulate the practice of law and to
oversee the conduct of lawyers.[109] They promulgate standards for
admission and disbarment, use codes of conduct to supervise lawyers,
and use these codes as a measure of professional standards in malpractice suits.[110]

Canon 5 of the 1969 *Code of Professional Responsibility* states that "a
lawyer should exercise independent professional judgment on behalf of
a client." And Disciplinary Rule 5-101(a) prohibits lawyers from
representing clients when doing so would adversely affect a lawyer's
independent judgment. Rule 1.7 of the *Model Rules of Professional Conduct* prohibits lawyers from representing clients if they will be limited

"by responsibilities to another client or to a third person or by the lawyer's own interests," except in limited circumstances. The policies implicit in these provisions are developed in numerous rules governing specific conflicts of interest.

Codes of conduct alternate between preventing situations that are prone to abuse and treating conflict-free representation as a right that clients can waive.[111] They allow lawyers to represent clients despite conflicts in some cases if the client is informed and consents. But they deem other conflicts severe enough to preclude lawyers from representing a client.[112] When codes allow representation despite conflicts, remedies exist if courts later decide that consent was not informed or voluntary. These include disallowing a lawyer from collecting a fee, compensating clients with damages, and overturning a conviction.

Allowing lawyers with conflicts of interest to represent clients may be appropriate if three conditions are present: (1) the risk of abuse of trust is low and can be controlled in other ways; (2) prohibiting lawyers with this kind of conflict from representing clients imposes greater social costs than expected benefits; and (3) clients are in a position to decide whether the risk is worth bearing. When one or more of these conditions is absent, it is more appropriate to disqualify a lawyer, despite disclosure and the client's consent.

When codes allow lawyers to represent clients despite conflicts of interest, the lawyer must still follow certain rules. Clients must give informed, intelligent, and explicit consent.[113] The lawyer may not proceed unless he or she is able to represent the client adequately. The lawyer must inform the client of the conflict, describe the possible effect on the exercise of the lawyer's independent judgment, and discuss the other risks involved. Often lawyers are required to counsel clients to seek independent professional advice.

Enforcement

One way of enforcing conflict-of-interest rules is the adversary system of resolving disputes. As part of their power to regulate the practice of law, judges can prevent lawyers or law firms from representing a client. In litigation, a lawyer is expected to use all substantive and procedural devices to advance the interests of his or her client.[114] This includes requesting that the court bar a particular lawyer from representing the opposing party when conflicts of interest threaten the interests of the objecting lawyer's client.[115]

In addition, a lawyer's conflicts of interest are imputed to the lawyer's partners, associates, and colleagues.[116] When a lawyer is disqualified from representing a client, all affiliated lawyers are usually disqualified as well.[117] The conflict of interest of one lawyer may disqualify an entire law firm from representing a whole class of clients, thereby eliminating substantial opportunities for work. Well-managed law firms generally find it to their benefit to self-police by making conflict-of-interest inquiries before taking on a new client.

Sometimes courts allow lawyers to rebut the presumption of disqualification, due to imputed conflicts of interest, by showing that they had no access to confidential information.[118] Occasionally a lawyer can be screened off from the rest of the firm to prevent the sharing of information and profits that would present a conflict of interest. This approach, used most frequently with former government lawyers, has been criticized by legal commentators as ineffective.[119]

Aside from court supervision, the main means of enforcing conflict-of-interest rules are penalties imposed by state licensing boards. Sanctions may include private or public reprimand, fines, probation, suspension, supervised practice, and disbarment. In the past, most state boards that investigated and adjudicated cases of lawyer misconduct were dominated by lawyers. But now, following ABA recommendations, boards typically comprise up to one-third nonlawyers.[120]

Opinion is mixed on how effectively the bar has disciplined lawyers. A 1970 report for the ABA by former Supreme Court Justice Tom Clark called the situation "scandalous." There has been little serious research on the rates of compliance or the effectiveness of discipline. Courts and disciplinary agencies interpret ethical codes more freely and inconsistently than they do other laws.[121] Still, unlike medical codes of ethics, which do not contain explicit or detailed rules for responding to conflicts of interest, legal professional codes have defined norms. They have also established procedures to investigate and resolve conflicts.

A massive body of case law explains how these rules apply in specific situations and how courts have responded when they are violated. In addition, bar advisory opinions and a literature on legal ethics analyze conflicts of interest that arise in all areas of practice.[122] Bar association ethics committees can help in interpreting rules and often produce advisory opinions upon request. Every law school requires courses on professional responsibility; these familiarize students with the professional codes, legal rules, and norms for conflicts of interest.

Such courses cannot assure ethical conduct, but they offer guidance to lawyers.

Four Types of Conflict

Lawyers face four kinds of conflicts of interest: (1) conflicts between loyalty to clients and personal financial interests; (2) conflicts between loyalty to clients and to their *constituents*; (3) conflicts between loyalties to clients with differing interests; and (4) conflicts between duty to clients and obligations as officers of the court.[123]

Money helps define the four conflicts. The conflicts of interest involve the lawyer's personal financial interest directly in the first category. In the second, competing financial ties are indirect; the threat to loyalty emerges through related but distinct obligations. In the third, the division in loyalty stems from financial commitments made to different clients. In the fourth, the lawyer presumes to act as an agent (usually paid) of the client; but society—wanting lawyers to serve the judicial system—places restrictions on what clients can legitimately expect.

Conflicts between Loyalty to Clients and Personal Financial Interests. In advising clients, lawyers can often promote their own interests.[124] For example, they might recommend unnecessary legal work. When lawyers are paid by the hour, as doctors paid on a fee-for-service basis, they have an incentive to do more.[125] Lawyers might also advise clients on wills and business ventures while serving as beneficiaries or business partners. Codes regulate such merging of roles. In some cases, they disqualify the lawyer from representing the client. In others, they allow representation if the lawyer explains the conflict, advises the client to seek independent counsel, and the client still consents.[126] If, after the fact, clients object to a conflictual business transaction, lawyers shoulder the burden of proving that their conduct was fair. Unless they can, courts will rescind the transaction, provide monetary damages or equitable relief, or impose sanctions upon the lawyer.[127]

Conflicts Between Loyalty to Clients and Constituents. When lawyers represent organizations, agencies, or a group, or are paid by a third party, there is the potential for confusion between clients and what I will call *constituents*.[128]

Constituents are individuals, groups, or organizations with which lawyers work directly, or who pay them, but are not clients. Examples include advocacy associations that sponsor litigation of individuals to establish a legal precedent; government, when it pays for legal services of the poor; insurers, when they reimburse the defense of a business; corporate management, when it acts for a corporation; and employers, when financing representation of employees.

Constituents retain lawyers and often can influence their conduct in ways that clients may not approve. To address this problem, the law states that when a third party pays a lawyer's fee, the lawyer cannot accept instructions from the payer.[129] But some liability insurance contracts give the insurer the right to control the defense, in which case the law treats insurer and insured as dual clients and tries to accommodate their interests. If both parties do not consent to joint representation, each must be represented separately.[130] When advocacy organizations sponsor lawsuits, they may promote remedies that differ from those the plaintiffs favor. The Supreme Court has decided to allow such representation anyway because the likely alternative for such plaintiffs is often no legal representation at all.[131]

In medicine, third-party payers, like constituents in law, usually pay the bills; but the doctor is still supposed to act for the benefit of the patient. This conflict is recognized but not yet dealt with on an institutional footing. In recent years, third-party payers have used their financial clout to promote a more frugal style of practice, thereby reducing their financial burden. This will often protect patients from overuse of services but not from underservice. When third-party payers have leverage over physicians, it results in some loss of their accountability to patients.

Conflicts between Loyalties to Clients with Differing Interests. The legal profession is most concerned with conflicts of interest that arise when a lawyer's representing one client interferes with adequately representing another. These conflicts arise in many ways. For example, a lawyer representing a firm on one matter may be asked by another client to sue the firm on an unrelated issue. Courts generally prohibit lawyers from representing the second client in such circumstances.[132] Conflicts also occur when lawyers represent two or more clients simultaneously in litigation. The interests of the clients could differ.

Lawyers sometimes represent several parties or even a group of similarly situated individuals in so-called class action lawsuits.[133] Even though the plaintiffs share common interests, they may also have interests that clash. Some plaintiffs may want to settle for a smaller sum rather than risk the uncertain outcome of a trial. Others may not. Lawyers can represent multiple parties in business transactions if the interests of the clients coincide. But many business transactions involve dividing shares of limited resources, thereby making joint representation possible only with full disclosure and consent.

Lawyers sometimes can simultaneously represent clients with differing interests. The lawyer must inform both parties of the conflict and its possible ramifications, and the clients must consent. Initially it is up to the lawyer and clients to decide whether to accept simultaneous representation. But a court can intervene on its own initiative or at the request of a client who later believes that his or her rights have been compromised. If the court believes that simultaneous representation was impermissible, it can disqualify the lawyer, disallow payment for work performed, or even set aside a criminal conviction.[134] The rule for conflicts involving former clients is less strict. It bars representation only when a lawyer previously represented a client on a related matter and the interests of the two clients are adverse.[135]

Conflicts between Duties to the Client and Obligations as an Officer of the Court. Lawyers—as officers of the court—must conform to court rules, as well as promote their clients' interests. They must inform the court of any controlling legal authority detrimental to their client's interests and disclose any ongoing client fraud.[136] Furthermore, lawyers are expected to screen out frivolous lawsuits and may not use lawsuits for extortion, even if this could promote their clients' interest. The above are not considered legitimate interests for a lawyer to represent. Rule 11 of the Federal Rules of Civil Procedure and the Model Rules of Professional Conduct hold a lawyer signing a pleading (i.e., legal claims and defenses made in a lawsuit) accountable for an adequate factual and legal basis.[137] If a court finds the pleading baseless, it may impose sanctions on the lawyer. Courts and disciplinary agencies can impose sanctions on the party who initiates harassing suits and on the lawyer who brings them.

Implications for Physicians

Physicians are patients' *advocates* in the sense that they owe loyalty to patients and can promote their interests in gaining access to health care services. Both physicians and lawyers combine the roles of adviser and provider of services, a position subject to abuse. And some lawyers' conflicts resemble those of physicians. Like physicians, lawyers encounter conflicts of interest stemming from payment supervised by third parties rather than clients. The law has tried to insulate lawyers from influence by third parties but has accommodated it when necessary to achieve other public policy goals. In medicine, the practice in this respect is changing. Third-party payers in the past exercised almost no control over the provision of medical care, but they are now asserting increasing control over standards of practice. The question for the future is what kind of accommodation is acceptable to take account of other policy goals. This is not a parallel situation, however, because most medical care is financed through insurance, while only a small part of legal services is paid for by third parties.

Like physicians, lawyers have conflicts of interest when they engage in business ventures. For lawyers, this occurs when they become business associates of clients or receive gifts from them while providing them with legal services. In the case of physicians, the conflicts occur when doctors form business arrangements with third parties that can affect their provision of care and advice to patients. The rules are lax for both professions, but lower for physicians than for lawyers.

The lawyer's most common conflicts of interest—those between clients with competing interests—are foreign to most medical practice. But there are parallels, albeit in special situations. For example, when one physician is treating two patients, each of whom needs resources that are limited, the physician encounters a conflict of interest. This conflict also occurs when a physician is the doctor for both an organ donor and a recipient. In both situations, dual "representation" is not ethically feasible and, as in the law, should not be attempted by one person.

However, the main lessons for physicians from the legal profession are not specific rules for handling conflicts. Rather, they are the process and the institutional framework. The legal profession does not rely mainly on the practitioner's individual conscience or discretion. Lawyers adhere to explicit standards and public norms. Rules and cases help lawyers to apply these standards. Incentives exist for code enforcement. Lawyers are also subject to outside monitoring and sanctions for violation of conflict-of-interest rules. Such measures supervise and limit conduct. Medicine still lacks these safeguards.

Common Intervention Strategies
to Hold Fiduciaries Accountable

Fiduciaries command expertise or power that can be abused. Yet it is often difficult, if not impossible, for the fiducie, the party on whose behalf the fiduciary acts, to control the fiduciary. Fiduciaries have opportunities to exploit their fiducie's trust whenever they can act for their personal interest rather than on the fiducie's behalf; whenever they perform conflicting roles for fiducies or others; and whenever they try to honor obligations to fiducies with divergent interests.

In public service, business, and the legal profession, fiduciary loyalty is no longer treated solely as an individual responsibility dependent on the good will and moral integrity of each fiduciary. The development of policy has made public what was once a personal, ethical issue for the fiduciary. The main concerns underlying public policy are the preservation of fiduciary impartiality and independence, as well as accountability.

Three main strategies are used to address conflicts of interest in each field. The first approach is preventive: fiducies are protected by prophylactic measures, such as prohibiting fiduciaries from entering into situations in which serious conflicts of interest occur. For example, government officials cannot participate in decision making that affects their private financial interests. Their receipt of outside compensation and gifts is restricted. They may not use confidential information for profit. After they leave government, their employment is temporarily restricted. In business, self-dealing is generally prohibited, restricted, or subject to court or independent review. Pension fund managers cannot self-deal except in limited situations. Stock exchange members generally cannot trade on their own accounts. Lawyers with conflicting interests, and sometimes even their affiliated law firms, are disqualified from representing clients, even when the client is informed of a conflict and wants the lawyer to represent him or her. Law firms may isolate lawyers working on a particular matter from any contact with other attorneys in the firm. Disclosure is also used as a preventive device in these fields.

The second approach is to supervise the conduct of fiduciaries through regulation, thereby reducing the discretion that they could abuse. In government, the OGE oversees an administrative apparatus that monitors the disclosure of the personal finances of employees.[138] The office reviews requests for exemptions from prohibitions on a case-by-case basis. It promulgates rules that can affect assignment of tasks within a particular job and defines the scope of allowable conduct on and off the job. Courts have the power to review transactions of corporate officials that involve conflicts of interest. They may void transactions if these are improper. The Department of Labor exercises regulatory control over pension fund managers and may remove them if they engage in prohibited conduct. In the securities business, the SEC exerts broad regulatory authority that includes power to license and revoke the licenses of broker-dealers and advisers; to set the range of permissible prices; and to establish the manner and timing of advertising and sales of securities. The SEC monitors the volume and timing of sales of dealers, and has broad investigatory and supervisory powers. In the practice of law, courts can review the transactions between lawyers and clients. The adversary system, and actions of opposing counsel, also help to enforce compliance with conflict-of-interest policy.

The third approach is to provide remedies if fiduciaries abuse their trust or harm fiducies. This strategy seeks to deter misbehavior through sanctions and to provide restitution to fiducies. Corporate law allows shareholders to recover financial damages from corporations and officials that have violated their fiduciary obligations. Pension fund managers who violate their trust are subject to civil and criminal penalties. In the securities business, professionals are subject to civil and criminal sanctions, loss of license, disgorgement of illegal profits, and private suits for financial damages for violating conflict-of-interest rules. Investors who have lost money as a result of professionals engaging in prohibited conduct are entitled to compensation. Courts can impose a range of sanctions on lawyers who violate conflict-of-interest rules. These include disallowing lawyers from collecting fees for work performed, fines, public censure, suspension of the professional license, or disbarment. Criminal defendants who have received inadequate representation as a result of their attorney's conflicts of interest can have their conviction reversed. Clients can also recover financial damages from their lawyers.

Collectively, these intervention strategies can be applied across a range of circumstances. Government and private groups can intervene before any activity by fiduciaries, while fiduciaries perform their tasks, and after the fact, if fiduciaries abuse their trust. Table 7-1 displays these approaches along a continuum.

Table 7-1. Conflicts of Interest:
Points of Intervention and Major Policy Approaches

Before fiduciary acts	*While fiduciary acts*	*After fiduciary acts*
PREVENTION	REGULATION OF THE ACTION	SANCTIONS AND RESTITUTION
Prohibit fiduciaries from entering into situations with conflicts of interest and use other preventive measures.	Supervise the conduct of fiduciaries and limit their discretion.	Penalize fiduciaries for violation of trust. Compensate fiducies for harm caused if fiduciaries abuse their trust.

Some measures are tailored to each profession's unique aspects. The federal government makes use of public participation, politics, the media, and public advocacy groups to help enforce standards. Business makes use of both market price and regulatory mechanisms to detect self-dealing transactions and to gauge appropriate compensation for abuse of trust and rules of fair competition. The regulation of lawyers draws on an adversary system of justice to help enforce rules and make use of court power to monitor the profession.

Public, enforceable laws uphold standards in each field. They are backed by an administrative apparatus that oversees prevention, regulation, and, when necessary, the imposition of sanctions and restitution awards. In government, the OGE supervises the administrative apparatus, but executive branch regulation also plays a role. In business, the SEC controls the securities market, the Secretary of Labor supervises pension funds, and courts supervise corporate conflicts of interest. Courts are also the main institution overseeing lawyers' conduct.

And yet the existence of conflict-of-interest policy in all of these fields has not solved the problem. There are always difficulties in enforcing policies, with the efficacy of some measures probably questionable and certainly hard to gauge. In addition, new situations not anticipated by existing rules can develop and may undermine policies. It is far more appropriate to speak of coping with conflicts of interest than of eliminating them.

Indeed, conflicts of interest are so prevalent that not all are worth eliminating. Many public policies reflect or take account of competing considerations and accept some conflicts to preserve other socially desirable goals. But save for medicine, policies at the very least address conflicts of interest and establish public standards backed by sanctions. These often influence behavior and provide some remedies.

Lessons for Physicians

Physicians often act as traditional fiduciaries and espouse a fiduciary ethic. In a few situations, courts apply fiduciary law principles to doctors.[139] But aside from these limited circumstances, physicians—as clinicians—are not held to fiduciary standards, especially with respect to financial conflicts of interest.[140]

Courts typically deter trustees from entering into conflict-of-interest situations and need not show harm to beneficiaries or unjust enrichment to invoke preventive measures limiting trustee freedom.[141] When behavior is questionable, courts require fiduciaries to prove that they have not violated their trust. Such is not the case for physicians. For example, unlike typical fiduciaries, who cannot accept gifts that may influence their professional decisions, doctors frequently accept gifts from pharmaceutical firms and medical suppliers.[142] Regulatory institutions can penalize doctors for misconduct, and can attempt to stop overuse and underuse of medical services and ensure quality of care. But they are woefully inadequate, and they do not explicitly address physicians' conflicts of interest. The experience of government, business, and the legal profession suggests a need for outside groups to evaluate professional conduct, set standards, and exercise disciplinary control. The fiduciary ideal, implicit in much of medical ethics and some medical law, needs reinforcement.

The day when doctors rely on their individual clinical judgment alone is passing. The medical profession is now developing criteria to hold physicians to standards of technical performance.[143] Third-party payers and others are developing practice guidelines for diagnosis and treatment. This trend is sometimes called the *outcomes movement*.[144] No such standards, however, have yet emerged for clinical medical ethics especially for financial conflicts of interest. In ethics physicians are still relatively unconstrained. The lack of standards has led to a proliferation of practices that, at the very least, create risk for patients while offering little or no benefit.

The development of clinical standards and measures of outcome may reduce the need for standards of financial conduct; it will enable the evaluation of physicians based on how well they care for patients. But technical performance standards alone will never suffice. A very large sphere of medicine is fraught with uncertainty. Within this zone, doctors will necessarily retain great discretion. This makes it important to develop financial practice standards that will preserve physicians' fidelity to patients.

8

What Needs to Be Done?

Lawmakers make the citizen good by inculcating [good] habits in them,
and this is the aim of every lawgiver; if he does not succeed in doing that,
his legislation is a failure. It is in this that a good constitution differs
from a bad one (Aristotle).[1]

Economists often propose to deal with unethical or antisocial behavior
by raising the cost of that behavior rather than by proclaiming standards
and imposing prohibitions and sanctions. The reason is probably that
they think of citizens as consumers with unchanging or arbitrarily
changing tastes in matters of civic as well as commodity-oriented
behavior. This view tends to neglect the possibility that people are
capable of changing their values. A principal purpose of publicly
proclaimed laws and regulations is to stigmatize antisocial behavior
and thereby influence citizens' values and behavior codes. This
educational, value-molding function of the law is as important as its
deterrent and repressive functions (Albert Hirschman).[2]

The medical profession and the country must rethink the ways
they deal with physicians' conflicts of interest. The problem is long
standing and systematically impairs medicine. Chapter 7 examined the

diverse measures developed to address conflicts of other professionals. This chapter considers what should be done. It starts by considering two misguided remedies: relying on disclosure of conflicts and using state employment of doctors. Then it reviews recommendations for addressing the seven kinds of conflict of interest this book examined. It also proposes various institutional means to bring about needed changes and concludes with reflections on the relations between incentives, ethics, law, and social policy.

The Limits of Disclosure as a Remedy

Many medical groups and commentators shun the idea of public intervention as a way to address physicians' financial conflicts of interest and advocate disclosure to patients as an alternative.[3] As we saw in Chapters 2 and 4, in recent years the American Medical Asociation (AMA) relied almost exclusively on disclosure as a remedy for conflicts of interest. It has, however, advocated more restrictive ethical strictures for gifts since 1990 and for self-referral since 1992, but its resolve on these conflicts wavers and there are many exceptions to these restrictions.

In relying on disclosure, the organized medical profession is drawing on just one of the two ethical norms that formed the basis for its traditional opposition to commissions and fee splitting. Early in this century doctors opposed these practices partly because patients were not informed. But they also opposed them because they compromised the physician's loyalty and judgment, a problem that remains even with disclosure. In banking so heavily on disclosure, the AMA puts the onus on individuals to solve a problem that actually requires enforceable public policy.[4]

Though often recommended, the rationale for disclosure is rarely articulated. Nor are its expected effects. There has been far too little discussion of precisely what information will be disclosed, to whom, when and how the information will be presented, and what measures— if any—will be necessary to ensure compliance. Nor have advocates discussed what role institutions will play in making disclosure helpful. Therefore, before examining other policy options, let us consider the experience of disclosure in various contexts and its limitations as a way to cope with physicians' conflicts of interest.

The experience of addressing conflicts of interest in government, business, and law suggests that to the extent that disclosure is helpful, standards must be set and certain activities prohibited; the institutional context must reinforce and amplify it; and the public and the press must support compliance with substantive rules. If disclosure is to help cope with physicians' conflicts of interest, then we will need (but do not have) equivalent conditions and institutions. Under the circumstances the chances that physicians' disclosure of conflicts of interest can help patients is greatly diminished.

Disclosure by Physicians in Informed Consent

Current law requires that physicians obtain their patients' informed consent before treating them.[5] To ensure that consent is informed, physicians must disclose the risks and benefits of alternatives, including nontreatment, to any medical intervention they propose.[6] Ideally, disclosure promotes communication and fosters trust between patients and physicians. When informed of the risks or choices, patients can confide their own concerns, values, and wishes to physicians; this feedback may modify the physicians' recommended treatment.[7] Here, the aim of disclosure is to facilitate the participation of patients in medical decision making. Physicians recommend the medical care they believe to be most appropriate, while patients retain the authority to decide whether to accept it—or an alternative.

Since the 1970s, when courts started holding physicians liable for failing to obtain their patients' informed consent, medical institutions and medical ethics have promoted disclosure of risks to patients. There is no doubt that attitudes and practices have changed and that patients are likely to receive more information today than in the past. Nevertheless, because of difficulties of enforcement, studies have shown that disclosure occurs relatively infrequently and not as envisioned by the law.[8] One observer has suggested that physicians sometimes couch their disclosure in terms designed to promote more costly procedures.[9] Psychological studies also indicate that even with accurate disclosure, patients may not understand the information provided or its implications.[10] Patients misunderstand, too, because of poor communication by physicians.[11] New information often does not lead patients to reconsider proposed treatments.[12] The detailed, written forms used in obtaining consent sometimes obscure understanding. Patients often treat them as meaningless and do not even remember what they have signed.[13] Even when doctors avoid making explicit decisions, patients typically choose what their physicians wish or suggest.[14]

The lack of clear standards and the discretion accorded to physicians in deciding what to disclose reduce the efficacy of disclosure.[15] Dependence of patients on physicians limits the ability of patients to use information effectively. In other words, disclosure in obtaining informed consent does not always give the patient either understanding or control; and without supervision, physicians generally do not disclose all pertinent information to patients.

We can expect similar problems to crop up when physicians disclose their financial interests to patients. Worse still, the disclosure of financial interests alone is insufficient to inform most patients. To understand the implications of these disclosures, patients need to know that virtually every major study indicates that physicians who make referrals to medical facilities that they either own or have a financial interest in, recommend more (or more expensive) medical tests and procedures than do physicians without a financial interest.[16] This occurs even in states that require disclosure of financial interests.[17] Patients also need to know that many physicians perform unnecessary medical services that can harm patients, and that physicians with risk-sharing arrangements in Health Maintenance Organizations (HMOs) and other managed-care providers tend to provide fewer services than those in fee-for-service practice.[18]

But even this information is not enough. Doctors who disclose conflicts of interest are unlikely to provide patients with other meaningful options. Patients of doctors in fee-for-service practices will still have difficulty choosing and evaluating the services of experts. And, unless they pay for the cost of the consultation, patients who are in HMOs or are insured through other managed-care providers cannot consult physicians outside a closed panel that is subject to similar financial arrangements. The problem is that *despite* disclosure, conflicts of interest can cloud physicians' judgment and affect their assessment of whether a medical service is needed—not just who should provide it. Patients need an opinion from a physician who is not compromised. And, as a rule, it makes sense to disqualify physicians who have significant conflicts of interest. An alternative that is not wholly adequate is for physicians to recommend that their patients seek a second opinion from a physician without a conflict of interest.

Disclosing financial ties to patients is unlike revealing the risks and benefits of proposed treatment as part of the process of obtaining informed consent. It warns not of the risks of a procedure or test, but of the limits of the physician as loyal agent or fiduciary. It is as if the physician were to invoke the principle of *caveat emptor* and to characterize patient and physician as adversaries. Rather than increase communication, trust, and participation in medical decision making, this information, if properly communicated, is likely to provoke doubts about the value of this medical advice.

Consumer Protection

Some people believe that disclosure can help patients become better consumers of medical care. Just as purchasers of consumer products are helped by accurate information, advocates of disclosure believe patients can be helped if doctors disclose information on conflicts of interest. But the experience of business with disclosure of information to consumers suggests serious limitations in the presumed analogy.

Federal and state consumer protection laws prohibit firms from using deceptive practices—such as omitting pertinent information—to sell goods or services.[19] In effect, businesses are often required to disclose any information that may loom large in a buyer's decision.[20] Similarly, the Food, Drug, and Cosmetic Act prohibits mislabeling of food, and federal regulations require that ingredients and nutritional content be listed.[21] Disclosure sometimes lowers consumers' costs in evaluating products and promotes allocative efficiency. When information is too voluminous or complex for the average consumer to interpret, outside groups—such as consumer associations or professional assessors—can evaluate the data. But studies show that purchasers are less likely to search for alternative products and services when time is critical or when they are ill-equipped to distinguish between crucial, deferrable, and unnecessary services.[22]

Despite efforts to foster competition in the health care market, patients remain particularly vulnerable.[23] They are frequently involuntary consumers; they cannot plan their purchases or assess alternatives carefully. They often have little opportunity to learn from personal experience, or else the cost of doing so is high. Constraints distort their choices and increase their reliance on physicians. Laypeople generally have some familiarity with government, law, and financial matters, since they deal with the law and markets in the course of their daily lives. Although this knowledge may be quite limited, it is much greater than their comparable medical knowledge and is more easily obtainable. The asymmetry of information availability in the patient-physician relationship renders patients dependent on physicians, and constraints prohibitively raise the cost to patients of obtaining and evaluating information.[24]

In the last decade, self-help groups and publications have provided advice to patients.[25] But patients still have great difficulty in assessing physicians or choosing ancillary medical care facilities. In a 1989 survey conducted by the Consumer Federation of America, more than half of the persons interviewed indicated that they found it somewhat difficult or very hard to shop for doctors and hospitals, and nearly three-quarters found it somewhat or very hard to shop for medical services.[26] Consumers even have a hard time determining physicians' specialties and training.[27] There is no equivalent of *Consumer Reports* to assess the competence and integrity of physicians and their advice, and institutions to perform these functions will not evolve easily.[28] The large number of physicians and the generally decentralized market for most medical care make such evaluations costly. Consumers who are considering elective surgery can obtain second opinions, but shopping for advice is often hit or miss or simply impractical. The disclosure of financial conflicts of interest will not ensure that patients can depend less on physicians.

Making more information available can help patients as consumers. But without careful guidelines, sellers often present information in a way that counteracts its beneficial effects. For example, some labels stress that foods contain no cholesterol but don't mention that they contain hydrogenated oils, which have similarly undesirable cardiovascular effects.[29] Studies show that the mandated warnings of health hazards on cigarette packages and advertisements are overshadowed by other material and often are not assimilated.[30] Manufacturers of cigarettes and other products have also used their disclosure of health risks as a way to limit their liability.[31] Disclosure can protect the seller rather than the purchaser. Some physicians may manipulate disclosure to limit their obligation to patients. Even well-intentioned physicians may disclose their financial interests in ways that encourage passive acceptance rather than increased patient awareness and scrutiny.

Disclosure by Public Officials, Financial Professionals, and Lawyers

Other professionals use disclosure to address conflicts of interest but in a manner quite different from the way it is likely to be used by doctors.

In government, disclosure is used as a tool to monitor conduct, publicize violations of conflict-of-interest laws, and deter any ethically dubious activities. Financial interest reports allow departmental supervisors and Office of Governmental Ethics (OGE) officials to keep abreast of employees' extragovernmental activities and to oversee their governmental work. Managers can use information on employees' personal finances to point out borderline activities before rules are violated. Disclosure reports help managers to reassign work, thereby preventing employees from participating in governmental matters that may affect their financial interests. Reports on the source and amount of outside income also help officials to identify individuals who have violated laws. In addition, failure to file accurate financial interest reports is itself subject to penalties, whether or not one has violated substantive prohibitions.

There is another important feature of disclosure in the federal government: it is *public*—reinforced by the press, watchdog groups, and the political process. The press as well as organizations such as Ralph Nader's Public Citizen and Common Cause can obtain information and publicize it, even if regulators fail to do their job.[32] Members of Congress, too, as part of the political process, often disclose embarrassing conflicts of interest of their opponents. Together these groups can arouse concern, ignite the electorate, and perhaps even oust administrations or officials from office.

In business, disclosure is used mainly as a preventive measure. Many state laws permit corporate officers and directors to enter into self-dealing transactions with their corporation if they disclose the conflict of interest to the board of directors, provide information that allows the board to assess the fairness of the transaction, and receive the board's approval. Shareholders must ratify the agreement. The rationale for allowing directors to enter into these transactions, despite the conflict of interest, is that disclosure will alert the board, which can assess the transaction's fairness. To the extent that the board errs, courts can void self-dealing transactions or award monetary damages, despite disclosure, if they deem transactions unfair.[33] In other areas of business, such as pension fund management, there is less reliance on disclosure because greater value is placed on reducing risk and because court supervision of self-dealing transactions is difficult and costly.

In the securities market, disclosure is employed as a preventive measure. In transactions between clients and broker-dealers, disclosure of conflicts of interest alerts investors, who may then protect themselves. Such disclosure is a halfway measure and does not provide a high level of protection. But its use is justified as a compromise necessary to preserve for all participants important economic gains that arise from merging the function of broker and dealer.

At a minimum, lawyers must always disclose conflicts of interest and explain the risk to clients. Often they must counsel clients to seek independent advice. While such disclosure does not eliminate conflicts, it does bring them into open view, warning and "arming" clients.[34] However, in some situations, lawyers may continue to represent clients, despite conflicts of interest, if clients have given independent, intelligent, and informed consent. Legal codes and courts nevertheless deem some conflicts of interest nonconsentable and prohibit lawyers without exception from representing clients.

Disclosure may prove effective for lawyers' conflicts of interest because of the unique institutional context in which it is used. Although disclosure by lawyers is usually conducted in private, the process is regulated by courts that specify its content, manner, and timing.[35] Lawyers who fail to disclose conflicts of interest do so at their peril. Courts can promote compliance with conflict-of-interest rules through a range of measures, including fines, disallowing lawyers from collecting fees for work performed, and other penalties.[36]

The adversarial nature of the American judicial system helps to enforce disclosure and other conflict-of-interest rules. In litigation, lawyers are expected to use every substantive and procedural device to advance the interests of their clients.[37] This includes asking the court to disqualify an opposing party's lawyer when conflicts of interest threaten the interests of the objecting lawyers' client. It also includes imputing one lawyer's conflicts to all affiliated lawyers.[38] Lawyers working in private firms therefore have an incentive to police themselves, since if they do not, they will collectively bear the stigma, financial loss, and possible threats of malpractice.[39]

In sum, disclosure can help address conflicts of interest, but only if it is part of a coordinated policy that sets high standards of ethical conduct, clearly delineates the permissible from the unacceptable, develops institutions to monitor behavior, and imposes meaningful sanctions to ensure compliance. Many institutional mechanisms that make disclosure helpful in other contexts are missing in medicine today.

The Limits of Public Intervention

There are also limits to what government intervention can achieve as an employer of physicians. This needs to be stressed because some people think that the federal government could eliminate all physicians' conflicts of interest by creating government health services that employ physicians on salary and purchase supplies and equipment. That view is mistaken. For although employing physicians would eliminate conflicts of interest arising from fee-for-service payment, as well as most of the conflicts of interest stemming from incentives to increase services, it still leaves open the possibility of other conflicts.

Many medical practices and commercial ties that lead to conflicts of interest thrive in the private sector and are typically associated with for-profit medicine. Yet these practices exist in the nonprofit sector as well. Nonprofit hospitals and providers can and do provide kickbacks and gifts and engage in joint ventures with physicians. Such practices encourage physicians to increase services. Many nonprofit HMOs have risk-sharing plans that offer doctors incentives to reduce services.

Just as nonprofit medical providers can engage in practices that promote conflicts of interest, so can the government if it employs physicians. When seeking to limit expenditures, government agencies may offer doctors financial incentives to limit services, just as HMOs do today with risk-sharing plans. They may also pursue other policies using means that compromise physicians' loyalty to patients.

Still, the government is likely to develop stricter conflict-of-interest policies than the private sector. There is already a well-established tradition of conflict-of-interest regulation for federal employees. In fact, physicians employed by the Veterans Administration (VA) are subject to conflict-of-interest rules from their own agency, and regulations that apply to all federal employees. The National Institutes of Health (NIH) regulates some conflicts of interest of physicians who perform research on human subjects.[40] In 1989 the NIH proposed and later withdrew guidelines to regulate the financial conflicts of interest of researchers.[41] It has since announced its intent to promulgate conflict-of-interest regulations.[42] These are the seeds of financial conflict-of-interest regulations for federally employed physicians.

If the government employs physicians, it will also prove easier to eliminate or discourage some kinds of physicians' conflicts of interest than it is when physicians are privately employed. It is relatively easy for government agencies to bar employed physicians from receiving gifts or kickbacks or developing compromising financial ties to suppliers, manufacturers, and hospitals. Such policies must be enforced, of course, but this is easier to do as an employer that exercises financial and managerial control over physicians than as an external regulator with only indirect means to oversee private individuals and businesses. Similarly, if a governmental authority purchased supplies and owned capital equipment (hospitals, offices, expensive medical equipment), private suppliers and manufacturers would not be able to tempt doctors easily with inducements, as they do now.

Even so, enforcement could present a challenge. A Veterans Administration investigation conducted between 1984 and 1987 indicates that Smith Kline & French, a major pharmaceutical firm, violated government conflict-of-interest policies and spent approximately $750,000 to hire as consultants Veterans Administration physicians who served on hospital formulary committees. Smith Kline & French paid honoraria, offered gratuities, and sponsored symposia.[43] Senate investigations revealed that some Veterans Administration physicians admitted that they had recommended changes to hospital formulary committees. They also found that some doctors had engaged in practices that were criminal violations—not only conflicts of interest—by getting paid for making speeches for the pharmaceutical firms while on government time.[44] The investigation, which resulted in three doctors being suspended and numerous others being reprimanded, revealed that several other pharmaceutical firms, including Merck, Sharp & Dohme; Ciba-Geigy; Eli Lilly; and Abbott Laboratories, may also have engaged in similar practices, which led to further investigations by the Office of the Inspector General. The supposed aim of these payments was to get the physicians to place their products on the hospital formulary. If government physicians can influence what products the government authority ordered, medical suppliers might still try to sway key physicians with various financial inducements.

More significant, physicians as employees (whether working for the government or for a private employer such as an HMO) have an *indirect* financial interest in their own continued employment. A government agency could offer its employed doctors financial incentives to limit services to patients. These practices may be enticing from a social point of view because they curb expenditures and help the public sector live within budget constraints. But from the point of view of patients, they are even less desirable than budget constraints that would limit available resources.

Physicians employed by a governmental agency may be unable to provide their best clinical advice if it conflicts with the government's policies, especially if the government penalizes them financially, blocks their advancement, or even dismisses physicians who make decisions conflicting with government policy. The physician as employee serves two masters: employer and patient. An example was the experience of physicians working at family planning clinics receiving federal funds during the administration of President George Bush. The Department of Health and Human Services had promulgated a gag rule that prohibited offering information about abortions, and doctors were not allowed to discuss this family planning option with patients.[45] In this case, the government used its financial leverage over the institutional recipient of funds, but the same principle applies.

Sociologist Mark Field, in his study of physicians in the former Soviet Union, coined the term *structured strain* to describe the kind of divided loyalty in physicians who work for the state.[46] However, physicians may also experience such conflicts when employed by a third party in the private sector. Although the public often regards physicians as independent practitioners they are increasingly employees of HMOs, hospitals, nursing homes, group practices, and corporations that provide medical care for their employees.[47]

Governmental employment of physicians would suspend some financial conflicts of interest, make others easier to control (if political consensus permitted it), and create still others. If a governmental agency replaces physicians as the owners and purchasers of medical equipment, it also assumes many of their conflicts of interest. Providers and suppliers may no longer be in a position to offer physicians incentives to practice in ways that benefit them. But the purchasing and budgeting decisions of government agencies may be influenced by their own financial concerns, which can conflict with those of patients. When proposing policies that reduce physicians' conflicts of interest, patients' advocates need to be careful not to replace them with government, provider, or third-party payer conflicts of interest. These institutions need policies to hold them accountable as well.

Policies for Physicians' Financial Conflicts of Interest

Alternative Strategies

To review, seven kinds of activities lead to significant conflicts of interest among physicians: (1) kickbacks to and from medical suppliers and providers for referrals; (2) physician self-referral (income earned from physicians referring patients to facilities in which they invest); (3) physician dispensing of drugs, selling medical products, and performing ancillary medical services that doctors themselves prescribe; (4) hospital purchase of physicians' private practice; (5) payments made by hospitals to recruit and bond physicians; (6) gifts to physicians from medical suppliers; and (7) physician risk sharing in HMOs and hospitals.

The first six practices generally create incentives to provide services, and the seventh creates incentives to withhold them. However, the second, fourth, and fifth practices can also create incentives to decrease services when physicians have financial ties to hospitals, home health care providers, or nursing homes. This is due to Medicare's fixed hospital payment per case which creates incentives to reduce services.

How should we cope with these conflicts of interest? Let us consider the issue first in general, then in relation to each of the conflicts.

Economists suggest that one can gauge the effect of a conflict of interest by the strength and directness of the financial incentive it offers doctors: as incentives become stronger or more direct, physicians are more likely to respond. The economist's prescription: target financial incentives that are direct or strong, rather than develop regulations to address broad categories of conflicts of interest.

There is merit in this view. Certainly not all conflicts of interest are equally compromising. And examining the effect of conflicts rather than the categories of activity also makes sense. From the perspective of preventing or otherwise addressing conflicts, it matters little whether a financial incentive that may prompt doctors to act contrary to the patient's interest arises from physicians selling a product, receiving a kickback, referring patients to medical facilities in which they invest, receiving gifts, participating in a risk-sharing plan, or maintaining other financial ties. The legal form or the financial arrangement may change, yet still produce the same effect. Thus there are risks in addressing conflicts of interest through rules for categories of activities.

There is, however, still a problem with this strength-of-incentive approach from the perspective of ensuring workable responses. Designing legal remedies based on the strength of incentives would be too time consuming and even impossible to administer. Within each of the seven categories of conflict of interest, there will be a range from weak and diffuse to strong and direct. For example, the strength of the financial incentive to refer patients to physician-owned facilities will vary depending on the number of investors and the way the investment is organized. Both factors affect the probability and amount of earnings. Self-referral arrangements, too, can have incentives varying from indirect and weak to direct and strong. They can resemble kickbacks where the payoff is nearly certain, or investments with an uncertain payoff. Earnings from the sale of drugs or other products can be small or large, creating proportionate incentives to prescribe or sell them. So, too, for kickbacks, gifts, hospital recruitment and bonding incentives, and other kinds of financial payments. Without some general rules, policymakers would have to review each arrangement or transaction to assess the strength and directness of the incentive.

Furthermore, even when we know the strength of a financial incentive and its predicted payoff, this alone will not tell us whether it will entice a physician to act inappropriately.[48] That depends on the particular circumstances and the possible risks for patients. For example, if the physician has an interest in a clinical lab that analyzes blood, making a referral can cause no direct harm to the patient's health, although the patient may lose some money.[49] If a doctor has a financial interest in a surgical center, and refers a patient for an invasive procedure when it is not needed, the patient faces increased risk of bodily harm. Physicians who encounter and respond to economic incentives may be more likely to make unnecessary referrals in the first situation because the patient's health is not at risk. Policymakers must distinguish between protecting a patient's pocketbook and his or her health.

Finally, the risk posed by a conflict of interest is only one part of the equation. It is important to know the potential benefits from the activities that may be subject to regulation. As the social value of activities increases it makes sense to bear greater risk from conflicts of interest. And for activities that have little social value, society may want to curb conflicts of interest that create even small levels of risk. We would also want to know if the desirable activity could take place even with regulation.

The experience of other professions reveals three regulatory approaches to conflicts of interest: to prohibit certain kinds of activities; to monitor and regulate conduct; and to provide penalties for improper conduct. The mix of tactics used should vary, depending on market conditions and individual circumstances. Often market mechanisms cannot be used to address conflicts of interest. Adequate legal remedies for misbehavior sometimes exist. But it may be preferable to regulate physicians when there is a risk of misconduct producing irreparable harm, if remedies for misconduct would be inadequate or if it is hard to detect misconduct. When regulatory supervision would be too costly or would reduce the value of the work physicians perform, it is usually preferable to prohibit certain transactions as a preventive measure.

So many transactions take place between patients and physicians in the United States that regulating conduct through rules for specific transactions would be cumbersome and expensive. Monitoring compliance with detailed rules would also be costly, as would reviewing physicians' performance to determine whether proper clinical decisions were made. The experience of reviewing the clinical decisions of physicians through PROs, utilization review programs, and quality assurance programs indicates that supervision is costly and difficult. Extending such review to physicians' conflicts of interest would add yet more administrative burdens and might not be very effective. The use of courts to review the appropriateness of individual transactions on a case-by-case basis would also involve great cost and clog the court system. Therefore, it appears simpler and more efficient to prohibit broad classes of conduct through legislation than to adopt policies that regulate the details of physicians' behavior or provide sanctions for misconduct.

This strategy may be less appropriate for certain conflicts of interest, however. Prohibiting activities can sometimes impose high social costs. Moreover, we may need to rely on other approaches for purely practical or political reasons. We might then prohibit the seven practices but allow a regulatory authority to grant exemptions in special circumstances. Those seeking the exemptions would carry the burden of proving that it was in the interest of patients. When exceptions are made, we could still rely on regulatory approaches and penalties for misconduct. It is from this perspective that we shall review the seven questionable practices.

Kickbacks

The aim of kickbacks is to promote the financial interests of the kickback payer and receiver; in general, the patient receives no benefit. Kickbacks directly link physicians' clinical decisions and advice to their financial interest and that of the payer. When doctors receive kickbacks, even though they outwardly profess to serve patients, they are toiling partly for another master. This is especially true of kickbacks from medical suppliers and manufacturers to physicians in return for referral of patients or use of the provider's services or products. While physicians may pay or receive kickbacks and still perform good clinical work for patients, the practice compromises the physicians' loyalty and judgment and should be prohibited.

The federal government already prohibits kickbacks and any payments that induce referrals in the Medicare and Medicaid programs, and statutes in 36 states prohibit physicians from receiving kickbacks for patient referrals.[50] Yet the history of fraud and abuse in the Medicare program shows that kickbacks thrive despite prohibitions and providers have devised means to disguise kickbacks. Nor do the states adequately enforce these laws, and they can impose only small sanctions. Prohibitions on kickbacks should cover doctors in whatever jurisdiction they practice and for whatever patients they treat. We also need more effective mechanisms to identify subterfuges and enforce prohibitions. Stopping kickbacks, however, will require additional resources for monitoring the financial practices of physicians and providers as well as for enforcement and prosecution.

Physician Self-Referral: Desirable and Undesirable Forms

Physician self-referral is analogous to physicians receiving kickbacks for steering business to third parties. Both activities present the same conflict of interest in different guises. Physicians can act as stronger advocates for their patients if they do not refer patients to medical facilities in which they invest. Independent physicians are also more likely to provide neutral advice. Independent medical care facilities are apt to be more sensitive to the needs of patients if they have to earn their referrals through their reputation for quality.

As a whole, patients would be better off if society prohibited physician self-referral. Physician self-referral, strictly defined, has no inherent social value, biases the judgment of physicians, and compromises their loyalty. In most cases, third parties can provide the same services without physician investment, and capital for most legitimate ventures can be obtained from other investors. Exceptions to a ban might be made for self-referral in rural areas. But self-referral should not be allowed even in such situations unless it can be shown that there is no other practical way to provide the services and unless the activity is regulated.

There are articulate defenders of physician self-referral to free-standing medical facilities in which physicians invest.[51] To restrict self-referral here, they argue, is inconsistent, since we allow physicians working in large group practices to refer patients to each other and share the profits.[52] And many other incentives to increase services, though not strictly self-referral, are similar in that physicians reward third parties in return for the third party's returning the favor. Physicians who are paid on a fee-for-service basis self-refer, broadly defined, every time they recommend and perform a procedure or service or even ask a patient to return for a checkup. Defenders of self-referral claim that it makes no sense to restrict self-referral to free-standing facilities in which physicians invest but not restrict self-referral—broadly defined—across the board. They say that there is no principled way to distinguish between such activities.

The argument can be carried further. Prohibitions against physicians referring patients to free-standing medical facilities in which they have a financial interest might merely shift the locus of self-referral in-house by encouraging the growth of group practices as a way to recoup lost self-referral income. Physicians in large group practices might purchase diagnostic and laboratory equipment to provide these services in-house. Would in-house self-referral be any better than the practice it replaced? If not, can we justify banning outpatient self-referral or the existence of such a common phenomenon as group practices? Would it be wise or even possible to prevent self-referral within group practice? And how is self-referral different from the conflicts of interest implicit in fee-for-service payment?

At first, it appears that prohibiting self-referral to free-standing facilities in which physicians invest might be a rule easily bypassed by changing the legal form of an organization, or, it could be that the prohibition constitutes too strict a policy. But the arguments of critics have less merit than at first appears.

There are several reasons to distinguish between physician self-referral within an office and self-referral to facilities in which physicians are limited partners. When physicians who are limited partners refer to facilities in which they invest, they have no control over the day-to-day management of such facilities. Their financial liability is limited to a small investment, and limited partners are not legally liable for the negligence of those operating the facility. Their investment is passive. These limited partners bear little financial risk, and no legal responsibility, and exercise no operational control, yet reap profits from referrals.

However, when physicians refer to in-house facilities, they earn their income not just from their investment and referrals, but from providing or supervising a service as well. Patients benefit because the referring physician can exercise some control over the provision of care, and presumably take measures to ensure high quality. Physicians who own a group practice have an incentive to be prudent and greater justification for earning profit, because they bear the financial risk and are legally liable for any negligence in the use of the equipment. Although these circumstances cannot eliminate all abuses, they significantly reduce the risk and provide far better justifications for physicians earning income from such referrals than passive investments in limited partnerships.

A ban on self-referral to physician-owned free-standing facilities is also likely to be more effective than critics claim. While some self-referral to free-standing medical clinical labs or diagnostic facilities might be brought in-house by group practices, much of it could not. Free-standing facilities often require expensive equipment. For these facilities to be profitable, they need to provide a high volume of services and could not survive on in-house referrals alone. Many of the activities could be brought in-house only in the largest group practices, and even these might also have to offer their services to unaffiliated physicians to make the investment profitable.

To the extent, too, that prohibitions on physician self-referral spur the growth of large group practices, this is a welcome side effect. Group practice can provide continuity and coordinate patient care. It is more efficient than solo practice. It often includes peer review and administrative oversight of doctors. Conflicts of interest remain, but they will be far easier to regulate in a few large group practices than in many solo or small group practices. Shifting the locus of self-referral will promote important health policy goals and make it easier for governmental authorities to address remaining conflicts of interest.

Prohibiting self-referral to free-standing facilities while leaving in-house self-referral untouched is not a complete solution; still it does restrict the practice most easily regulated. The proposal has merit because it provides some protection to patients, even though it does not eliminate all risks. At the moment, we lack means for a more comprehensive remedy.[53]

It makes little sense, however, to prohibit all self-referral broadly construed. If a ban on self-referral were carried to its logical conclusion, some activities that one person could perform would have to be split up between two or more parties. For example, physicians could not recommend and perform an inoculation if they were paid for the serum or recommended the need for an inoculation. And doctors could not recommend that patients continue or extend their ongoing medical therapy. Such broad restrictions would not be practical or desirable. Indeed, the cure would be worse than the problem. That is not the case for the restrictions proposed here.

Dispensing Drugs, Selling Medical Products, and Performing Ancillary Services

There are physicians who now dispense drugs and medical products they prescribe. They benefit directly from the kind and volume of prescriptions they write and the products they sell. This practice, a classic conflict of interest, is long-standing, if not widespread. Except for a few situations, as in rural areas where access to pharmacies and other providers is limited, there is no strong reason, medical or otherwise, to allow the practice. Pharmacies can dispense just as well as physicians—if not better and more cheaply—and even provide a check on doctors' errors. It may be more convenient for patients to purchase drugs in a doctor's office in some situations. But it will usually be more convenient to refill prescriptions in a pharmacy since they are open for longer hours. A prohibition against physicians dispensing drugs would eliminate situations in which physicians overprescribe due to financial incentives or dispense a less desirable product merely because they have it in stock. It would also help to defuse another conflict of interest. As we have seen, pharmaceutical firms often offer physicians gifts in an effort to change their prescribing habits. This conflict of interest is exacerbated when physicians have a direct financial interest in the drugs and products they prescribe. Some allowance may be necessary for physicians performing certain laboratory tests in their offices or dispensing certain drugs for medical emergencies. But a broad prohibition against physicians dispensing products they prescribe is feasible and warranted.

*Hospital Purchase of Medical Practices, Bonding Programs,
and Physician Recruitment*

Doctors often form financial ties to providers, insurers, and other parties. These ties encourage physicians to provide or limit services to patients for the benefit of doctors or third parties. There are three main examples of such arrangements: (1) hospitals purchasing the private practice of physicians; (2) hospitals recruiting physicians and subsidizing their private practices; and (3) hospital bonding programs that aim to acquire physician loyalty by providing a range of financial support, either directly or through participating in lucrative joint ventures.

It is true that physicians and hospitals have bonds that transcend direct financial incentives. Physicians may be loyal to institutions where they have affiliations even in the absence of the direct financial ties and inducements discussed previously. Some physicians may be employed by hospitals. Others have long-standing affiliations related to their medical training, colleagues, or location. Moreover, some physicians have privileges at only one hospital and thus may not be able to offer a choice to patients. These factors, too, can limit the options for patients and bias physicians' advice concerning which hospital is most appropriate. Constraints therefore exist on the extent to which physicians can act as ideal neutral advisers in recommending hospitals. Nevertheless, promoting clinical neutrality and loyalty to patients is a worthy ideal, even if it can never be fully achieved. We ought to offset, not add, to these problems.

Advocates of hospital recruitment payments, practice subsidies, and bonding programs sometimes claim that such practices are necessary to attract physicians to rural areas, many of which are underserved. But these practices are not used only or even primarily in rural and underserved areas. There are also other ways to address the rural problem. The state or federal government could provide incentives to encourage doctors to locate in rural or underserved areas. Such programs would not make physicians beholden to a particular hospital or encourage physicians to accept hospital payments in order to repay their debts. If individual hospitals are left instead to develop their own recruitment incentives, hospital growth will be spurred more by marketing than by health care needs.

Strong arguments can be made against hospital purchase or subsidy of physicians' practices, and against many bonding programs that create financial conflicts of interest for physicians. Usually not needed, such programs increase the risk that physicians will promote their own interests, or those of particular hospitals, at the expense of patients. Most hospital subsidies of physicians' private practices should be eliminated. Short of prohibiting all such practices, state or federal governments could regulate them by limiting the kind, amount, and manner of financial inducements, thereby eliminating the worst abuses.

Not all financial ties between physicians and providers create conflicts of interest. Some that do may have social value. Selected joint ventures between hospitals and physicians should, in fact, be exempted from strict prohibitions. In addition, some financial ties between hospitals and physicians may not be easily eliminated without significant social costs. It is impossible to anticipate all of the financial arrangements that may grow up between physicians and hospitals, let alone survey all existing arrangements. However, we need defensible criteria to justify exceptions. Moreover, those who wish to engage in such arrangements should have the burden of proving that an exemption is warranted.

The aim of these policies must be to restrict practices that make physicians beholden to providers, suppliers, and other third parties. We should start with a presumption that payments between physicians and providers that are not for services rendered or exceed market rates are the functional equivalent of kickbacks. Physicians and third parties who make or receive such payments should be required to demonstrate that they have legitimate objectives that cannot be met through other means except at greater cost.

Gifts from Medical Suppliers

Gifts can indebt physicians and often corrupt or subtly influence their judgment. This is especially the case for gifts received from medical care suppliers and manufacturers, particularly those whose products can be recommended to patients or whose services physicians use. As in the case of kickbacks, little social loss would ensue if physicians could not receive gifts from medical suppliers, manufacturers, and providers. The example of federal executive branch employees is a useful model. Federal employees are generally forbidden to accept gifts from people who might benefit from their official decisions. Likewise, public policy should prohibit physicians from receiving gifts from individuals working in the health care field who stand to benefit from clinical choices these physicians might make. Exceptions might be made for gifts of nominal value or involving limited business entertainment, such as paying for modest dinners or lunches. But policymakers might even discourage such practices by amending the tax code to disallow deducting such costs as business expenses and by requiring recipients to declare such gifts as income.

Risk Sharing in HMOs and Hospitals

Many HMOs, managed-care providers, and a few hospitals use risk-sharing plans to hold affiliated physicians financially responsible for the costs of the medical services they recommend. The purpose of such plans is to limit the expense of clinical decisions made by physicians. When separated from other considerations, the aim seems harmless. But like self-referral, risk sharing compromises the loyalty and judgment of physicians. It allies physicians with budget cutters rather than with patients. Physicians can enrich themselves by denying services.

Proponents of risk sharing allege that when the risk borne by physicians is limited, the incentive will not lead physicians to limit service inappropriately. The argument is plausible. But we do not know it to be true or, if true, what level of risk is acceptable, and we cannot as yet adequately measure medical underuse. Proponents of volume incentives also contend that when physicians are offered incentives to reduce services they will first cut unnecessary or marginally useful ones. And when physicians are offered incentives to increase services they will first offer useful rather than unnecessary ones. The problem, of course, is that volume incentives do not reward physicians for making such distinctions, and they operate regardless of the value of the service provided or denied.[54] Consequently they reward inappropriate choices just as much as those that are suitable. Even if risk sharing does not, in general, cause underuse of medical services, the practice should be shunned; it tempts physicians to do just that.

Health providers cannot plausibly argue that risk sharing is necessary to their operation or provides important social benefits not otherwise available. The best that can be said for risk sharing is that it can be used to limit inappropriate overuse of medical services. But there are many other ways to address overuse.

Why not eliminate financial incentives for both increasing and decreasing services? Paying primary care physicians by salary or on a per capita basis for each of their patients (capitation) approximates a neutral position more closely than any other existing payment mechanism, since there is no direct incentive to increase or decrease services.[55] However, it may be necessary to regulate capitation payments because this too can be a limited form of risk sharing under certain conditions.[56] Another way to limit inappropriate services is to provide incentives for appropriate use and impose fines for inappropriate use. The incentive would be linked to the correctness of clinical decisions, not general volume targets.

Should the prohibition of risk sharing be politically unacceptable, the next best tactic would be to strictly regulate the amount of risk individual physicians could bear. Restricting the financial risk would reduce the strength of perverse incentives and would probably reduce the degree of harm to patients. The most practical way to do this would be to cap physicians' financial gain or loss to a small percentage of their baseline pay. This would provide a rule easy to monitor, with effects that would be easy to gauge. For example, a statute might restrict profit or loss under risk-sharing plans to between 1% and 2% of baseline income or to a fixed dollar amount. Such a restriction would prevent providers from tempting physicians to change their behavior.[57] Although we cannot be sure that small financial incentives would not produce inappropriate conduct, strictly controlled risk sharing would be preferable to risk sharing with stronger incentives.

Another tactic to discourage inappropriate risk sharing would be to place legal liability on organizational providers for the malpractice caused by underuse of services by their affiliated physicians. (Currently, hospitals and other organizational providers usually are not liable for the negligence of doctors who are hired as independent contractors; and proving that risk sharing caused negligence is difficult.) Providers would then examine more carefully the amount of risk sharing imposed on physicians. They would also devise quality-of-care policies with a reduced risk of patient harm. The liability approach is far from ideal, however, because only a small amount of medical malpractice actually results in an award, thereby reducing the deterrent effect.[58] Some doctors believe that fear of medical malpractice already causes doctors to perform inappropriate tests in order to reduce the risk of liability. Although there are no solid data indicating whether or to what extent this occurs, this also may be a drawback of the liability approach.

The Job Ahead

The Need for Fiduciary Standards

The medical profession and society can and should create new institutions and rules to hold physicians to fiduciary standards that already exist in other fields. This is best done by legislatures. Courts might also play a role.

In theory, courts could develop fiduciary standards through the slow process by which they make common law, declaring rules of law while adjudicating cases. The California Supreme Court recently declared, in *Moore v. California*, that doctors are obligated to disclose financial conflicts of interest to human research subjects as part of a requirement to obtain informed consent.[59] Conceivably, this disclosure requirement could be extended to physicians in clinical practice; courts might even develop rules disqualifying physicians with certain conflicts of interest from performing services.

Professor E. Haavi Morreim, a philosopher specializing in medical ethics, has advocated similar court involvement for addressing inappropriate physician self-referral. Under her proposal, courts would award patients attorney's fees, compensation for emotional distress, and even punitive damages if they could show that a physician self-referred in bad faith.[60] Presumably, such a court-made rule would discourage bad faith self-referral while allowing legitimate or other self-referral.

Relying on courts to develop common law for physicians' conflicts of interest has significant drawbacks, however, for it relies on patients to initiate lawsuits. Patients are unlikely to bring suit even if they are aware of financial improprieties, since most are insured and thus protected from the overwhelming share of out-of-pocket costs. Indeed, they may not have legal standing to bring such suits. In addition, most patients won't act unless they are significantly harmed. In other cases, they are unlikely to suspect that their physician acted inappropriately. Courts will therefore play a role only in cases of malpractice or adverse medical outcomes. But clinical practice standards and malpractice law are already established. What is lacking are preventive rules for financial conflicts of interest that reduce the risk of inappropriate conduct.

Both patients and third-party payers face another obstacle if courts do award punitive damages for bad faith breach of obligations. Proving bad faith is difficult. In the presence of medical uncertainty or differences of opinion among experts, patients and payers will usually be unable to show bad faith. If they can, such cases are better addressed through existing laws preventing kickbacks, fraud, or other violations of legal norms. Bad faith suits are unlikely to be helpful in dealing with financial conflicts of interest that bias the judgment of physicians in subtle ways.

An approach that holds more promise is for courts to impose strict liability on physicians (i.e., liability without regard to fault or negligence) if patients are injured when a physician has engaged in self-referral or other financial conflicts of interest.[61] Physicians might then hew more closely to fiduciary standards to increase their insulation from liability. But this approach has drawbacks, too. Under a strict liability standard, patients could bring suit only if harmed. Many clinical or diagnostic tests add expense, inconvenience, or discomfort. This approach would only discourage those financial conflicts of interest that might put patients at risk of physical harm that patients eventually detect. Still, the specter of strict liability for malpractice might reduce conflicts of interest.

Another weakness of the proposal is that the trend today is to propose malpractice reforms that provide greater protection for physicians, limit awards to patients, or use a no-fault system. In today's political climate, legislative proposals to increase liability for physicians are apt to be defeated. Although courts could develop such a strict liability rule, there is no reason to believe they will anytime soon. Strict liability is usually reserved for inherently dangerous activities.

There is also the issue of fairness. A strict liability approach might deter physicians from entering into conflict-of-interest situations, but it is more severe and punitive for bad outcomes than are rules that regulate or prohibit certain forms of conduct outright. Such measures would penalize a few physicians whose patients may have died or taken a turn for the worse through no fault of the physician; the measures would also ignore all other physicians with conflicts of interest.

Legislatures are probably in a better position than courts to lay the groundwork for fiduciary standards. Their statutes can declare policies and rules. Courts can then grant remedies when rules are breached. Legislatures need not require proof of harm to patients. They may develop preventive rules and standards. Regulatory agencies, third-party payers, state attorney generals, federal authorities, or other parties could enforce them.

Legislatures have imposed fiduciary standards on selected groups: explicitly, as in the case of the Employee Retirement Income Security Act (ERISA), the Investment Advisors Act, and state legislation regulating trustees; or implicitly, when regulating, for example, the conduct of insurers—even though the legislation does not use the term *fiduciary*. And, of course, many professionals are now subject to these standards: government officials, lawyers, corporate officers and directors, and such financial specialists as money managers, advisers, and broker-dealers, as well as trustees and agents. Why not doctors as well?

If physicians were answerable to patients under a strict fiduciary standard for their financial conflicts of interest the legal framework would not need to specify all the details. Once the fiduciary principle is established, it will be much easier for regulatory agencies and courts to develop specific rules for the large variety of financial conflicts of interest. Both regulatory agencies and courts can use fiduciary principles to address new kinds of conflicts as they arise, yet their policies and rules are likely to be more coherent and consistent when developed in the context of a statutory scheme.

Establishing legal fiduciary standards would also allow existing institutions to address conflicts of interest in ways currently not possible. Malpractice law—which holds physicians responsible for their negligence—could hold physicians liable for departing from the standards. Since fiduciary law for doctors is now all but nonexistent, malpractice law focuses mainly on physicians' technical clinical competence. Similarly, state medical licensing boards—which have the power to grant and revoke licenses and discipline physicians, and which currently focus only on egregious acts that violate ordinary standards of conduct— might also discipline physicians for breaching fiduciary standards.[62]

Create New Institutions or Use Existing Ones?

No one can end by edict commercial practices that lead to physicians' conflicts of interest. Legislation cannot anticipate all future problems. Legislating specific prohibitions will provide only partial ad hoc solutions. Soon after the enactment of any legislation that restricts certain activities, medical care providers, suppliers, and physicians are likely to develop new financial arrangements, giving rise to unforeseen conflicts of interest. Further, some activities that cause conflicts of interest may be so highly valued as to discourage outright prohibition.

What we need are institutions—organizations and processes—to enforce prohibitions, supervise conduct, monitor problems, and develop and implement new rules or policies as the need arises. The odds are that we will rely as much as possible on existing institutions and encourage them to develop measures to deal with physicians' conflicts of interest. But we will also need new institutions.

It is easier and often more acceptable to rely on existing institutions and to initiate small-scale reforms than to create major institutional changes. Many organizations already regulate physicians or medical care. They could develop conflict-of-interest policies. State and federal governments are more likely to bolster the authority of existing institutions than to establish a new regulatory authority. If existing institutions are used, problems can be tackled in stages. Legislators at both the federal and state levels can devise reforms for one or two conflicts of interest and leave others for future deliberation. Similarly, one state can develop policies before a political consensus exists to develop policies in other states.

With small-scale reform, it is also possible to encourage laboratories for experimentation with different policies. Congress, state legislatures, administrative agencies, and maybe even courts can address various aspects of conflicts of interest. Each can learn from and build on the experience of the others. If state or federal legislatures address conflict-of-interest issues in legislation, courts can expand their reach through interpretation of the law and adjudication of cases.

Yet small-scale reforms have drawbacks. They would address conflicts of interest only partially. Existing institutions generally have other goals. Conflict-of-interest policies may receive low priority and remain vulnerable when at odds with the main objectives of the sponsoring institution. Efforts by such a wide variety of authorities with limited jurisdiction also produce policies that are often uncoordinated, inconsistent, and difficult to enforce. Without effective linkages between different authorities, there are sure to be inconsistencies or policy gaps. A piecemeal approach is apt to yield only partial remedies to even simple conflict-of-interest problems.

New institutions designed to address physicians' conflicts of interest are less likely to neglect them, but they may still lack the regulatory authority needed. This is because existing agencies already claim jurisdiction over some areas of medical practice that affect physicians' conflicts of interest and are unlikely to cede their powers to new institutions.

For instance, the Internal Revenue Service (IRS) has much leverage over physicians' conflicts of interest, but the extent to which it will use this leverage is uncertain. Consider two examples. The IRS is now considering adopting a policy that would define as an impermissible private benefit many payments hospitals often make to physicians as part of recruiting and bonding programs. This would jeopardize the charitable tax status of many hospitals or require them to change their practices. If the IRS adopts such a policy, it would discourage nonprofit hospitals from offering doctors a wide range of financial incentives, thereby eliminating a major area of physicians' conflicts of interest.

The IRS could also discourage other payments by for-profit institutions. Currently, firms that give gifts and hospitals that subsidize the practices of doctors are encouraged to do so because their expenditures are tax deductible as necessary business expenses. Typically, these expenses are not declared as income by the physicians who receive them, partly due to the ambiguity of the law and partly due to the IRS's lackluster enforcement. If we do not disallow such practices altogether, the least we can do is not subsidize them. Changes in the Internal Revenue Code or IRS regulations could disallow such expenditures as business expenses. IRS enforcement policy could make physicians declare the services they receive as income based on the fair market value of the services and thereby discourage gifts and other compromising subsidies by hospitals.

The IRS's interest in adopting such policies stems from a mission to preserve the charitable purposes of hospitals, not from concern over physicians' conflicts of interest. Furthermore, the IRS often shies away from making policy explicitly, and so is unlikely on its own to consider disallowing the deduction of certain business expenses.[63] So, although the IRS has powerful tools to deter conflicts of interest, it is likely to use them sparingly.

Sooner or later, to achieve significant change, either local jurisdictions must adopt uniform or at least similar policies, which is unlikely, or the federal government must develop appropriate policies, which is far more plausible. The federal role could evolve gradually as an extension of one or more federal health programs, such as Medicare and Medicaid, the Veterans Administration, and the Civilian Health and Medical Program of the Uniformed Services. These programs, however, do not cover all patients and physicians.

If the federal government decides to develop conflict-of-interest policies that apply to all physicians, Congress will have to pass appropriate legislation or use its revenue-granting authority as leverage. For example, the federal government might make state receipt of Medicaid funds conditional upon states adopting and enforcing certain conflict-of-interest policies. Such an approach would have states incorporate standards and might require that they create agencies to enforce such laws. Alternatively, the Medicare program might require that physicians who participate in the program follow conflict-of-interest policies for all their patients.

Medicine as a Regulated Industry

Another model of how physicians' conflicts of interest might be addressed is provided by the experience of regulated industries, such as the securities market. Congress established the Securities and Exchange Commission (SEC) to oversee the industry, license and revoke the licenses of financial professionals in the industry, and oversee the manner in which the industry operates. Currently, the medical industry is regulated by a patchwork of state and federal programs and laws. No single agency oversees medical care activities as the SEC does, and existing regulation is much less extensive than in the securities industry. At present, and perhaps even in the future, it is unlikely that the federal government will be given regulatory authority over the medical care industry equivalent to its control over the securities industry. The reasons are rooted in the political traditions of the United States and in problems associated with centralized controls and the traditional image of medicine. Nevertheless, President-elect Bill Clinton has made clear his interest in health care reform and many observers believe that there may be major policy changes in the next decade. One may, therefore, speculate about how such authority might emerge.

If, in the future, the federal government develops a national health insurance program, it might well create a new federal agency to oversee the program, and such an agency could also be given authority to regulate physicians' conflicts of interest.[64] Small-scale reforms over time have increased the federal government's powers over the financing and delivery of medical care; these powers already provide the starting point for a national health insurance program.

An important source of regulatory supervision of medical practice and conflicts of interest could be federal licensing of physicians. Traditionally, medical licensing is a state function, performed in cooperation with the medical profession. In 1990, however, Representative Pete

Stark (D.-California) proposed that Medicare certify physicians on a periodic basis to monitor the quality of medical care it provides.[65] Federal certification in the Medicare program would put the federal government in a position to enforce conflict-of-interest regulations and standards of financial conduct for doctors and hospital. Working with the medical profession, the federal government might also codify or develop practice standards. There are other benefits of federal licensing. It would also allow greater control over physicians' qualifications and a means to intervene if doctors were incompetent or impaired.

There would be certain advantages in treating the practice of medicine as a regulated industry along the lines of the securities industry. If federal legislation created a Medical Regulatory Commission (MRC) to oversee the business and practice of medicine and physicians' conflicts of interest, it would presumably cover all physicians. Many physicians' conflicts of interest arise from the practices of hospitals, insurers, suppliers, and other institutions. The most effective solution would be to change the practices of the institutions that give rise to the conflicts of interest, rather than place the onus on physicians to change their conduct. To pursue such a strategy, an agency is needed to regulate the medical industry as a whole. Unlike approaches that divide authority between multiple state and federal agencies, a federal authority could address physicians' conflicts of interest, the market conditions that produce them, and even problems in accountability and consistency that exist due to the lack of a single authority.

Just as the securities industry belongs in the private sector but is subject to SEC control, medical care could remain a private sector activity while subject to oversight by the MRC. The MRC would address physicians' conflicts of interest without becoming an employer of physicians. Nor would it own medical facilities or capital equipment.

The commision would need to control the conditions under which physicians, medical providers, and suppliers conduct their trade and practice. It could accomplish this task by licensing medical personnel, providers, and suppliers, and by setting policy with respect to medical care financial practices and conflicts of interest. It might prohibit some activities, supervise others, and require disclosure for still more. Like the SEC which allows self-regulatory organizations to implement some policies (under its supervision), the MRC could delegate some of its implementing functions to professional organizations. It might even share costs with the organizations undertaking these tasks in compliance with MRC standards.

Just as the SEC was once fiercely resisted, the suggestion that such a medical commission be created is certain to distress the medical profession, providers, and suppliers. Even if not politically realistic in the short run, the idea of such a commission highlights the current problems of confronting physicians' conflicts of interest through government policy.

Examples of New Organizations: The Independent Hospital Auditor and the Conflict-of-Interest Review Board

Whether or not conflicts of interest are addressed through a federal authority or small-scale reforms using existing institutions, we can help deal with them by adapting some well-known processes, such as auditing and review boards.

One of the major areas in which physicians' conflicts of interest arise is physician-hospital relations. Some conflicts could be dealt with by prohibiting certain kinds of financial arrangements, such as physician self-referral to facilities that physicians own jointly with the hospital. However, if this occurs, some hospitals will develop new arrangements to induce physicians to act for their mutual interests in ways that may threaten loyalty to patients. Still other financial arrangements between hospitals and physicians other than joint-ownership cause conflict-of-interest problems not easily dealt with through prohibitions. Hospital-physician relations already are, and in the future will be, an important area to monitor. While a standard approach to the problem would be to assign a government agency direct authority to regulate hospitals and for courts to enforce their regulations, more sensitive, less costly, and more effective approaches exist. For example, the government could develop standards of financial practice for the relations between hospitals and physicians. It could require hospitals to let an independent auditor assess their financial practices—with respect to physicians' conflicts of interest—and to make the findings public.[66]

The American College of Surgeons (ACS) reported that when the Columbus Surgical Society audited the financial records of physicians, fee splitting declined sharply.[67] IRS auditing of books also bolstered the reform program. Monitoring financial relations can constrain certain kinds of commercial conduct. Moreover, the auditor/controller approach is used by many financial institutions. At mutual funds, compliance officers monitor financial conduct. Banks have controllers. Both ensure compliance with financial standards.

If such an approach were used for health care institutions, it would require federal legislation that would set standards for financial relations between hospitals and physicians. The standards would specify which practices were prohibited and the manner in which other activities would be performed. The legislation could require hospitals to see that an auditor files periodic reports. These would facilitate enforcement by allowing outsiders to detect prohibited or suspect activities. They would also allow hospital administrators to monitor the practices of doctors affiliated with their institutions. In addition, they would generate data that could enable the government to identify practices that might be subject to additional controls.

The auditor position would have to be independent or semi-tenured, well-paid, and prestigious. Auditors would need to be vested with authority to review all of the hospital's financial records, patient complaints, assessment of physician performance, organizational files relating to hospital/physician relations, and other hospital records. The reports would be public, auditors would be accountable for their findings, and all hospitals would have an auditor.

The auditor approach has several merits. Much of the cost of monitoring would be borne by financial institutions (albeit eventually the public). At the same time, institutions would be subject to closer scrutiny than if regulated by an outside agency. The practice would help to instill a vigilant attitude within a hospital and help to prevent conflict-of-interest problems.

A variation on the auditor model is the hospital review board. The federal government requires that institutions receiving federal funds for research on human subjects have Institutional Review Boards (IRBs) assess research proposals to ensure that certain criteria are met. A review board could be used to examine the financial arrangements made between hospitals and affiliated physicians. Physicians who proposed to enter into contracts with third parties or providers would have to have their arrangements approved by such a board.

As yet, no basis exists for the federal government to require hospitals to have such a board, nor does authority exist for such boards to exercise control over physicians. Congress would have to pass legislation to create the authority. Also, since hospitals have interests that differ from those of patients, it is unclear how hospitals or hospital review boards can presently effectively monitor physicians' conflicts of interest. Detailed federal standards of conduct would be needed, and some governmental authority would probably have to study the performance of the hospital review boards. The experience with hospital IRBs, which review the ethics of research proposals, supports cautious optimism about the possibilities for hospital review boards.

Institutionalized Conflict-of-Interest Assessment

The government can take other measures short of prohibiting or regulating activities that cause physicians' conflicts of interest. Government can promote health policies and finance medical care in ways that avoid exacerbating present conflicts of interest or creating new ones. It can also devise policies that mitigate conflicts of interest. Faced with alternative health care policies, government can choose one that creates fewer or less serious conflicts of interest.

To do this, government must assess the effect of policies on conflicts of interest by using or requiring conflict-of-interest impact statements. Government should consider how its programs, administrative rules, and proposed policies affect the financial interests of physicians in ways that compromise loyalty to patients. When health policymakers currently assess a policy, they consider its effect on physicians' practice patterns, cost containment, and a host of other factors. What they do not consider are the implications for financial conflicts of interest, and as a result, many government programs fuel these conflicts.

Assessing the conflict-of-interest effect of policies would provide a useful antidote for a major misconception in health policy today: the idea that society can provide physicians with financial incentives to reduce or increase services with only minor ill effects. Current federal health policy assumes that doctors are economically driven and encourages self-interested behavior, while ignoring, in general, the perverse effects of incentives. In some circumstances, economic incentives can be a useful policy tool. In others, economic incentives can and do create conflicts of interest. Governments, third-party payers, and providers should either modify policies to reduce their undesirable effects or establish institutional mechanisms to manage them.

Of course, many other important factors besides conflicts of interest should be considered in designing health care policies. The creation of conflicts of interest may be the dominant consideration in some situations but not in others. Conflict-of-interest impact assessment would not necessarily cause government to adopt policies based only on conflict-of-interest criteria. However, if two programs had roughly similar effects in other respects, yet had significantly different effects on physicians' conflicts of interest, then this might tip the balance. Even if conflicts of interest did not frequently trump other concerns, simply including them as an issue to consider would encourage policymakers to develop programs and policies that fared better in this respect.

Ideally, government should institutionalize conflict-of-interest assessment as part of its policy making process.[68] Government agencies are now required to assess the environmental impact of any major project they fund. The Office of Management and Budget requires a cost-benefit analysis of any proposed federal regulation. In a similar vein, the federal government could require a conflict-of-interest assessment before funding any health program or adopting any health care regulation. Providers and third-party payers could also make conflict-of-interest assessment a standard procedure in developing their own programs and policies.

Incentives, Ethics, Law, and Social Policy

Although financial incentives can play a useful role in promoting desirable physician behavior, there are problems with private or public policies that use incentives to guide clinical choices of doctors. Incentives work best in markets that adjust prices automatically rather than through cumbersome or bureaucratic regulation. But, in fact, any incentives to promote particular clinical choices will not be automatic. They will be set and administered by some management team or agency and will involve all the problems of prices set by a regulatory agency: bureaucracy, uncertainty as to what the correct inducement is or should be, and inducements that lag behind or do not account for changes in practice and thereby send inappropriate signals.[69] Even if it were possible to calibrate such an incentive system, it would be unstable since the world is in flux. For the incentives to have their intended effect, managers and policymakers would have to revise them constantly to account for changes.

The main drawback of relying heavily on financial incentives is that they may encourage undesirable attitudes, which in turn will adversely affect patients. An important element of medicine—one not easily quantifiable—is caring. Studies have shown that physicians and other caregivers can promote a placebo effect in their patients. Though not a substitute for medical or surgical interventions, this placebo effect can trigger measurable biochemical and psychosocial changes that affect a patient's health.[70]

If we want to tap this psychosocial aspect of medicine, we need to encourage commitment and caring; yet these values may be undermined when we rely heavily on explicit financial incentives for doctors. Such incentives stimulate physicians to think of their own financial well-being, rather than promote a fiduciary ethic. By encouraging self-serving actions, incentives play down compassion and caring, and compromise the patient-centered ethos, which in turn may diminish the physician's power to heal.[71] Ultimately, no incentive (or regulatory) system will function well if it undermines the ethos that promotes desired behavior.

Medicine today is practiced in a market environment, which already disposes physicians to think of their own welfare. There is a need to balance this trend and to guard physicians from being influenced by self-serving incentives which may affect adversely the patient.[72] Regulations that restrict physicians' conflicts of interest can bolster professionalism by shielding physicians from these corrupting influences. Although they impose restrictions on permissible conduct in certain spheres, their more enduring effect will probably be to encourage an ethic that promotes conduct beneficial to patients. Herein lies their irony: law and rules are sometimes needed to promote an ethos that is deeper, stronger, and more important than the rules themselves.

Yet medical ethos, personal integrity, and individual conscience, however admirable and necessary, are insufficient for dealing effectively with conflicts of interest. In medicine, as in government, business, and law, evidence of abuses and the inadequacy of self-regulation justifies public intervention. We need to develop explicit public standards.

The transformation needed is similar to the change that occurred in medical practice as a result of *informed consent*, the legal doctrine specifying that physicians have an obligation to tell patients the pros and cons of alternative medical choices. Traditionally, what a physician told a patient about the risks and benefits of surgery was considered a matter to be decided by the individual physician. The physician presumed to act *for* the patient. In the 1970s, courts started to declare physicians liable if they did not obtain the informed consent of patients.[73] Court intervention made what was previously a private matter a subject of public policy. In effect, courts supervised the patient-physician relationship to protect the rights of patients and created public standards.[74]

A similar transformation for conflicts of interest could also benefit patients. Courts, legislation, or regulatory institutions could transform conflicts from personal issues into policy matters, holding physicians to public norms and restricting behavior that places patients at risk.[75]

Many physicians say that transforming medical ethical issues into legal problems, a process that could be termed *legalizing medical ethics*, would only make matters worse.[76] They argue that morality cannot be legislated—that ethical issues are too subtle and personal to be dealt with through the law.[77] It is true that legalizing issues does not solve them. But law can transform social issues by making them a subject of public policy and amenable to response through collective action. Such changes can buttress important values, curb objectionable behavior, and provide more effective remedies or compensation. Over 150 years ago Alexis de Tocqueville wrote that in the United States nearly all important social issues were resolved, sooner or later, as legal questions.[78] The same is true today. Whatever the limitations of the law in the United States, recasting social issues as legal ones is often a prelude to addressing them effectively.

Transforming issues of personal ethics into public policy questions does not necessarily diminish their ethical component; it often reinforces it. The law can and does embody norms and make them public. When courts and legislatures announce policies, they support public norms with the prestige and clout of the law. The public may hold the law in disrepute or even flout it, as in the case of the prohibition on alcohol in the 1920s, or the current disputes about a patient's right to elect abortion or euthanasia. More frequently, however, the law helps promote public norms and elicit public support. The Supreme Court's decision in *Brown v. Board of Education* helped alter attitudes about racial discrimination.[79] Even in less ethically charged situations, the law provides moral weight. Legalizing conflict-of-interest issues may even stimulate the medical profession to recast its views. In the case of biomedical research on human subjects, ethical norms were neglected when the medical profession dealt with these issues on its own. But following the development of federal regulations through the NIH, which funded most biomedical research, the literature on the ethics of human subject research blossomed. New legal standards and public policy for physicians' conflicts of interest are likely to have a similar effect on medical norms for patient care.

Traditionally, medical culture has encouraged physicians to act in the best interests of patients. But today, the lure of incentives promotes financially driven conduct, deflecting this intent. By developing conflict-of-interest policies, government may prompt new thinking in medical ethics and rein in undesirable medical practices. The profession can supplement such changes through educational efforts, but these are likely to be most effective if supported by, and linked to, public policy.

There are limits, of course, on the effects that policies can have on attitudes and motivations. However, law has other important influences. It can alter people's actions even if their attitudes remain unchanged. Quite often, we conform to legal standards because penalties and stigmas punish those caught violating the law. Public policy need not legislate morality to be effective. It will also be effective if it changes conduct.

We should seek to empower patients and the public as well. Despite their disadvantages as consumers of medical care, patients, insurance beneficiaries, and HMO members should play a larger role in holding government and providers accountable when they do not perform their monitoring roles adequately. The women's health movement and the disability rights movement have shown that activism and self-help by affected individuals can be a powerful force for desirable change.[80] Consumer self-help alone will not hold physicians accountable. But neither will institutions designed to protect consumers function effectively without the presence of some kind of consumer or patient rights movement. Grass-roots efforts deserve the support that would ensue from changes in institutions, laws, and the organization of medicine at the state and national levels.[81]

American society's failure to face physicians' conflicts of interest squarely has led to major distortions in the way medicine is practiced, compromised the loyalty of doctors to patients, and resulted in harm to individual patients, society, and the integrity of the medical profession. Today medicine, money, and morals are often in dangerous conflict. They need not be. Many of these conflicts can often be reduced or rendered harmless through social policies. Designing new policies and institutions that hold physicians accountable to patients will be difficult. Yet we should not shrink from the challenge. For the difficulties of the status quo are far worse.

Acronyms

ABA	American Bar Association
ACP	American College of Physicians
ACS	American College of Surgeons
AHA	American Hospital Association
AHM	American Healthcare Management
AMA	American Medical Association
CIGNA	CIGNA Health Care Plan
CHAMPUS	Civilian Health and Medical Program of the Uniformed Services
CRF	Comprehensive Referral Fund
DRG	Diagnosis Related Groups
ERISA	Employee Retirement Income Security Act
ESOPs	Employee Stock Option Plans
FTC	Federal Trade Commission
GAO	Government Accounting Office
GHS	Group Health Services of Michigan
HCA	Hospital Corporation of America
HMO	Health Maintenance Organization
IOM	Institute of Medicine
IPAs	Independent Practice Associations
IRB	Institutional Review Board
IRC	Internal Revenue Code
IRS	Internal Revenue Service
MeSH	Medical Staff Hospital
MRC	Medical Regulatory Commission
NIH	National Institutes of Health

NME	National Medical Enterprises
NCCH	National Council of Community Hospitals
OGE	Office of Governmental Ethics
PCN	Physician Computer Network, Inc.
PCS	Physician Clinical Services
PMA	Pharmaceutical Manufacturers Association
PPO	Preferred Provider Organization
PRF	Pooled Risk Fund
PROs	Peer Review Organizations
PSROs	Physician Standard Review Organizations
RICO	Racketeer Influence and Corrupt Organizations Act
SEC	Securities and Exchange Commission

APPENDICES

A

The Concept of
Conflict of Interest

The notion of conflict of interest is generally known and widely used. But it has not been subject to careful analysis.[1] The idea may be so basic that we use it to conduct analysis rather than subject it to analysis.[2] Law texts and court decisions frequently either do not explain the term or define it perfunctorily. Few philosophers have written about conflicts of interest; most who have analyze the term without carefully examining the way it is used in law.[3]

Joseph Margolis identifies conflicts of interest with a person performing two incompatible roles simultaneously.[4] Yet he does not explain what makes two roles incompatible or link conflicts of interest to legal or moral obligations. Ruth Macklin has distinguished three types of interests that can conflict in a conflict of interest: (1) the actor's personal interests; (2) interests of the actor's organization; (3) society's or the public's interests.[5] Her analysis does not refer to legal obligations or distinguish conflicts of interest from general moral conflicts. Joseph McGuire draws on models of conflicts of interest from systems theory. He compares conflicts of interest to a clash between an individual or organization and the system in which these operate.[6] McGuire, also, ignores the legal tradition that is the source of concept.

The Lack of An Analytic Framework

Most writers characterize physicians' conflicts of interest as an exception to the norm. An extensive sampling of the existing literature indicates no sense that conflicts of interest are problems embedded in the nature of contemporary practice. As yet, no efforts have been made to identify systematically the existing range of physicians' conflicts of interest, to analyze their similarities and differences, or to suggest which of these are of particular concern to society. The literature generally assumes that these issues should be left to the individual physician and resolved through informal means or through professional self-regulation. No sustained discussion occurs about social policies that could or should govern these issues, the groups or authorities who should be responsible for controlling them, or how society should balance the competing benefits and costs of any policies that address the problem. Moreover, no studies have compared the problems of physicians with the experience of other professionals or with policies and problems in other countries. The lack of a generally accepted analytic framework for approaching physicians' conflicts of interest hampers the development of effective social policy.

Discussions of physicians' conflicts of interest typically address only one kind, rather than presenting a generic view of the problem. Some writers address only a specific clinical situation, such as experimentation;[7] or a particular practice situation, such as referrals;[8] or a particular activity, such as dispensing drugs.[9] Some writers have linked the problem to "for profit" medicine.[10] Others explore problems in the use of payment based on a fixed fee but ignore problems arising from payment based on fee-for-service,[11] physician ownership of health facilities,[12] and managed care.[13] Many discussions of the patient-physician relationship allude to physicians' conflicts of interest and plead for a patient-centered ethic.[14]

A few philosophers have analyzed the concept of conflict of interest or have examined the problem in other professions, such as business. Joseph McGuire views conflicts of interest as conflicts between an individual or organizational entity and the system in which these operate.[15] Joseph Margolis distinguishes between conflicting interests and conflicts of interest. The former occur in any situation where competing considerations are presumed to be legitimate. Conflicts of interest, on the other hand, are characterized by an individual occupying dual roles which should not be performed simultaneously. Because of the potential for abuse, performing both roles simultaneously is considered inappropriate, even if the individual has good intentions, never exploits the conflict, and does not harm anyone.[16] Ruth Macklin elucidates the concept of conflict of interest by distinguishing the kinds of "interests" involved.[17] Michael Davis argues that codes of legal ethics provide a basis for regulating conflicts of interest among other professionals.[18] Norman Bowie believes that in some activities, such as financial auditing, loyalty to a client can conflict with loyalty to the public, and suggests that society may want to insulate professionals so they can play a neutral role. He wants the auditor to disclose information that the public needs and that the employer often seeks to conceal.[19] Bowie also notes that professional roles can define a physician's moral obligations.[20] But none of these writers have analyzed such issues in depth or have related them to physicians. One of their common refrains, in fact, is the paucity of existing analysis.[21]

B

Note on Physicians' Divided Loyalties

Physicians have many conflicts of interest arising from divided loyalties that do not involve financial conflicts of interest. These conflicts of interest evoke issues and problems similar to those discussed in the book. This note describes some of these other types of conflicts.

Physicians' judgment or loyalty to patients can be compromised by their performing roles other than patient care, by working on behalf of or being paid by groups other than patients, or by serving two or more patients with diverging interests.[1] In these situations, physicians' loyalty to patients is threatened by pursuing legitimate roles but acting in the interests of others.[2]

Physicians in teaching hospitals perform many roles. They care for patients but often conduct research and teach residents, interns, and medical students as well; they may also be involved in quality assurance programs or hospital management. Commitment to a research protocol can color physicians' judgment of patients' needs and prompt physicians—often inadvertently and in good faith—to recommend an experimental or relatively new therapy over one that is safer or in other ways better for the patient.[3] Residents need clinical experience—not necessarily in the patient's interest—and physician-teachers also may seek to demonstrate clinical skills to their students. As participants in hospital management, physicians may act to advance the hospital's financial situation and other goals, which can impair their clinical judgment or loyalty to patients.

Psychiatry presents an example of the conflict between physicians' loyalty to patients and physicians' legal obligations to the public.[4] Psychiatrists owe loyalty to their patients but are also expected to institutionalize dangerous patients in order to protect society. Likewise, leading court decisions have held psychiatrists liable for failing to divulge the confidences of their clients when doing so was necessary to protect an identifiable third party at risk of serious immediate harm.[5] Physicians' role in promoting public health requires that they report certain contagious diseases, which in turn creates conflicts with the traditional legal and ethical presumption that physicians protect the confidences of their clients.[6] In the case of the human immunodeficiency virus (HIV) infection the law is unresolved, but the American Medical Association and the American Psychiatric Association state that physicians are ethically obligated to divulge a patient's confidences and warn sexual partners known to be at risk of contagion.[7]

Physicians often act as gatekeepers. In this role, they ration medical resources for the benefit of providers, insurers, government, or society at large. Primary care physicians in Health Maintenance Organizations and other managed-care settings act as gatekeepers when they control the flow of patients to specialists or deny marginally beneficial services to patients to promote the institutions' interests.[8] Physicians also work for government, certifying eligibility for disability income and insurance benefits.[9] Physicians limit beneficial services to patients in disaster triage.[10] They may also consider the needs of other patients in deciding whether to place a patient in an intensive care unit, and they can consider criteria other than medical need.[11] In all these situations, physicians have conflicts of interest because fulfilling these legitimate roles can conflict with their role in promoting the best interests of their patients.

Occupational physicians who treat workers in a business are subject to pressures from their employers, who often have interests that differ from those of patients.[12] Physicians who work for the armed forces[13] or for sports teams face similar conflicts of interest.[14] In each of these settings, physicians must serve the enterprise that hires and pays them as well as their patients.

Physicians sometimes care for patients whose interests conflict with each other. The physician who treats a dying patient and a potential transplant recipient of human organs works for two different patients with interests that can conflict.[15] Some writers suggest that physicians who care for a pregnant woman have both the woman and the fetus as patients, and that their interests can sometimes conflict.

These are but a few of the divided loyalties that can compromise physicians' loyalty to patients.

C

Bioethics and
Medical School Ethics Education

The Origins of Bioethics[1]

Traditionally, medical ethics evolved separately, relatively unaffected by other intellectual trends.[2] As late as 1954, Joseph Fletcher noted that, with the exception of Catholic theologians, philosophers and other theologians had discussed "almost every conceivable phase of personal and social ethics *except medicine and health*."[3] Fletcher and those who followed introduced the perspectives of outsiders into medical ethics. Fletcher challenged the paternalism of physicians and examined medical ethics from the point of view of the patient. Other social, political, and legal developments in the 1960s also contributed to the development of bioethics.

Powerful new medical technologies shaped new vistas and capabilities. These ranged from immune suppressing drugs and surgical techniques that facilitated organ transplants to the artificial heart, new forms of contraception, reproductive technologies such as in vitro fertilization, the increased use of respirators, neonatal intensive care units, and other technologies that could extend life. Physicians now had clinical choices previously unavailable. Many people thought that these technologies were being used in a dehumanizing way. Bioethics scholars began to analyze the values inherent in the new choices.

The 1960s also saw the growth of the civil rights struggle and of movements to empower women, students, homosexuals, children, and people with disabilities. Disaffected groups wanted to participate in decision making and politics. The public and affected individuals questioned the authority of institutions. Professionals, in particular, were criticized by groups on whose behalf they acted. This questioning of authority affected schools, government, social work, religious institutions, hospitals, and prisons. Clinical researchers were not immune from this questioning, and when the press revealed a series of scandals in which researchers had risked the health of human subjects without their consent, a movement developed to hold clinical researchers accountable. Subjects of research are not a discrete group that can easily organize to protect their interests, but self-appointed spokesmen and the government sought legal and procedural rights to protect them. This led the National Institutes of Health (NIH) to develop guidelines and later regulations requiring institutions to establish Institutional Review Boards (IRBs) to review proposals for research involving human subjects.[4]

By the late 1970s, IRBs had become institutionalized and had generated interest in the ethics of clinical research and medicine. The federal government had sponsored several important commissions to study ethical problems in biomedical research, medicine, and health policy. Bioethics had become a staple in medical schools, and had its own professional journals and associations.

Bioethics

Early bioethics scholars were united in viewing traditional medical ethics as provincial and lacking in intellectual content. Bioethics differs from traditional medical ethics in several respects. It is broader in scope. It goes beyond issues of individual medical care, encompassing social issues as well as biology, health, and health policy. The field thrives on systematic analysis of concepts, examination of assumptions, and the like.[5]

In the 1970s and 1980s, much of the writing in bioethics drew on philosophy. Scholars searched for "principles," "foundations," and ethical "theory."[6] Moral philosophers entered the bioethics field, and those who were Kantians or utilitarians or had other theoretical commitments used medicine as a testing ground for illustrating and arguing their doctrinal differences. Medical issues were translated into the language and categories of moral philosophy and analyzed accordingly.[7] Typical texts in bioethics discuss the conceptual foundation of bioethics, ethical theories such as utilitarian and rights-based theories of ethics, and the various moral principles and theories under the categories of autonomy, paternalism, nonmaleficence, beneficence, justice, virtues, the concept of personhood, the right to health care, rationing, the just allocation of medical care resources, contract keeping, honesty, confidentiality, and avoiding killing.

The theoretical writing of the late 1970s and early 1980s precipitated a reaction. Many physicians believed that the abstract discussions did not help them with the practical problems they faced. They were more interested in deciding particular cases than in coming to agreement on principles. Two new approaches arose to address these concerns. First, physicians at the University of Chicago and elsewhere started their own programs in *clinical* medical ethics.[8] With an additional fellowship in ethics, these programs trained physicians to become specialists who could provide ethics consultations, serve on ethics committees, or in other ways provide advice to physicians on clinical ethical issues. Second, some philosophers and other ethics scholars shifted their focus to *applied* ethics.[9]

By the end of the 1980s, the field of bioethics was in ferment. However, some rough generalizations are possible. Bioethics scholars address four kinds of problems. First, they analyze individual moral dilemmas. Their discussions often portray physicians contemplating theoretical alternatives and examining the pros and cons of each difficult choice. A second problem bioethics scholars address involves resource allocation, either for individual patients or for institutions, so called micro-allocation issues. A third issue involves macro- or societywide allocation of health and medical resources. And a fourth issue discussed is the social implication of changes in the practice and finance of medicine for society and individuals.[10] A more recent trend in bioethics draws on political theory and considers the role of physicians in the community or the liberal state.[11]

Bioethics textbooks often present difficult clinical choices.[12] Medical ethics cases often start with a description of a clinical situation and end with the need for the physician to make a choice or resolve a problem. Students are faced with a dilemma and are required to explain how and why they would resolve the case.

Typical anthologies and textbooks in bioethics cover the ethics of withholding life-sustaining treatment, euthanasia, fetal research, genetic engineering and counseling, and new reproductive technologies. Other concerns include patients' rights, privacy, confidentiality, and truth telling; paternalism, informed consent, and research on human subjects; decision making for children and patients who are incompetent; organ transplants, and the artificial heart; and for-profit medicine.

Although the field of bioethics has addressed many important social and ethical issues since its inception, it has left certain areas and topics undisturbed. There has been great attention to the way physicians make decisions, the grounds for them, and the involvement of patients in decision making through informed consent. But there has been hardly any concern with physicians' personal conduct or their financial conflicts of interest. Until recently, conflicts of interest was not even listed as a separate category for study, and those articles that have recently addressed such issues are at the periphery of the field.

Ethics Teaching in Medical Schools

In recent years, medical schools have introduced medical ethics and humanities into their undergraduate curriculum and into their internship and residency training programs. They have even offered postgraduate fellowships in ethics.[13] Started in the late 1960s, these programs varied widely, but there is now some standard subject matter.[14] A key aim is to ensure that practitioners are aware of ethical issues and are trained to analyze them.

Medical ethics and humanities programs frequently address issues surrounding death and dying, termination of medical treatment, informed consent, do-not-resuscitate orders, allocating intensive care, euthanasia, care of newborns with a poor prognosis, organ donation and transplants, the duty to treat HIV-infected patients, and cost containment.[15] Some programs teach ethical theory and principles of biomedical ethics; others concentrate on case discussions;[16] still others use literature, films, philosophy, and related subjects to encourage physicians to think critically about medicine and clinical choices. A few programs consciously try to set an example of ethical practice that students can emulate.

Still other programs emphasize humanistic qualities and the ability of students to empathize with patients. Most attempt to raise the consciousness of physicians, to help them clarify their values, to refine their ability to analyze ethical issues critically, to enhance their communication and relations with patients, and to improve their clinical decision making. Often programs want to improve the moral reasoning of medical students, and one evaluation suggests that they do.[17]

These programs often assume that physicians will act in the interests of patients, even without guidelines or constraints on acceptable conduct. One limitation of this approach is seen by what the standard curriculum neglects: financial conflicts of interest.[18]

D

The Sources and Data Used

Since the 1960s, health service researchers have produced voluminous
studies and created enormous sets of statistical data. This has been
complemented in recent years by data on finances from the Medicare and
Medicaid programs. Yet despite the enormous amount of information
available on the American health care system in general and medical care
finance in particular, there are little data on kickbacks, gifts, or physician
ownership of medical facilities. This kind of information, of course, is not
systematically recorded or dutifully collected for any governmental
purpose, and few studies have attempted to unearth it.

Physicians and medical suppliers do not generally furnish such data
or talk freely about physician dispensing, kickbacks, gifts, or self-dealing
practices. One might have expected information about physician
ownership of medical facilities to be more readily available, but here, too,
much remains cloaked in mystery. The reason often given is that much
of this information constitutes trade secrets, the release of which would
allow competitors to gain the upper hand or at least an even hand—not
an attractive prospect. Obtaining data on physician ownership is also
difficult because physicians often hide ownership through shell corporations. These make it appear that a medical care facility, such as an
imaging center or a diagnostic laboratory, is owned and operated by an
autonomous company. But the company that owns the facility is itself

often owned and operated by other companies, each of which is owned by one or more physicians.[1]

In some respects, the researcher is not much better off than patients in obtaining, deciphering, or disentangling information on this subject. I have resorted to a sort of ethnographic sampling of trade publications, prospectuses, government reports, and other documents. These do not yield numbers on distribution and frequency that would satisfy the appetite of scholars trained in sophisticated statistical techniques and sampling. But the lack of good data sets is a common problem. It means that we have to squeeze what we can from other kinds of evidence, partial as it may be. When data exist from other studies that bear on the problem, I have relied on them as well.

Many of my sources are not traditionally tapped in social science research. I have used court records (pleadings and depositions, and trial records have supplemented reported cases). Congressional investigations into kickbacks in the Medicare program have provided numerous documents and much testimony. Other government agencies have also provided reports. The trade press, newspaper articles, and other published materials have provided other sources of information. To understand current financial practices that create conflicts of interest and gain access to source materials, I interviewed physician recruiters, lawyers, physicians, health care entrepreneurs, and other professionals working in the field. Some physicians I have interviewed provided examples of gifts they received from pharmaceutical firms.

For information on physician investments and self-referral, three sources were particularly helpful. In 1988-89 the Department of Health and Human Services Inspector General, who has responsibility for overseeing the department's enforcement of its fraud and abuse statute prohibiting kickbacks, announced his intent to promulgate regulations interpreting the statute. Many medical providers had criticized the statute for defining kickbacks too broadly. The Inspector General's regulations were to create safe harbors that would give some guidance to health care providers in interpreting the statute. As in all formal federal government administrative rule making, affected parties have an opportunity to comment on the proposed regulations. In response to the notice of intent to propose a rule, and then in response to the proposed rule, health providers and their attorneys submitted massive comments. (Together the comments make up six 5-inch binders, and each person's or institution's comment is numbered.)

I obtained copies of these comments under the Freedom of Information Act. Many providers gave details of financial arrangements they used or wanted to put into effect and requested that the safe harbors protect these arrangements. Others used the comments to report on the activities of competitors and argued that these practices should be prohibited. These comments are a rich source of examples of the health care financial practices that are often not reported. (In footnotes, I cite the Health and Human Services comment number, the date of the letter, and the name of the individual and/or institution submitting the comments.)

A second source of data was prospectuses and private placement memoranda given to potential investors. These documents provide detailed information on the proposed ventures, who would finance them, how the business would be run, a business plan, copies of contracts and legal documents, financial forecasts, and so forth. I have obtained copies of some of these prospectuses and private placement memoranda from the Office of Representative Pete Stark (D.-California). He has introduced legislation to restrict physicians participating in Medicare from referring patients to health care facilities in which they have a financial interest. Still other examples were obtained from lawyers and health care organizations. Many physicians who opposed this kind of venture turned over these documents to organizations opposed to physician ownership and to Representative Stark. They are not an unbiased sample. I have made partially successful efforts, however, to obtain a few other prospectuses from organizations that defend physician ownership, and I do discuss these in the study. But not many proponents of physician-owned ventures have been willing to provide samples of prospectuses. Results from a study of all providers in Florida indicate that many of the patterns I identify are in line with what transpires generally in that state.[2]

A third source of data was information on recent kickback trials and investigations into conflicts of interest of physicians employed by the Veterans Administration. I obtained numerous documents on these subjects, under the Freedom of Information Act, the Department of Health and Human Services, and the Veterans Administration.

There are very few secondary sources on the history of the medical profession's response to fee splitting and other financial conflicts of interest. I relied heavily on records of the American Medical Association (AMA), the American College of Surgeons (ACS), and the Joint Commission on Accreditation for Health Care Institutions. I also used reports from the AMA's House of Delegates, its Council on Ethical and

Judicial Affairs, and other organizational reports as the backbone of my history. The ACS does not make public any such internal reports. But its *Bulletin* provides a fertile source, as does the history of the organization. Its opposition to AMA policies in the past provides a counterpoint and helps document disputes within the medical profession. Minutes of the meetings of the Joint Commission help fill in some history because this organization took over the hospital standardization program that had been run by the ACS until the 1950s. I supplemented these sources with articles in medical journals, popular journals, and medical histories.

My study of conflicts of interest in other professions was based largely on a voluminous literature. I also consulted original statutes, cases, and professionals in the field. I relied on my own experiences in facing conflicts of interest as a lawyer, and I drew, too, on the insights I gleaned from private practice in addressing conflict-of-interest issues that arose in business and government services.

In citing books, articles, and other materials, I use a full citation the first time I note the source in each chapter. After that I use an abbreviated citation.

E

Excerpts from
Medical Codes of Ethics

Hippocrates. 1923. (trans. W. H. Jones), The Lode Classical Library. Cambridge: Harvard University Press.

> I will use treatment to help the sick according to my ability and judgment but never with a view to injury and wrong-doing. . . . Into whatsoever houses I enter, I will enter to help the sick, and I will abstain from all intentional wrong-doings and harm, especially from abusing the bodies of man or woman. . . . And whatsoever I shall see or hear in the course of my profession. . . if it be what should not be published abroad, I will never divulge. . . .

World Medical Association Declaration of Geneva Adopted by the General Assembly of The World Medical Association at Geneva, Switzerland, September 1948. Reprinted from *World Medical Association Bulletin*. 1949. 1:109-111.

> The health of my patient will be my first consideration; I will respect the secrets which are confided in me. . . .
> *Duties of Doctors in General*
> .
> .
> .

A doctor must not allow himself to be influenced merely by motives of profit.

The following practices are deemed unethical:

.

.

.

... (c) To receive any money in connection with services rendered to a patient other than the acceptance of a proper professional fee, or to pay any money in the same circumstances without the knowledge of the patient.
Duties of Doctors to the Sick

.

.

A doctor owes to his patient complete loyalty and all the resources of his science. Whenever an examination or treatment is beyond his capacity he should summon another doctor who has the necessary ability.

A doctor owes to his patient absolute secrecy on all which has been confided to him or which he knows because of the confidences entrusted to him.

A doctor must give the necessary treatment in emergency, unless he is assured that it can and will be given by others.

American Medical Association: First Code of Medical Ethics. Proceedings of the National Medical Convention 1846-1847. pp. 83-106.

Article 1-Duties of Physicians to Their Patients.
1.... Physicians should ... minister to the sick with due impression of the importance of their office; reflecting that the ease, the health, and the lives of those committed to their charge, depend on their skill, attention and fidelity....
2. Every case committed to the charge of a physician should be treated with attention, steadiness and humanity. Reasonable indulgence should be granted to the mental imbecility and caprices of the sick. Secrecy and delicacy, when required by peculiar circumstances, should be strictly observed; and the familiar and confidential intercourse to which physicians are admitted in their professional visits, should be used with discretion, and with the most scrupulous regard to fidelity and honor. The obligation of secrecy extends beyond the period of professional services;—none of the privacy of personal and domestic

life, no infirmity of disposition or flaw of character observed during professional attendance, should ever be divulged by him except when he is imperatively required to do so. . . .

American Medical Association Principles of Medical Ethics (1957)
Section 5
A physician may choose whom he will serve. In an emergency, however, he should render service to the best of his ability. Having undertaken the care of a patient, he may not neglect him; and unless he has been discharged he may discontinue his services only after giving adequate notice. . . .

Section 6
A physician should not dispose of his services under terms or conditions that tend to interfere with or impair the free and complete exercise of his medical judgment and skill or tend to cause a deterioration of the quality of medical care.

Section 7
In the practice of medicine a physician should limit the source of his professional income to medical services actually rendered by him, or under his supervision, to his patients. His fee should be commensurate with his service rendered and the patient's ability to pay. He should neither pay nor receive commission for referral of patients. . . .

Section 9
A physician may not reveal the confidences entrusted to him in the course of medical attendance . . . unless he is required to do so by law or unless it becomes necessary in order to protect the welfare of the individual or of the community.

Chapter 1

[1]Etziony, M. B. 1973. "The Prayer of Moses Maimonides." (Markus Herz) in *The Physician's Creed: Anthology of Medical Prayers, Oaths and Codes of Ethics Written and Recited by Medical Practitioners Through the Ages.* Springfield, Il.: Charles C. Thomas. pp. 28-31.

[2]Shaw, George Bernard. 1913. "Preface on Doctors." *The Doctor's Dilemma: A Tragedy.* Baltimore: Penguin Books. p. 35.

[3]Jonsen, Albert R. 1990. *The New Medicine and the Old Ethics.* Cambridge: Harvard University Press.

[4]The March 9, 1929, cover has the girl with the doll; the March 15, 1958, cover has the boy undressing to receive an injection.

[5]Rothman, David J. 1991. *Strangers at the Bedside: A History of How Law and Bioethics Transformed Medical Decisionmaking.* New York: Basic Books.

[6]Shaw, George Bernard. *The Doctor's Dilema.* 1913. p. 17. The play was first performed in 1911 but published in 1913.

[7]Shaw, George Bernard. 1913. *The Doctor's Dilema.* p. 10.

[8]Shaw, George Bernard. 1913. *The Doctor's Dilema.* p. 9.

[9]Source on physician income: AMA, Fall 1990, *Physician Market Place Statistics.* The "average" used is the mean income.

Source on U.S. per capita income: U.S. Bureau of the Census, Current Populations Reports, Series P-60, No. 174. *Money Income of Households, Families and Persons in the United States: 1990.* Washington, D.C.: U.S. Government Printing Office, 1991.

Although U.S. census statistics are not yet available for 1991, it is likely that the difference between physicians' and average income is even greater than in 1990. The *average* annual income of doctors after expenses and before taxes in 1991 was $164,300. Source on physician income: AMA. Fall 1991. *Physician Market Place Statistics.*

[10]The title of the article featured on the cover page is "Group Practices Tie Hospital, Physician Objectives."

[11] Parsons, Talcott. 1951. *The Social System* Glencoe, Ill.: Free Press. Chapter 10.

Parsons, Talcott. 1975. "The Sick Role and the Role of the Physician." *Milbank Memorial Fund Quarterly* 53(3):257-78.

[12]The patient-physician relationship is often seen as one between principals and agents. Buchanan, Allen. 1988. "Principal/Agent Theory and Decision-making in Health Care." *Bioethics* 2(4):317-333.

[13]A selection of medical ethics codes is reprinted in Reiser, Stanley Joel, Arthur J. Dyck, and William J. Curran. 1977. *Ethics in Medicine: Historical Perspectives and Contemporary Concerns*. Cambridge: MIT Press. Appendix E includes some excepts.

[14]Jonas, Hans. 1969. "Philosophical Reflections on Experimenting with Human Subjects." *Daedalus* 98(2):219-247, at 239.

[15]Fried, Charles. 1976. "The Lawyer as Friend: The Moral Foundations of the Lawyer-Client Relation." *The Yale Law Journal* 85(8):1060-1089. The analogy is not suggested offhandedly. Charles Fried has written extensively on medical ethics as well. The theme of the essay is illustrated by the following passage:

> The lawyer-client relation is a personal relation, and legal counsel is a personal service. This explains directly why, *once the relation has been contracted,* considerations of efficiency or fair distribution cannot be allowed to weaken it. The reaction itself is not a creature of social expediency . . .; it is the creature of moral right, and therefore expediency may not compromise the nature of the relation. This is true in medicine because the human need creates a relation of dependence which it would be a betrayal to compromise. In the lawyer-client relation the argument is more complex but supports the same conclusion. . . . Once the relation has been taken up, it is the client's needs which hold the reins— legally and morally. (p. 1077)

[16]Advertising by broker-dealers, to the public and within the trade, stresses the great trust that can be placed in the firm's recommendations, often comparing the obligations of the broker-dealer to those of the doctor or lawyer. These claims would impart a fiduciary quality to the relations of broker-dealers with their customers even if the fiduciary responsibilities of broker-dealers were not, at least in part, codified in law.

Meyer, Martin. 1980. "Broker Dealer Firms," in *Abuse on Wall Street: Conflicts of Interest in the Securities Markets*. Report to the Twentieth Century Fund Steering Committee on Conflicts of Interest in the Securities Markets. Westport, Conn.: Quorum Books. p. 433.

[17]Patients have all sorts of interests. Consider three basic kinds: (a) medical (receiving high-quality medical care, reducing their exposure to medical risk, being healed or relieved of suffering, participating in treatment decisions, and

receiving medical care in a convenient and pleasant manner); (b) financial (reducing their payments for medical care through direct out-of-pocket payments or copayments and through insurance premiums or taxes to pay for public financing); and (c) general (having a system that distributes medical care resources justly and respects patients' rights to privacy and autonomy).

One can expand the analysis of conflicts of interest to include these and other factors. But traditional conflict-of-interest law has slighted these conflicts because of the difficulty of measuring many of these factors.

[18]There is a voluminous literature in philosophy, economics, and psychology devoted to examining the concepts of interest, self-interest, and altruism. Some writers have taken the position that any person's free acts necessarily increase his or her welfare or utility, even if the act appears to be done for the sake of others. These writers attempt to rule out the possibility of altruism and of actions taken for the sake of others by explaining any action by the actor's desire to increase his or her own utility. My distinction between interests and commitments acknowledges the possibility of individuals taking altruistic action.

[19]The law distinguishes between a *malum in se* and a *malum prohibitum*. The former is the *act* that is wrong in itself; the latter is wrong because society prohibits it to prevent some *malum in se*. Law or ethics may prohibit certain conflicts of interest as a way to reduce the risk of breach of trust. This distinction arises in constitutional law as well. See, Grano, Joseph D., 1985. "Prophylactic Rules in Criminal Procedure: A Question of Article III Legitimacy." *Northwestern University Law Review* 80(1):100-164.

[20]The distinction between personal interests and divided loyalties reflects usage in fiduciary law and legal ethics. Kenneth Kipnis states it most clearly in his essay on conflicts of obligation and conflicts of interest. These are not mutually exclusive categories. Personal conflicts may be a special case of divided loyalties (loyalty to self versus loyalty to the party on whose behalf one acts). Loyalty to a third party often reflects a financial tie to that party.

Personal conflicts of interest include situations in which the party with a conflict does not receive benefits directly. For example, when the individual's relatives or friends may benefit from his or her actions, it is harder for them to be objective and they may not fulfill their obligations. Moreover, there is a sense in which family and friends are an extension of a person: emotional and financial ties bind them. A parent also benefits when a son or daughter receives money or a promotion. Even when individuals do not receive a tangible benefit directly, they may try to help a friend to repay a debt owed or to help a relative in the anticipation that the relative will return the favor later.

See Kipnis, Kenneth. 1986. *Legal Ethics.* Englewood Cliffs, N.J.: Prentice-Hall. Ch. 3. Conflict of Interest and Conflict of Obligation. pp. 40-62.

Finn, P. D. 1977. *Fiduciary Obligations.* Sydney: Law Book Co.

[21]"Conflict of interest . . . denotes a situation in which two or more interests are legitimately present and competing or conflicting. . . . The individual (or firm) making a decision that will affect those interests may have a larger stake in one of them than the other(s) but he is expected—in fact, obligated— to serve each as if it were his own, regardless of his own actual stake."

Schotland, Roy A. 1980. "Introduction," in *Abuse on Wall Street: Conflicts of Interest in the Securities Markets*. Report to the Twentieth Century Fund Steering Committee on Conflicts of Interest in the Securities Markets. Westport, Conn.: Quorum Books.

[22]*Black's Law Dictionary*, which first included an entry for the term in its fifth edition in 1979, ignores divided loyalties in its definition.

> **Conflict of Interest**. Term used in connection with public officials and fiduciaries and their relationship to matters of private interest or gain to them. Ethical problems connected therewith are covered by statutes in most jurisdictions and by federal statutes on the federal level. Generally, when used to suggest disqualification of a public official from performing his sworn duty, term "conflict of interest" refers to a clash between public interest and the private pecuniary interest of the individual concerned.

Webster's Third International Dictionary defines a conflict of interest as "a conflict between the private interests and the official responsibilities of a person in a position of trust (as a government official)."

Manning's study of conflict of interest in government uses the term to refer to "only two interests: one is the interest of government official (and of the public) in the proper administration of his office; the other is the official's interest in his private economic affairs. A conflict of interest exists whenever these two interests clash, or appear to clash." Manning, Bayless. 1964. *Federal Conflict of Interest Law*. Cambridge: Harvard University Press. p. 2.

A similar approach is taken by Davis, Michael. 1982. "Conflict of Interest." *Business & Professional Ethics Journal* 1(4):17-27.

[23]*The Random House Dictionary of the English Language* (2nd ed., 1987) includes both personal interests and divided loyalties in its definition.

> **Conflict of interest** 1. The circumstances of a public officeholder, business executive, or the like whose personal interests might benefit from his or her official actions or influence: The senator placed his stocks in trust to avoid possible conflicts of interest. 2. The circumstance of a person who finds that one of his or her activities, interests, etc. can be advanced only at the expense of another of them.

[24]Self-referral may be defined more broadly to include any referral from which physicians gain financially. This would include referral to medical facilities that employ physicians and recommendations physicians make for the use of their own services. The context indicates whether the term is used in a broad or narrow sense.

[25]A physician's loyalty to the patient is still compromised when their interests coincide if there are structural factors that compromise the physician's loyalty. If the physician acts in a patient's interest only as a way to promote his or her own economic welfare, the patient's well-being will depend on what promotes the physician's gain. This is an unreliable basis for trust.

[26]Bursztajn, Harold. 1990. *Medical Choices, Medical Chances: How Patients, Families, and Physicians Can Cope with Uncertainty*. New York: Routledge.

[27]Ginzberg, Eli. 1984. "The Monetarization of Medical Care." *The New England Journal of Medicine* 310(18):1162-1165.

[28]Information provided by John Roberts and Brian Gordon of The MR Cooperative, Solana Beach, California, and by the American Hospital Association, *Hospital Statistics*, 1989 edition.

[29]Statistics are estimates provided by John Roberts of The MR Cooperative, Solana Beach, California, and Susana Hoppszallern, Technology Department, American Hospital Association. Fees paid for scans are "global" fees, including both the fee paid to the technician for professional services and the fee paid to the owners of the equipment.

[30]The term was first used by Barbara Ehrenreich and others in the book: Health PAC. 1970. *The American Health Empire: Power, Profits & Politics: A Report from the Health Policy Advisory Center*. New York: Random House.

[31]Relman, Arnold S. 1983. "The Future of Medical Practice." *Health Affairs* 2(2):5-19.

[32]Most historians date the start of medical insurance to the Baylor Health Plan in 1929. Twelve hundred Dallas, Texas, school teachers were guaranteed limited hospital benefits at the Baylor Hospital in return for subscribing to a plan under which they paid a premium of $.50 a month. In the 1930s and 1940s prepaid group practice, Blue Cross/Blue Shield plans, and commercial insurance spread. But it was not until the 1950s that approximately one-half of all Americans had health insurance coverage. See Fein, Rashi. 1986. *Medical Care, Medical Costs: The Search for a Health Insurance Policy*. Cambridge: Harvard University Press.

[33]Our insurance system is far from universal. Approximately 12%, or 37 million people, lack health insurance.

[34]For an early analysis of this literature, see Fein, Rashi. 1967. *The Doctor Shortage: An Economic Diagnosis*. Washington, D.C.: The Brookings Institute. A variety of studies measured the shortage, using different means. A constant theme was the need to increase the supply of physicians to meet current demand for services.

Ginzberg, Eli. 1966. "Physician Shortage Reconsidered." *The New England Journal of Medicine* 275(2):85-87.

For a more recent assessment, see Reinhardt, Uwe E. 1991. "Health Manpower Forecasting: The Case of Physician Supply," in *Health Services Research*, Eli Ginzberg, ed. Cambridge: Harvard University Press. pp. 234-283.

[35]Ginzberg, Eli, and Miriam Ostow, eds. 1984. *The Coming Physician Surplus: In Search of a Policy*. Ottowa: Rowman & Alanheld. p. 117.

AMA. 1992. *Physician Characteristics and Distribution in the U.S. 1991*. Chicago: AMA.

[36]Altman, Stuart H. 1984. "The Growing Physician Surplus: Will It Benefit or Bankrupt the U.S. Health System?" In Ginzberg, Eli, and Miriam Ostow. 1984. *The Coming Physician Surplus*. p. 9.

[37]Ginzberg, Eli, and Miriam Ostow. 1984. *The Coming Physician Surplus*.

[38]Levit, Katherine R., Helen Lazenby, Daniel R. Waldo, and Lawrence M. Davidoff. 1985. "National Health Expenditures, 1984." *Health Care Financing Review* 7(1):1-35. These statistics are adjusted for inflation.

[39]Vladeck, Bruce C. 1984. "Medicare Hospital Payment by Diagnosis-Related Groups." *Annals of Internal Medicine* 100(4):576-590.

[40]Heniz, John. 1986. "The Effects of DRGs on Patients." *Business and Health* (July-August):17-20.

[41]Prospective Payment Assessment Commission. 1990. *Medicare Prospective Payment and the American Health Care System: Report to Congress*. Washington, D.C.

Kahn, Katherine L., David Draper, Emmett B. Keeler, et al. 1992. *The Effects of DRG-Based Prospective Payment System on Quality of Care for Hospitalized Medicare Patients*. Santa Monica: Rand Corporation.

[42]AMA Council on Medical Education and Hospitals. 1925. "Hospital Service in the United States." *Journal of the American Medical Association* 13(84):961-967.

The survey lists ownership under the term individuals or partnership rather than physician-owned. Rules against the corporate practice of medicine made it difficult, if not impossible, for nonphysicians to own proprietary hospitals then. This inference is supported by other categories of ownership listed: religious denominational, fraternal, industrial, independent association, and governmental (federal, state, country, city).

[43]Source: AMA Council on Medical Education and Hospitals. 1952. "Hospital Service in the United States." *Journal of the American Medical Association* 152(2):143-151.

The 1952 data use a slightly different classification than in 1925. The 1952 survey refers to "proprietary hospitals," while the 1925 survey refers to hospitals owned by individuals or partnerships. I assume that in both cases these hospitals are owned by physicians or that this statistic is a good proxy for physician ownership. In 1952 there were 6,665 hospitals and 1,541,615 beds.

[44]Steinwald, Bruce, and Duncan Neuhauser. 1970. "The Role of the Proprietary Hospital." *Law and Contemporary Problems* 35(4):817-838. The data are based on a survey published in *Hospitals* on August 1, 1969.

[45]There is a dearth of data on physician ownership of hospitals. Neither the AMA nor the American Hospital Association tracks such statistics. But reports in trade publications indicates that this trend is increasing.

[46]*Issues Related to Physician "Self-Referrals"*: Hearings before the Subcommittee on Health and the Subcommittee on Oversight of the Committee on Ways and Means, House of Representatives, 101st Congress, 1st Session, on H.R. 939. Testimony of Richard P. Kusserow. March 2, June 1, 1989. (Serial No. 101-58). pp. 124-144.

State of Florida Health Care Cost Containment Board and Department of Economics and Department of Finance, Florida State University. 1991. *Joint Ventures Among Health Care Providers in Florida: Volumes I—III.*

The principal results of these studies are summarized in Mitchell, Jean M., and Elton Scott. 1992. "New Evidence on the Prevalence and Scope of Physician Joint Ventures." *Journal of the American Medical Association* 268(1):80-84.

Mitchell, Jean M., and Elton Scott. 1992. "Evidence on Complex Structures of Physician Joint Ventures Under Existing Regulation." *Yale Journal of Regulation* 9(3):489-520.

[47]Hillman, Bruce J., George T. Olson, Patricia E. Griffth, Jonathan H. Sunshine, Catherine A. Joseph, Stephen D. Kennedy, et al. 1992. "Physicians' Utilization and Charges for Outpatient Diagnostic Imaging in a Medicare Population." *Journal of the American Medical Association* 268(15):2050-2054.

Mitchell, Jean M. and Jonathan H. Sunshine. 1992. "Consequences of Physicians' Ownership of Healthcare Facilities-Joint Ventures in Radiation Therapy." *New England Journal of Medicine* 327(21):1497-1501.

Mitchell, Jean M. and Elton Scott. 1992. "New Evidence of Complex Structure of Physician Joint Ventures." *Yale Journal on Regulation* 9(3):489-520.

Mitchell, Jean M. and Elton Scott. 1992. "Evidence on the Prevalence and Scope of Physician Joint Ventures." *Journal of the American Medical Association* 268(1):80-84.

Mitchell, Jean M. and Elton Scott. 1992. Physician Ownership of Physical Therapy Services: Effects on Charges, Utilization, Profits, and Service Characteristics. *Journal of the American Medical Association* 268(15):2055-2059.

Swedlow, Alex, Gregory Johnson, Neil Smithline, Arnold Milstein. 1992. "Increased Costs and Rates of Use in the California Workers' Compensation System as a Result of Self-Referral by Physicians." *New England Journal of Medicine* 327(21):1502-1506.

Hemenway, David, Alice Killen, Suzanne B. Cashman, Cindy Lou Parks, and William J. Bicknell. 1990. "Physicians' Response to Financial Incentives from For-Profit Ambulatory Care Centers." *New England Journal of Medicine* 322(15):1059-1062.

Hillman, Bruce J., Catherine A. Joseph, Michael R. Mabry, Jonathan H. Sunshine, Stephen Kennedy, and Monica Noether. 1990. "Frequency and Costs of Diagnostic Imaging in Office Practice—A Comparison of Self-Referring and Radiologist-Referring Physicians."*New England Journal of Medicine* 323(23):1604-1608.

Inspector General. 1989. *Financial Arrangements Between Physicians and Health Care Business: Report to Congress.* Washington, D.C.: Office of the Inspector General. (OAI-12-88-01410).

Medical Affairs Division. 1984. *A Comparison of Laboratory Utilization and Payout to Ownership.* Blue Cross and Blue Shield of Michigan.

Department of Health and Human Services, Health Care Financing Administration, Division of Health Standards and Quality, Region V. 1983. *Diagnostic Clinical Laboratory Services in Region V.* (No. 2-05-2004-11).

Medical Services Administration, State of Michigan. 1981. *Utilization of Medicaid Laboratory Services by Physicians With/Without Ownership Interest in Clinical Laboratories: A Comparative Analysis of Six Selected Laboratories.* Michigan Department of Social Services, Medicaid Monitoring and Compliance Division.

Childs, Alfred A., and E. Diane Hunter. 1972. "Non-Medical Factors Influencing Use of Diagnostic X-ray by Physicians." *Medical Care* 10(4):323-335.

Childs, Alfred W., and D. W. Hunter. 1970. *Patterns of Primary Medical Care—Use of Diagnostic X-Ray by Physicians.* Berkeley: Institute of Business and Economic Research and the School of Public Health, University of California.

[48]AMA. 1991. *Physician Characteristics and Distribution in the U.S. 1990.* Chicago: AMA.

However, many physicians affiliated with HMOs have private practices in which they see patients not affiliated with the HMO.

[49]Marder, William D., David W. Emmons, Phillip R. Klecke, and Richard J. Willke. 1988. "Physician Employment Patterns." *Health Affairs* (Winter):137-145 at 138.

[50]Havlicek, Penny L. 1993. *Medical Groups in the United States: A Survey of the Practice Characteristics.* Chicago: AMA, Division of Survey and Data Resources. p. 44.

Chapter 2

[1]"Shall the Consultant Pay the General Practitioner for Cases Referred to Him?" 1898. *Journal of the American Medical Association* 31 (17 December): 1480-1481.

[2]AMA Council on Ethical and Judicial Affairs. 1989. "Opinion 8.03." *Current Opinions.* Chicago: AMA.

[3]Reports from the AMA *Proceedings of the House of Delegates* (abbreviated as AMA *Proceedings*) are published each year and available at major medical libraries. Summaries and excerpts of many of the proceedings cited are more easily found in several volumes of the American Medical Association *Digest of Official Actions* (abbreviated as AMA *Digest*). The AMA also periodically publishes *Principles of Medical Ethics* and *Judicial Council Opinions and Reports* (after 1985 renamed *Opinions of the Council on Ethical and Judicial Affairs*).

[4]OBRA Act of 1989, P.L. 101-239, Title 6.

Iglehart, John K. 1990. "Congress Moves to Regulate Self-Referral and Physicians' Ownership of Clinical Laboratories." *The New England Journal of Medicine* 322(23):1682-1687.

[5]AMA. By-laws 2.115.

[6]Hirsh, Bernard D. 1984. *he History of the Judicial Council of the American Medical Association*. (This is an unpublished paper commissioned by James H. Sammons, executive vice-president of the AMA. The author was the legal counsel for the Council on Ethical and Judicial Affairs for 25 years.)

[7]Fishbein, Morris. 1947. *A History of the American Medical Association 1847 to 1947*. Philadelphia: W.B. Saunders. p. 949.

[8]Proceedings of the National Medical Convention 1846, 1847, reprinted in Reiser, Stanley Joel, Arthur J. Dyck, and William J. Curran. 1977. *Ethics in Medicine: Historical Perspectives and Contemporary Concerns*. Cambridge: MIT Press. pp. 26-34.

[9]Article 1 (4) states that it is "derogatory to professional character . . . , for a physician to hold a patent for any surgical instrument, or medicine. . . ."

[10]Burns, Chester. 1978. "Medical Ethics, History of: North American: Seventeenth Century to Nineteenth Century," in *Encyclopedia of Bioethics*, Warren T. Reich, ed. London: Free Press. pp. 963-968, at 966.

Konold, Donald E. 1962. *A History of American Medical Ethics 1847-1912*. Madison: University of Wisconsin Press.

[11]*American Medical Association v. Federal Trade Commission*, 638 F. 2d 448 (1980); 101 S.C. 3102 (1982).

Berland, Jeffrey Lionel. 1975. "Medical Ethics and Monopolization." *A Study of Medicine in the United States and Great Britain*. Berkeley: University of California Press.

Goldfarb v. Virginia State Bar Association 421 U.S.773 (1975).

Arrow, Kenneth J. 1973. "Social Responsibility and Economic Efficiency." *Public Policy* 16(2):303-317.

Stevens, Rosemary. 1971. *American Medicine and the Public Interest*. New Haven: Yale University Press.

Kessel, Reuben A. 1958. "Price Discrimination in Medicine." *Journal of Law and Economics* 1:20-53.

Friedman, Milton, and Simon Kuznets. 1945. *Income from Independent Professional Practice*. New York: National Bureau of Economic Research.

[12]Konold, Donald. 1978. "Codes of Medical Ethics: History," in *Encyclopedia of Bioethics*, Warren T. Reich, ed. London: Free Press. pp. 162-170.

Veatch, Robert M. 1978. "Code of Medical Ethics, Ethical Analysis," in *Encyclopedia of Bioethics*, Warren T. Reich, ed. London: Free Press. pp. 172-180.

[13]Konold, Donald E. 1962. *American Medical Ethics*. p. 65.

[14]AMA. *Proceedings*. 1913. (June):12-15.

[15] AMA. *Proceedings*. 1913. (June):12-15.

AMA Judicial Council. 1965. "Fee-Splitting Defined." *Opinions and Reports* Section 7, No. 19, at 45. Chicago: AMA.

[16]AMA. *Proceedings*. 1929. (June):24-25.

[17]One popular article used both terms in 1953. See Whitman, Howard. 1953. "Why Some Doctors Should Be in Jail." *Collier's* (October 30):23-27. By 1960 the terms were used interchangeably in the medical profession.

See Meyers, Robert S. 1960. "The Surgeon, the General Practitioner, and Medical Ethics." *Bulletin of the American College of Surgeons* 45(6):473-475, 500, at 474.

By the 1980s, medical literature made it clear that what physicians called fee splitting in the past was the same thing regulated as kickbacks under the Medicare fraud and abuse statute.

See Jurkiewicz, M. J. 1985. "Fee-splitting: College Bylaws Clarified." *Bulletin of the American College of Surgeons* 70(11):19-20. ("Fee-splitting, a covert kickback arrangement as an inducement to refer patients, remains an evil and cannot be condoned.")

For a series of articles that link the ACS's anti-fee-splitting policy with the Medicare antikickback statute, see the article and two statements in the April 1986 issue of the *Bulletin of the American College of Surgeons*.

Gebhard, Paul. 1986. "Lithotripsy Referral Fees: Medicare Fraud and Abuse?" *Bulletin of the American College of Surgeons* 71(4):16, 25.

Hanlon, C. Rollings. 1986. "Fee-Splitting." *Bulletin of the American College of Surgeons* 71(4):1.

"Regents Issue Statement on Fees for Lithotripsy." 1986. *Bulletin of the American College of Surgeons* 71(4):21.

[18]Vaughan, Fred W. 1910. *A Complete Exposé of the Doctor Drumming Evil at Hot Springs, Arkansas*. Little Rock.

Dr. Lydston defines drumming as such: "As I understand the matter a 'drumming doctor' is a man who has paid agents upon whom he depends wholly or in part for his 'business.' The medical drummer is the man who takes his business to him."

Lydston, G. Frank. 1900. "Further Remarks on the Bisection of Fees, Surgical Drummers and Drumming Surgeons." *The Philadelphia Medical Journal* 6(23):1075-1078.

[19]Lord, J. P. 1911. "The Secret Commission Evil." *Journal of the American Medical Association* 61(10):725-727, at 726.

[20]AMA. *Proceedings.* 1926. (April):28.

[21]AMA. *Proceedings.* 1952. (December):97, 110. The matter was referred back for further study.

[22]AMA. *Proceedings.* 1947. (June):39-41, 89, 90.

[23]AMA. *Proceedings.* 1935. (June):63.

AMA. *Proceedings.* 1936. (May):45, 56, 63-64, 67.

[24]AMA. *Proceedings.* 1915. (June):12, 60, 61.

[25]Lydston, G. Frank. 1899. "The Surgical Commission Man and Surgical Canvassing." *The Philadelphia Medical Journal* 4(1a):837-840.

Lydston, G. Frank. 1900. "Further Remarks."

[26]Lydston, G. Frank. 1900. "Further Remarks." p. 1076.

[27]Lydston, G. Frank. 1899. "The Surgical Commission." p. 840.

[28]Lydston, G. Frank. 1900. "Further Remarks." p. 1076.

[29]AMA. *Proceedings.* 1913. (June):12-15. The Judicial Council sent letters to 6,000 physicians and received replies from over 3,000.

[30]Lydston, G. Frank. 1899. "The Surgical Commission."

[31]AMA. *Proceedings.* 1913. (June):2-16.

[32]AMA. *Proceedings.* 1915. (June):12.

[33]AMA. *Proceedings.* 1915. (June):12.

[34]AMA. *Proceedings.* 1915. (June):12.

[35]AMA. *Proceedings.* 1924. (June):21.

[36]AMA. *Proceedings.* 1924. (June):22.

[37]AMA. *Proceedings.* 1930. (June):23, 37.

[38]Hirsh, Bernard D. 1984. *History of the Judicial Council.* p. 91. Citing the 1939 St. Louis Meeting of the House of Delegates.

[39]House of Delegates Report. 1934. Reprinted in Judicial Council. 1965. *Opinions and Reports.* Chicago: AMA.

[40]AMA. *Proceedings.* 1942. (June):65, 70.

[41]Bleakley, William F., and Herman T. Stichman. 1944. *Administration of the Workmen's Compensation Law in the State of New York.* Report to the Honorable Thomas E. Dewey (Moreland Commission Report authorized under Section 8 of the Executive Law).

[42]Evans, C. L. 1912. "Sic Vos Non Vobis." *Journal of the Missouri State Medical Association* 8(April):405-406.

[43]Lydston, G. Frank. 1899. "The Surgical Commission."

[44]"Hawking Physicians." 1898. *Journal of the American Medical Association* 31(17 December):181 ("County doctors frequently go about from surgeons to surgeons seeking the highest bidders.")

[45]Bowman, John G. 1919. "General Hospitals of 100 or More Beds." *Bulletin of the American College of Surgeons* 4(4):8-9. ("[F]ee-splitting makes for unnecessary surgical operations.... Much of the unnecessary surgery in our present day is due directly to fee splitting."

ACS. 1918. "Standard of Efficiency for the First Hospital Survey of the College." *Bulletin of the American College of Surgeons* 3(3):5. ("The consequence of the division of fees are, first, incompetent medical care and surgical services; second unnecessary surgical operation . . .")

Lydston, G. Frank. 1900. "Further Remarks." p. 1076.

Brettauer, J. 1911. "The Secret Division of Fees." *New York State Journal of Medicine* 11(6):301-303, at 302. ("No surgeons who employs agents, be they doctors or others, to bring cases to him, can avoid doing unnecessary, illegitimate, and dishonest work.")

Morris, R. T. 1911. "Secret Division of Fees." *New York State Journal of Medicine* 11(8):387-390, at 388. ("Surgeons who try to be responsible may not operate upon more than half the patients sent to them, and who are ready if the surgeon so decides. What are the chances of such patients in the hands of rebaters?")

Pryor, John H., M. D. Mann, Bernard Bartow, et al. 1911. "Report of the Committee Appointed by the Erie County Medical Society to Investigate the 'Division of Fees, and Its Causes and Remedies.'" *New York State Medical Journal* 11(2):92-97, at 93. ("The practice [of fee-splitting] may lead to unnecessary operating and junk surgery.")

[46]Vance, A. P. Morgan. 1899. "Where Are We At?" *Journal of the American Medical Association* 32(10):1033-1038.

[47]Lord, J. P. 1911. "The Secret Commission Evil."

[48]Morfit, John C. 1906. "Graft in Medicine." *Journal of the Michigan State Medical Association* 2(May):771-776.

[49]See AMA. 1965. *Judicial Council Opinions and Reports* Chicago: AMA.

AMA. 1969. *Judicial Council Opinions and Reports* Chicago: AMA.

[50]*Journal of the American Medical Association* 34(24):1553, 1557, 1559 (June 16, 1900).

[51]*Journal of the American Medical Association* 38(25):1661 (June 21, 1902).

[52]AMA. 1903. *Principles of Medical Ethics*. Chicago. Chapter 2, Article I, Section 8 states that it is derogatory to professional character to accept rebates, patent surgical instruments or medicines, or use or promote secret nostrums. Article VI, Section 4 condemns giving, soliciting, or receiving commissions.

[53]Konold, Donald E. 1962. *American Medical Ethics*. p. 69.

"1903 Principles of Medical Ethics." *Journal of the American Medical Association* 40(20):1379-1381 (May 16, 1903).

[54]Konold, Donald E. 1962. *American Medical Ethics*. pp. 69-70.

[55]Davis, Loyal. 1938. *J. B. Murphy: Stormy Petrel of Surgery*. New York: G. P. Putnam's Sons. Ch. 15, pp. 211-220.

[56]Link, Arthur Stanley and William M. Leary, Jr. 1969. *The Progressive Era and the Great War: 1896-1920*. New York: Appleton-Centry-Crufts.

Wiebe, Robert H. 1967. *The Search for Order: 1877-1928*. New York: Hill and Wang.

57Lord, J. P. 1911. "The Secret Commission Evil." p. 725.

58Vance, A. P. Morgan. 1899. "Where Are We At?" p. 1038.

Evans, C. L. 1912. *"Sic Vos Non Vobis."*

59Mayo, William J. 1906. "The Medical Profession and the Issues Which Confront It." *Journal of the American Medical Association* 46(23):1737-1740, at 1740.

60AMA. 1912. *Principles of Medical Ethics.* Chicago: AMA. Article VI, Section 3.

61Konold, Donald E. 1962. *American Medical Ethics.* p. 71.

AMA. *Proceedings.* 1912. (June). The AMA acted at its meeting in Atlantic City in 1912.

62Fishbein, Morris. 1947. *American Medical Association.* p. 277.

AMA. *Proceedings.* 1912. (June):11, 45.

AMA. *Proceedings.* 1913. (June):12-16, 49.

63Discussions about fee splitting emphasize two objections: (a) its secrecy, which deceived patients, and (b) the distorting effect fees had on referrals. Although the ACS said that the secrecy was the lesser of two evils, the AMA objected primarily to "secret" fee splitting. It is hard to square the concern over secrecy with other standards of disclosure at the time. Medical ethics and practice did not promote disclosure in other areas. There was no tradition of disclosing the risks and benefits of surgery. Physicians were counseled not to reveal disagreements among colleagues.

64Davis, Loyal. 1960. *Fellowship of Surgeons: A History of the American College of Surgeons.* Springfield, Ill.: Charles C. Thomas. p. 415.

65Konold, Donald E. 1962. *American Medical Ethics.* p. 66.

Proceedings of the Medical Society of the County of Erie, December 19, 1910, in *New York State Journal* 11 (February 1911):93.

66Garceau, Oliver. 1961. *The Political Life of the American Medical Association:* Hamden, Connecticut: Achon Books.

67Davis, Loyal. 1960. *Fellowship of Surgeons.* p. 481. Today members still have to pledge not to split fees.

68Davis, Loyal. 1960. *Fellowship of Surgeons.* pp. 207, 258.

69Davis, Loyal. 1960. *Fellowship of Surgeons.* pp. 264, 492-494.

70Meyers, Robert S. 1955. "The Rise and Fall of Fee-splitting." *Bulletin of the American College of Surgeons* 40(6):507-509, 523, at 508.

MacEachern, Malcolm T. 1948. "College Continues Militant Stance Against Fee-Splitting and Rebates." *Bulletin of the American College of Surgeons* 33(2):65-67, at 65.

71Davis, Loyal. 1960. *Fellowship of Surgeons.* p. 414.

72Stevens, Rosemary. 1971. *American Medicine.* p. 91.

73Williams, Greer. 1952. "The Columbus Five-year Cure for Fee-splitting." *The Modern Hospital* 78(6):67-69, 94-95. Reprinted in *Bulletin of the American College of Surgeons* 37(2):153-158, 168, at 154.

74Williams, Greer. 1948. "The Truth About Fee-splitting." *The Modern Hospital* 70(2):43-48, reprinted in *Readers Digest.* July 1948.

Williams, Greer. 1952. "The Columbus Five-year Cure." pp. 94-95.

[75]Williams, Greer. 1952. "The Columbus Five-year Cure." pp. 94-95.

[76]AMA. *Proceedings.* 1948. (November-December):61.

[77]MacEachern, Malcolm T. 1948. "Fee-splitting." p. 65.

[78]MacEachern, Malcolm T. 1948. "Fee-splitting." p. 65.

[79]Hamilton, Edwin B. 1992. "Columbus Surgical Society." *Columbus Physician* 58(2):78-79.

[80]AMA. 1947. *Principles of Medical Ethics.* Chapter 1, Section 6 (Patents, Commission, Rebates and Secret Remedies) and Chapter 3, Article VI, Section 5 (Commissions).

[81]AMA. 1947. "Report of the Judicial Council." *Journal of the American Medical Association* 143(2):178.

[82]Stevens, Rosemary. 1971. *American Medicine.* p. 84.

[83]Davis, Loyal. 1960. *Fellowship of Surgeons.* p. 435.

[84]*Lilly v. Commissioner of Internal Revenue Service,* 343 U.S. 90, 72 S Ct. 497 (1952).

[85]Whitman, Howard. 1953. "Why Some Doctors Should Be in Jail." 23-27, at 27.

[86]"Eight-Point Program Seeks to Prevent Fee-Splitting." 1967. *Bulletin of the American College of Surgeons* 62(3):146.

[87]Jesillow, Paul, and Henry Pontell. (forthcoming). *Prescription for Profit: How Doctors Defraud Medicaid.* Berkeley: University of California Press.

House of Representatives Report No. 393, 95th Congress, 1st Session, reprinted in *U.S. Code, Congressional and Administrative News,* 1977:3039.

Fraud and Abuse in the Medicare and Medicaid Programs: Subcommittee on Health, Committee on Ways and Means and Subcommittee on Health and the Environment, Committee on Interstate and Foreign Commerce. U.S. House of Representatives. 1977. Washington, D.C.: U.S. Government Printing Office.

Medicare-Medicaid Anti Fraud and Abuse Amendments. 1977. Joint Hearings Before the Subcommittee on Health, Committee on Ways and Means and the Subcommittee on Health and the Environment, Committee on Interstate and Foreign Commerce, U.S. House of Representatives, 95th Congress, 1st Session, Serial 95-7.

Fraud and Abuse Among Practitioners Participating in the Medicaid Program. Subcommittee on Long-Term Care, Special Committee on Aging, U.S. Senate. 1976. Washington, D.C.: U.S. Government Printing Office.

House Report No. 231, 92nd Congress, 2nd Session, reprinted in *U.S. Code Congressional and Administrative News.* 1972:4989.

[88]Hyman, David, and Joel V. Williamson. 1988. "Fraud and Abuse: Regulatory Alternatives in a 'Competitive' Health Care Era." *Loyola University of Chicago Law Journal* 19(4):1131-1196.

[89]Brennan, Troyen A. 1991. *Just Doctoring: Medical Ethics in the Liberal State.* Berkeley: University of California Press.

[90]Mayo, William J. 1906. "The Medical Profession." p. 1740.

Lord, J. P. 1911. "The Secret Commission Evil." pp. 725-727.

[91]AMA. *Proceedings.* 1952. (December):97.

[92]Hawley, Paul R. 1952. "American College of Surgeons Restates Principles of Financial Relations." *Bulletin of the American College of Surgeons* 37(3):233-236, at 233.

[93]AMA. "Resolution on Clarification of Section 5 of Principles of Medical Ethics." *Proceedings.* 1954. (June):45.

AMA. "Report of Reference Committee on Amendments to Constitution and Bylaws." *Proceedings.* 1953. (June):52.

[94]AMA. *Proceedings.* 1953. (December):79.

[95]Williams, Greer. 1948. "The Truth About Fee-splitting." pp. 45-46.

[96]AMA. "Report of the Committee on Medical Practice." *Proceedings.* 1955. (June 6-10):12-13.

[97]Daseler, Edward H. 1955. ". . . For the Triumph of Evil." *Bulletin of the American College of Surgeons* 40(1):22, 55-56.

Whitman, Howard. 1953. "Why Some Doctors Should Be in Jail." pp. 23-27.

Williams, Greer. 1952. "The Columbus Five-year Cure." pp. 94-95.

Williams, Greer. 1948. "The Truth About Fee-splitting." pp. 43-48.

Deutsch, Albert. 1947. "Unnecessary Operations." *Woman's Home Companion* (July):32-33, 123-126.

[98]Whitman, Howard. 1953. "Why Some Doctors Should Be in Jail." pp. 23-27.

[99]Quoted in Whitman, Howard. 1953. "Why Some Doctors Should Be in Jail." pp. 23-27.

[100]Davis, Loyal. 1960. *Fellowship of Surgeons.* pp. 424-428.

AMA. *Proceedings.* 1953. (June 1-5): 34, 35, 36, 38, 40-44, 57-58.

[101]*U.S. News and World Report.* 1953. "Too Much Unnecessary Surgery: Interview with Dr. Paul Hawley. " (February 20):48-55.

AMA. *Proceedings.* 1953. (June):26.

[102]See, e.g., AMA. "Resolution on Dr. Paul R. Hawley, Resolution of Robert B. Homa, Jr. and Resolution on Public Relations." *Proceedings.* 1953. (June 1-5):36, 43, 34.

[103]AMA. "Resolution on Controlling Public Expression of Members." *Proceedings.* 1953. (June):44.

[104]AMA. *Proceedings.* 1954. (June):31.

[105]See, e.g., AMA. *Proceedings.* 1961. (November 27-29):201-203.

AMA. *Proceedings.* 1962. (June 24-28):30-32.

[106]The AMA previously urged local medical societies to support state legislation.

AMA. *Proceedings.* 1948. (November-December):61, 71.

[107]Davis, Loyal. 1960. *Fellowship of Surgeons.* p. 435.

Between 1914 and 1953, 22 states had passed statutes making fee splitting illegal. Wisconsin led the way by enacting legislation making fee splitting a misdemeanor punishable by forfeiture of diploma of any surgeon who gave a commission. Stevens, Rosemary. 1971. *American Medicine.* p. 84.

Davis, Loyal. 1960. *Fellowship of Surgeons.* p. 435. Davis reports that 22 states had some kind of legislation in 1953.

[108]Hirsh, Bernard D. 1984. *History of the Judicial Council.* p. 94. Citing the AMA's December 1950 Cleveland meeting.

[109]AMA. *Proceedings.* 1952. (December):97.

[110]AMA. *Proceedings.* 1953. (December):58.

[111]AMA. *Proceedings.* 1954. (June):29-30.

[112]AMA. *Proceedings.* 1954. (June):29-30.

[113]"It is not unethical for a physician to prescribe or supply drugs, remedies, or appliances as long as there is no exploitation of the patient." AMA. *Proceedings.* 1955. (June):52.

AMA. *Proceedings.* 1954. (November-December):81, 100, 101.

AMA. *Proceedings.* 1955. (June): 37, 38, 39, 40, 42, 46, 48, 52, 53.

In 1959, the Judicial Council held that physicians could own stock in pharmaceutical companies "unless the patient was exploited." AMA. *Proceedings.* 1962. (June):36-45.

This was broadened in 1961 to allow physicians to own or operate a pharmacy. Hirsh, Bernard D. 1984. *History of the Judicial Council.* AMA. p. 105. Citing the AMA's November 1961 Denver meeting.

AMA. 1959. "Ownership of Pharmacies." *Proceedings.* (December 1-4):135-136.

[114]AMA. *Digest of Official Actions 1846-1958.* p. 276.

[115]Lydston, G. Frank. 1899. "The Surgical Commission."

[116]Bowman, John G. 1920. "General Hospitals of 100 or More Beds: Report for 1920." *Bulletin of the American College of Surgeons* 5(1):6. ("Sometimes the fee is divided with the explanation to the patient that the physicians 'assist the surgeon' or gives the anaesthetic.")

MacEachern, Malcolm. 1930. "Round-table Conference. Professional Problems in Hospitals." *Bulletin of the American College of Surgeons* 14(1):51-57, at 53. ("The 'trusted doctor' often accompanies his patient to the surgeon and frequently acts as a dummy assistant....")

"Principles of Financial Relations in the Professional Care of the Patient." Adopted 1942. Revised and reprinted in the October 1960 *Bulletin of the American College of Surgeons.*

Downing, W. L., and Paul R. Hawley. 1952. "Two Physicians Speak Their Minds on Fee-Splitting." *Bulletin of the American College of Surgeons* 37(4):388-390, 392-393.

Hawley, Paul R. 1952. "American College of Surgeons."

Meyers, Robert S. 1955. "Fee-Splitting."

Hirsh, Bernard D. 1984. *History of the Judicial Council.* p. 102.

AMA. *Proceedings.* 1961. (June): 24-31, 157.

AMA. *Proceedings.* 1962. (June):112-113; (November):219.

AMA. *Proceedings.* 1961. (June): 24-31, 156-157.

AMA. *Proceedings.* 1962. (November):219.

[117]Downing and Hawley. 1952. "Two Physicians Speak Their Minds." p. 393.

[118]McCann, James C. 1958. "Consideration of Deduction and Allocation of Surgical Fees by Blue Shield Plans." *Journal of the American Medical Association* 166(6):624-628.

[119]"Position of American College of Surgeons on Proration of Insurance Payments." 1959. *Bulletin of the American College of Surgeons* 44(1):5-8.

[120]Meyer, Robert S. 1960. "Medical Ethics."

[121]"Itinerant Surgery." 1960. *Bulletin of the American College of Surgeons* 45(3):116. "Policy on Itinerant Surgery." 1962. *Bulletin of the American College of Surgeons* 47(3):132.

[122]Hanlon, C. Rollins. 1989. "Itinerant Surgery: Outreach or Outrage?" *Bulletin of the American College of Surgeons* 74(10):6-8.

[123]Flexner, Abraham. 1910. *Medical Education in the United States and Canada.* New York: Carnegie Foundation for the Advancement of Teaching.

[124]MacLeod, Gordon K., and M. Roy Schwartz. 1986. "Faculty Practice Plans: Profile and Critique." *Journal of the American Medical Association* 265(1):58-62.

[125]Bogdanich, Walt, and Michael Waldholz. 1989. "Warm Bodies: Hospitals That Need Patients Pay Bounties for Doctors' Referrals." *The Wall Street Journal* (27 February):1.

United States of America v. Russell Furth. U.S. D.C.(S.D. Texas, Houston Division). Trial Transcript. Doc. No. H-85-721. March 11-14, 1986.

[126]Williams, Greer. 1952. "The Columbus Five-year Cure." p. 156.

[127]AMA. 1977. *Judicial Council Opinions and Reports.* Chicago. AMA.

AMA. 1969. *Judicial Council Opinions and Reports.* Chicago. AMA.

[128]Hirsh, Bernard D. *History of the Judicial Council.* 1984. p. 110. Citing the November 1965 meeting at Philadelphia.

[129]AMA. *Proceedings.* 1969. (November 30-December 3):243, 313 ("Physician Ownership of Stock in Corporations Operating Profit-making Hospitals").

[130]AMA. "Resolution 13." *Proceedings.* 1976. (June 27-July 1):372.

[131]AMA. "Physician Ownership of Expensive Equipment." *Proceedings.* 1977. (June 19-23):176.

[132]Altman, Stuart H., and Marc A. Rodwin. 1988. "Halfway Competitive Markets and Ineffective Regulation: The American Health Care System." *Journal of Health Politics, Policy and Law* 13(2):323-339.

[133]*American Medical Association v. Federal Trade Commission* 638 F.2d 448 (1980) affirmed, 101 S. Ct. 3107 (1982).

Hirsh, Bernard D. 1984. *History of the Judicial Council.* p. 7.

Koefoot v. American College of Surgeons, 652 F. Supp 882 (1986); 692 F. Supp. 843 (1988).

Goldfarb v. Virginia State Bar Association 421 U.S.773 (1975).

[134]Arquit, Kevin J. 1992. *A New Concern in Health Care Antitrust Enforcement: Acquisition and Exercise of Market Power by Physician Ancillary Joint Ventures* (Remarks Before the National Health Lawyers Association, January 30.)

Moreland, Judith A. 1992. Official Correspondence from the Office of Legal Counsel, Federal Trade Commission, to Edward B. Hirshfeld, Office of General Counsel, AMA, (January 27).

[135]Personal communication with Maureen Conklin and Dr. Peter Van Schoonhoven at the Joint Commission on Accreditation of Health Care Institutions.

[136]Relman, Arnold S. 1980. "The New Medical-Industrial Complex." *The New England Journal of Medicine* 303(17):963-970.

[137]Relman, Arnold S. 1985. "Editorial: Dealing with Conflicts of Interest." *The New England Journal of Medicine* 313(12):749-751.

[138]Relman, Arnold S. 1989. "Economic Incentives in Clinical Investigations." *The New England Journal of Medicine* 320(14):933.

Relman, Arnold S. 1988. "Salaried Physicians and Economic Incentives." *The New England Journal of Medicine* 319(12):784.

Relman, Arnold S. 1988. "Medicine as a Profession and a Business," in *The Tanner Lectures on Human Values,* Sterling M. McMurrin, ed. Salt Lake City: University of Utah Press. pp. 283-313.

Relman, Arnold S. 1987. "Doctors and the Dispensing of Drugs." *The New England Journal of Medicine* 317(5):311-12.

Relman, Arnold S. 1987. "Practicing Medicine in the New Business Climate." *The New England Journal of Medicine* 316(18):1150-1151.

Relman, Arnold S. 1985. "Cost Control, Doctor's Ethics, and Patient Care." *Issues in Science and Technology* (Winter):103-111.

Relman, Arnold S. 1983. "Investor-Owned Hospitals and Health-Care Costs." *The New England Journal of Medicine* 309(6):370-372.

Relman, Arnold S. 1983. "The Future of Medical Practice." *Health Affairs* 2(21):5-19.

[139]Committee on Implications of For-Profit Enterprise in Health Care, Institute of Medicine. 1986. "Physicians and Entrepreneurialism in Health Care," in *For-Profit Enterprise in Health Care,* Bradford H. Gray, ed. Washington, D.C.: National Academy Press.

Gray, Bradford H., ed. 1983. *The New Health Care for Profit: Doctors and Hospitals in a Competitive Environment.* Washington, D.C.: National Academy Press.

[140]Relman, Arnold S., and Uwe Reinhardt. "An Exchange on For-Profit Health Care," in *For-Profit Enterprise,* Bradford H. Gray, ed. 1986. Reprinted in *Health Affairs* (1986) 5(2):5-31.

[141]AMA. 1990. *AMA Policy compendium.* Chicago: AMA.

AMA. 1989. "Current Opinions of the Council on Ethical & Judicial Affairs." Chicago: AMA.

AMA. "C: Conflict of Interest: Update." *Proceedings.* 1989. (June):188-189.

AMA. 1986. "Report of the Council on Ethical and Judicial Affairs, Report A (I-86): Conflicts of Interest." Chicago: AMA. *Proceedings.* (December):216-228.

AMA. 1986. "Current Opinions of the Council on Ethical and Judicial Affairs." Chicago: AMA. Numbers 6 and 8.

AMA. "Concept of Gate Keeper." *Proceedings.* 1986 (June):294-297.

AMA. "Integration of the Health Care Sector: Definitions, Trends and Implications." *Proceedings.* 39th Interim Meeting, 1985:100-109.

AMA. "Physician Conflict of Interest." *Proceedings.* 1984. (June):87-88.

AMA. *Proceedings.* 38th Interim Meeting, 1984. (2-5 December):144-154.

AMA. 1983. "Commercialism in the Practice of Medicine." *Proceedings.* Washington, D.C.: Board of Trustees, AMA. 132nd Annual Meeting. pp. 101-102.

[142]AMA. "Report of the Council on Ethical and Judicial Affairs, Report A (I-86): Conflicts of Interest." *Proceedings.* 1986.

[143]AMA. "Report A (I-86): Conflicts of Interest." *Proceedings.* 1986.

[144]AMA. 1989. "Current Opinions of the Council on Ethical and Judicial Affairs of the American Medical Association." Chicago: AMA. No. 8.07.

[145]American Medical Association. 1987. *Physician-Hospital Joint-Ventures: A Resource Manual For Physicians and Physician Advisers.* Chicago: AMA.

[146]AMA. *Proceedings.* 1986:2. "Suggestions for resolving conflicts of interest are predicated on the fact that, at a minimum, they must be resolved in compliance with the law and public policy. Individual physicians may, of course, choose the strictest personal moral course. . . ."

[147]Rodwin, Marc A. 1989. "Physicians' Conflicts of Interest: The Limitations of Disclosure." *The New England Journal of Medicine* 321(20):1405-1408.

[148]*Cipollone v. Liggett Group Inc.*, 120 L. Ed. 407, 112 S. Ct. 2068 (1992); 789 F. 2nd 181 (3rd Cir. 1986).

[149]AMA. "Physicians' Involvement in Commercial Ventures—Status Report." *Proceedings.* 1989. (December):131-132.

AMA. 1989. "Physician Ownership of Health Facilities: Report on the AMA Socioeconomic Survey Effort." Chicago: Center for Health Policy Research, AMA. (September).

[150]Social Security Act. 1987. 42 U.S.C. Section 139 nn(b), as amended by Pub. L. 100-93; 101 Stat 680 1987); 42 U.S.C. Sections 1320a-7b(b).

[151]AMA. "Ethical Implications of Certain Physician-Hospital Profit-Sharing Arrangements." *Proceedings.* 1984. (June):242-244; (December):175-176.

[152]AMA. "AMA Initiative on Quality of Medical Care and Professional Self-Regulation: Review of Membership Rolls." *Proceedings.* 1987. (June):89-92.

[153]Personal Communication, Nancy Watson, AMA.

[154]Hirsh, Bernard D. 1984. *History of the Judicial Council.* p.18.

[155]OBRA Act of 1989, P.L. 101-239, Title 6.

Iglehart, John K. 1990. "Congress Moves to Regulate."

[156]State of Florida Health Care Cost Containment Board and Department of Economics and Department of Finance, Florida State University. 1991. *Joint Ventures Among Health Care Providers in Florida: Volumes I—III.*

Hemenway, David, A. Killen, S. B. Cashman, C. L. Parks, and W. J. Bicknell. 1990. "Physicians' Responses to Financial Incentives: Evidence from a For-Profit Ambulatory Care Center." *The New England Journal of Medicine* 322(15): 1059-1063.

Hillman, Bruce J., Catherine A. Josephs, Michael R. Mabry, Jonathan H. Sunshine, Stephen D. Kennedy, and Monica Noether. 1990. "Frequency and Cost of Diagnostic Imaging in Office Practice—A Comparison of Self-Referring and Radiologist-Referring Physicians." *The New England Journal of Medicine* 323(23):1604-1608.

Kusserow, Richard P. 1989. *Financial Arrangements between Physicians and Health Care Businesses: Report to Congress.* Office of Analysis and Inspections. OAI-12-88-01410.

Hillman, Alan L., Mark V. Pauly, and Joseph J. Kerstein. 1989. "How Do Financial Incentives Affect Physicians' Clinical Decisions and the Financial Performance of Health Maintenance Organizations?" *The New England Journal of Medicine* 321(2):86-92.

Hillman, Alan L. 1987. "Financial Incentives for Physicians in HMOs: Is There a Conflict of Interest?" *The New England Journal of Medicine* 317(27):1743-1748.

Blue Cross and Blue Shield of Michigan. 1984. *A Comparison of Laboratory Utilization and Payout to Ownership.* Blue Cross and Blue Shield of Michigan, Medical Affairs Division.

Department of Health and Human Services. 1983. Health Care Financing Administration, Division of Health Standards and Quality, Region V. *Diagnostic Clinical Laboratory Services in Region V.*, Report No. 2-05-2004-11.

Michigan Department of Social Services. 1981. *Utilization of Medicaid Laboratory Services by Physicians With/Without Ownership Interest in Clinical Laboratories.*

Childs, A. W., and E. D. Hunter. 1972. "Non-Medical Factors Influencing Use of Diagnostic X-ray by Physicians." *Medical Care* 10(4):323-335.

[157]Crane, Thomas S. 1992. "The Problem of Physician Self-Referral Under the Medicare and Medicaid Anti-Kickback Statute: The Hanlester Network Case and the Safe Harbor Regulation." *Journal of the American Medical Association* 268 (1):85-91.

Inspector General v. Hanlester Network et al. September 18, 1991. Final Decision on Review of Administrative Law Judge Decision, Department of Health and Human Services, Departmental Appeals Board; Appellate Division. Doc. Nos. C-186 through C-192, C-208, C-213. Doc No. 1275. *Commerce Clearing House Medicare and Medicaid Guide.* Paragraph 39, 566.

[158]AMA Council on Ethical and Judicial Affairs. 1991. *Conflicts of Interest: Physician Ownership of Medical Facilities.* Report C (I-91).

[159]AMA. *Proceedings.* 1989. (June):108–111.

[160]McCormick, Brian. 1992. "AMA, State Society on Opposite Sides." *American Medical News* (June 1):1, 11.

[161]AMA. *Proceedings.* 1992. (June):344.

McCormick, Brian. 1992. "Referral Ban Softened: Frustrated Physicians OK Self-Referral if Doctors Disclose Ownership of Interests." *American Medical News* (July 6/13):1, 52.

[162]Substitute resolution 4, adopted by the AMA House of Delegates, December 8, 1992.

[163]ACS. 1985. *Statements on Principles.* Chicago: ACS.

[164]McCormick, Brian. 1992. "AMA Reverses Self-Referral Stance." *American Medical News* (December 21):1, 29, 30.

[165]Fletcher, Joseph F. 1954. *Morals and Medicine: The Moral Problems of the Patient's Right to Know the Truth, Contraception, Artificial Insemination, Sterilization, Euthanasia.* Princeton, N.J.: Princeton University Press. pp. viii–ix.

[166]Rothman, David J. 1990. "Human Experimentation and the Origins of Bioethics in the United States," in *Social Science Perspectives on Medical Ethics,* George Weisz, ed. Dordrecht: Kluwer Academic Publishers. pp. 185–200.

Rothman, David J. 1991. *Strangers at the Bedside: A History of How Law and Bioethics Transformed Medical Decisionmaking.* New York: Basic Books.

[167]Beecher, Henry E. 1966. "Ethics and Clinical Research." *The New England Journal of Medicine* 274(24):1354–1360.

Pappworth, M. H. 1968. *Human Guinea Pigs: Experimentation on Man.* Boston: Beacon Press.

[168]The federal government's policies were revised and issued as regulations of the Department of Health and Human Services on May 30, 1974 IRB in 45 Code of Federal Regulations 46.

A history of IRBs is provided in Levine, Robert. J. 1988. *Ethics and the Regulation of Clinical Research* (2nd ed.). New Haven: Yale University Press, Ch. 14.

[169]Congress held hearings on conflicts of interest in research in 1988, and on September 15, 1989, the National Institutes of Health and the Alcohol, Drug Abuse and Mental Health Administration proposed conflict-of-interest guidelines for institutions receiving funds for biomedical or behavioral research. However, these were later withdrawn. Louis Sullivan, the Secretary of the Department of Health and Human Services, stated that he would issue regulations, but he has not done so yet. However, many universities have their own policies for financial conflicts of interest in research.

Ad Hoc Committee on Misconduct and Conflicts of Interest in Research. 1990. *Policy Statement and Guidelines.* Washington, D.C.: Association of American Medical Colleges.

Academic Health Centers Task Force on Science Policy. 1990. *Conflicts of Interest in Academic Health Centers.* Washington, D.C.: Association of Academic Health Centers.

Request for comment on proposed guidelines for policies on conflict of interest developed by the National Institutes of Health and the Alcohol, Drug Abuse, and Mental Health Administration. NIH guide for grants and contracts. 1989. 18(32):1-5 (September 15).

Federal Response to Misconduct in Science: Are Conflicts of Interest Hazardous to Our Health? Subcommittee on Human Resources and Intergovernmental Relations of the House Committee On Government Operations. 100th Congress, 2nd Session. Washington, D.C.: U.S. Government Printing Office. September 29, 1988.

[170]Commission for the Protection of Human Subjects of Biomedical and Behavioral Research. 1978. *The Belmont Report: Ethical Principles and Guidelines for the Protection of Human Subjects of Research.* DHEW Publication No. (OS) 78-0012.

[171]*President's Commission for the Study of Ethical Problems in Medicine and Biomedical and Behavioral Research* (15 volumes). 1983. Bethesda: U.S. Government Printing Office.

[172]These included the Society for Health and Human Values in 1969, The Hastings Center in 1969, and the Kennedy Institute of Ethics at Georgetown University in 1971.

[173]One of the most cogent summaries of the subject is Clouser, K. Danner. 1980. *Teaching Bioethics: Strategies, Problems, and Resources.* Hastings on Hudson: The Hastings Center.

Some important anthologies include Abrams, Natalie, and Michael D. Buckner. 1983. *Medical Ethics: A Clinical Textbook and Reference for the Health Care Professions.* Cambridge: MIT Press; Beauchamp, Tom L., and LeRoy Walters. 1982. *Contemporary Issues in Bioethics* (2nd ed.). Belmont, Calif.: Wadsworth; Reiser, Stanley Joel, Arthur J. Dyck, and William J. Curran. 1977. *Ethics in Medicine.*

The leading handbook is Jonsen, Albert R., Mark Siegler, and William J. Winslade. 1982. *Clinical Ethics: A Practical Approach to Ethical Decisions in Clinical Medicine.* New York: Macmillan.

One of the most influential textbooks (now about to be republished in the 4th edition) is Beauchamp, Tom L., and James P. Childress. 1979. *Principles of Biomedical Ethics.* New York: Oxford University Press.

Examples of journals include the *Hastings Center Reporter, Journal of Medical Ethics, Journal of Medicine and Philosophy,* and *Bioethics.*

The *Encyclopedia of Bioethics* was published in 1978 and is still highly regarded. A revised edition is planned for publication in 1994.

[174]A special edition of *Academic Medicine* in 1989 is devoted to teaching medical ethics. The journal includes a survey of the literature and articles on different programs. *Academic Medicine: Journal of the Association of American Medical Colleges.* 1989. Special Issue: Teaching Medical Ethics 64(12):1.

Some other relevant articles include:

Frader, Joel, Robert Arnold, John Coulehan, et al. 1989. "Evolution of Clinical Ethics Teaching at the University of Pittsburgh." *Academic Medicine* 64(12):747-750.

Perkins, Henry S. 1989. "Teaching Medical Ethics During Residency." *Academic Medicine* 64(5):263-266.

Puckett, Andrew C., Dole G. Graham, Lois A. Pounds, et al. 1989. "The Duke University Program for Integrating Ethics and Human Values into Medical Education." *Academic Medicine* 64(5):231-235.

Bickel, Janet. 1987. "Human Values Teaching Programs in the Clinical Education of Medical Students." *Academic Medicine* 62(5): 369-378.

Veatch, Robert M. 1987. "Medical Ethics Education," in *Encyclopedia of Bio-Ethics*, Warren T. Reich, ed. London: Free Press. pp. 870–875.

Culver, Charles M., K. Danner Clouser, Bernard Gert, et al. 1985. "Basic Curricular Goals in Medical Ethics." *The New England Journal of Medicine* 312(4):253-256.

[175]National standards for medical ethics programs were proposed by the Association of American Medical Colleges in consultation with the Society for Health and Human Values.

See Thomasma, David C. 1982. "Report of Group II on the Future of Medical Humanities Programs," in *The Humanities and Human Values in Medical Schools: A Ten-year Overview*. E. D. Pellegrino and T. K. McElhinney, eds. Washington, D.C.: Institute on Human Values in Medicine of the Society for Health and Human Values. pp. 66-79.

But a recent survey on teaching ethics in medical schools shows variations in approach and content. See *Academic Medicine: Journal of the Association of American Medical Colleges*. 1989. Teaching Medical Ethics. 64(12).

[176]Veatch, Robert M. 1986. "Challenging the Power of Codes." *Hastings Center Report* 16(2):14-15.

[177]See, e.g., Engelhardt, H. Tristram, Jr. 1986. *The Foundations of Biomedical Ethics*. New York: Oxford University Press. p. 7.

[178]For example, the *Encyclopedia of Bioethics* has only one entry under "conflict of interest," and this deals with general moral conflicts, not conflicts of interest. A leading handbook on bioethics does discuss conflicts of interest. But the focus is on role conflicts, particularly of physicians employed by organizations, rather than on financial conflicts of interest. See Jonsen, Albert R., Mark Siegler, and William J. Winslade. 1982. *Clinical Ethics*. p. 174.

[179]Lilla, Mark. 1981. "Ethos, 'Ethics' and Public Service." *The Public Interest* 63:3-18.

[180]An exception is the curriculum at the University of California, Los Angeles, School of Medicine, supervised by Dr. Michael S. Wilkes.

[181]Buchanan, Allan E., and Dan W. Brock. 1989. *Deciding for Others: The Ethics of Surrogate Decision Making*. Cambridge: Cambridge University Press.

President's Commission for the Study of Ethical Problems in Medicine and Biomedical and Behavior Research. 1982. *Making Health Care Decisions: A Report on the Ethical and Legal Implications of Informed Consent in the Patient-Practitioner Relationship*. Washington, D.C.: U.S. Government Printing Office.

Wickler, Daniel. 1991. "What Has Bioethics to Offer Health Policy?" *Milbank Memorial Quarterly* 69(2):233-251.

[182]Brennan argues for physicians adapting medical ethics to take account of existing legal institutions and tenets of liberalism. Emanuel argues for democratic communal decision making. May emphasizes the physician's covenant. Veatch stresses that physicians must share responsibility with patients and others.

Brennan, Troyen A. 1991. *Just Doctoring*. Berkeley. University of California Press.

Emanuel, Ezekiel J. 1991. *The Ends of Human Life: Medical Ethics in a Liberal Polity*. Cambridge: Harvard University Press.

May, William F. 1983. *The Physician's Covenant: Images of the Healer in Medical Ethics*. Philadelphia: The Westminster Press.

Veatch, Robert M. 1981. *A Theory of Medical Ethics*. New York: Basic Books.

May, William F. 1975. "Code, Covenant, Contract or Philanthropy." *Hastings Center Report* 5(6):29-38.

[183]Jonsen, Albert R. 1983. "Watching the Doctor." *The New England Journal of Medicine* 308(25):1531-1535.

Jonsen, Albert R. 1990. *The New Medicine and the Old Ethics*. Cambridge: Harvard University Press.

[184]Callahan, Daniel. 1987. *Setting Limits*. New York: Simon and Schuster.

Daniels, Norman. 1987. *Am I My Parent's Keeper? An Essay on Justice Between the Young and the Old*. New York: Oxford University Press.

[185]For example, a recent issue of *Academic Medicine* that reviewed nine medical school teaching programs on medical ethics does not even mention conflicts of interest in passing. However, an article reviewing the literature on medical ethics education does indicate four articles that discuss physicians and cost constraints or economic incentives. See Miles, Steven H., Laura Weiss Lane, Janet Bickel, et al. 1989. "Medical Ethics Education: Coming of Age." *Academic Medicine: Journal of the Association of American Medical Colleges* 64(12):705-714. But a reading of these articles reveals that they do not discuss conflicts of interest except in passing.

[186]Berenson, Robert A., and David A. Hyman, 1990. "When Opportunity Knocks." *Hastings Center Report* 20(6):33-35.

The author's comment on this case and the response of Drs. Hyman and Berenson appear in "Vested Interests." 1991. Hastings Center Reporter 21(6):43.

The ethics literature on physician self-referral is sparse, and these commentaries are good examples of how bioethics approaches such issues. Still, some writers mix ethics and policy. For example, E. Haavi Morreim argues that society should not prohibit self-referral but instead should impose legal sanctions for those who make unnecessary referrals in bad faith.

Morreim, E. Haavi. 1990. "Physician Investment and Self-referral: Philosophical Analysis of a Contentious Debate." *Journal of Medicine and Philosophy* 15(4):425-448.

Morreim, E. Haavi. 1989. "Conflicts of Interest: Profits and Problems in Physician Referrals." *Journal of the American Medical Association* 262(3):390-394.

[187]Dr. Berenson has written about conflicts arising from physicians' risk sharing in HMOs. Dr. Hyman has written about physician self-referral to medical facilities in which they invest.

Hyman, David A., and Joel V. Williamson. 1989. "Fraud and Abuse: Setting the Limits on Physicians' Entrepreneurship." *The New England Journal of Medicine* 320(19):1275-1278.

Hyman, David A., and Joel V. Williamson. 1988. "Fraud and Abuse. Regulatory Alternatives in a 'Comparative' Healthcare Era." *Loyola University of Chicago Law Journal*. 19(4):1131-1196.

Berenson, Robert A. 1987. "Dealing with Financial Risks and Ethical Dilemmas." *Consultant* 27(9):100, 103-105.

Berenson, Robert A. 1987. "Financial Confessions of a Sawbones: In a Doctor's Wallet." *The New Republic* (18 May):11-13.

Berenson, Robert A. 1987. "Hidden Compromises in Paying Physicians." *Business and Health* (July):18-19, 22.

Berenson, Robert A. 1986. "Capitation and Conflict of Interest." *Health Affairs* 5(1):141-146.

Chapter 3

[1]Luft, Harold S. 1983. "Economic Incentives and Clinical Decisions," in, Gray, Bradford, ed. *The New Health Care for Profit: Doctors and Hospitals in a Competitive Environment*. Washington, DC.: National Academy Press.

[2]The sources used in this chapter are unconventional. The most unusual are the comments made in response to the Inspector General's notice of intent to promulgate a rule on kickbacks and his proposed rule on kickbacks. For an explanation of the significance of these sources and how they should be interpreted, see Appendix D. In this chapter, I cite these comments using the number assigned to each by the Department of Health and Human Services, the date of the letter, and the name of the individual and the institution submitting the comments.

The other highly unusual sources are the prospectuses and private placement memoranda sent to potential investors. These documents provide detailed information on the finances of the proposed ventures. I cite the name and date of the prospectus or private placement memorandum.

[3]Numerous studies have shown that physicians paid fee-for-service perform many more services than physicians who are paid a set fee. For a review of this literature, see Luft, Harold S. 1982. *Health Maintenance Organizations: Dimensions of Performance*. New York: Wiley.

There is also evidence that variations in the volume of service physicians provide are not based on purely clinical factors or the health status of patients. Wennberg, John E., and A. Gittelshon. 1973. "Small Area Variations in Health Care Delivery." *Science* 183(117):1102-1108.

Other studies have shown that physicians adjust the volume of the services they provide, depending on the size of the fee. For example, during the Nixon administration's Economic Stabilization Program, from August 1971 to April 1974, the government imposed price controls on many physicians' services to limit health care spending. But during this period of time there was an increase in the volume and complexity of the services performed, so that payments to physicians increased. See Holahan, John, and William Scanlon. 1978. *Price Controls, Physicians' Fees, and Physician Incomes from Medicare and Medicaid*. Washington, D.C.: The Urban Institute.

Some analysts suggest that physicians induce the demand for their services and adjust the volume of procedures they perform to reach a target income. See, for example, the following articles:

Cromwell, Jerry, and Janet B. Mitchell. 1986. "Physician-Induced Demand for Surgery." *Journal of Health Economics* 5(4):293-313.

Reinhardt, Uwe W. 1985. "The Theory of Physician-Induced Demand: Reflections After a Decade." *Journal of Health Economics* 4(2):87-93.

Wilensky, Gail R., and Louis F. Rossiter. 1983. "The Relative Importance of Physician-Induced Demand in the Demand for Medical Care." *Health and Society* 61(2):252-277.

Rossiter, Louis F., and Gail R. Wilensky. 1983. "A Reexamination of the Use of Physician Services: The Role of Physician-Induced Demand." *Inquiry* 20(2):162-172.

Sweeney, George H. 1982. "The Market for Physicians' Services: Theoretical Implications and an Empirical Test of the Target Income Hypothesis." *Southern Economic Journal* 48(3):459-613.

Sloan, Frank A., and Roger Feldman. 1978. "Competition Among Physicians," in *Competition in the Health Care Sector: Past, Present, and Future*, Warren Greenberg, ed. Germantown, Pennsylvania: Aspen Systems.

Fuchs, Victor R. 1978. "The Supply of Surgeons and the Demand for Operations." *Journal of Human Resources* 13 (Supplement):35-56.

[4]In ordinary usage, kickbacks are a percentage of income—often paid secretly—to a person or organization that has made the income possible. (See *The Random House Dictionary of the English Language*, 2nd ed. 1987. New York: Random House.) However, the Medicare-Medicaid fraud and abuse statute uses a much broader definition, including as illegal payments any payment or money or in-kind services made to induce referrals. 42 U.S.C. Sections 1320a-7b.

[5]A smaller group of "attending" physicians are paid by hospitals as independent contractors. Residents and interns are usually employed by hospitals under a contract.

[6]*United States of America v. Russell Furth.* U.S. District Court, Southern District of Texas, Houston Division, Docket No. H-85-721. Trial transcript. 1986. Testimony of Dr. Spinks. March 11-14. vol. 3, p. 8.

[7]*Russell Furth.* Trial transcript. 1986. Testimony of McShane. vol. 5, p. 81.

[8]As will be discussed later, whether this practice is illegal depends on the patient's status and residence. The practice is illegal for Medicare patients, and many state laws prohibit it as well.

[9]The story was reported as part of a series in *The Wall Street Journal.* See Bogdanich, Walt, and Michael Waldholz. 1989. "Warm Bodies: Hospitals That Need Patients Pay Bounties for Doctors' Referrals." *The Wall Street Journal* (February 27):1, A4.

Waldholz, Michael, and Walt Bogdanich. 1989. "Warm Bodies: Doctor-Owned Labs Earn Lavish Profits in a Captive Market." *The Wall Street Journal* (March 1):1, A6.

Additional details of my discussion come from the trial transcript. *Russell Furth.* Trial transcript. 1986.

[10]In his opening statement, Furth's defense lawyer argued that the prosecution's contention that Furth paid kickbacks for Medicare patients was not credible, since Medicare reimburses hospitals at too low a rate. He admitted that Furth paid kickbacks but only for patients insured by Blue Cross and commercial insurers. In fact, the evidence presented on payment for Medicare patients was ambiguous and could support either conclusion. The jury may have reacted to the apparent unfairness of convicting Furth, who received no money himself, while Spinks and McShane, who were paid kickbacks and had gross earnings of about $700,000 a year, were granted immunity in return for their testimony.

[11]*Russell Furth* Trial transcript. 1986. vol. 3, p. 15; vol. 4, p. 16.

[12]McShane and Spinks were to count each patient admitted as an hour of consulting. They would submit bills for the days worked, rounding the reported time up to help disguise the payments. Any meetings, phone calls, and luncheons with other physicians were to be recorded in a diary and used as a pretext for initiating discussion of referrals. But both physicians testified that they spent no more than a couple of hours recruiting physicians and never succeeded in

recruiting. Taped conversations provide discussions of how to fake the records to disguise the basis of payment. *Russell Furth.* Trial transcript. 1986. vol. 3, p. 20.

[13]*Russell Furth.* Trial transcript. 1986. vol. 2, p. 26; vol. 2, p. 55.

[14]*Russell Furth.* Trial transcript. 1986. vol. 4, p. 100; vol. 4, p. 150.

[15]Walt Bogdanich and Michael Waldholz. 1989. "Warm Bodies: Hospitals That Need Patients."

[16]This practice may be widespread. Some individuals have requested that the Department of Health and Human Services create a safe harbor that exempts this practice from the Medicare antikickback statute. See Comment 77; December 17, 1987 letter of Donald S. Franke, of the law firm Dorsey & Whitney. ("We believe that it should be lawful for referral hospitals and specialists to make fixed payments to referring health care professionals in exchange for the referring professional's agreement to refer a set percentage of his or her patients who need the particular services to the referral provider." p. 3.)

[17]Walt Bogdanich and Michael Waldholz. 1989. "Warm Bodies: Hospitals That Need Patients."

[18]*Examination of the Pharmaceutical Industry 1973-74*: Hearings Before the Subcommittee on Health of the Committee on Labor and Public Welfare, United States Senate, 93rd Congress on S. 3441 and S. 966, part 3, March 8, 12, 13, 1974. See the statement of Gerald F. Laubach, Ph.D., president of Pfizer. March 12, pp. 793-867, especially p. 801.

[19]In the 1970s and 1980s, many firms provided gifts to physicians for participating in marketing studies.

[20]Information from interviews with Marek L. Laas, Assistant Attorney General, Medicaid Fraud Control Unit, Massachusetts Attorney General's Office; Lewis Morris, Special Prosecutor, Department of Health and Human Services, Office of the Inspector General's Criminal Investigations Divisions; and others.

Additional information provided from the following published sources:

Franklin, Karen. 1989. "The Pharmaceutical Tango." *The New Physician: Journal of the American Medical Student Association* 38(5):24-28.

"Outrage of the Month: Frequent Prescriber Equals Free-flying Doctor." 1989. *Public Citizen Health Research Group Health Letter* 5(5):12.

Arlie, Elie, and Joe Rosenblum. 1988. "Prescriptions for Profit." *Frontline* (March 28). Aired on the Public Broadcasting Service.

Graves, John. 1987. "Frequent-Flyer Program for Drug Prescribing."*The New England Journal of Medicine* 317(4):252.

For a response by Ayerst Laboratories see Mahady, Joseph M. 1987. "Frequent-Flyer Program for Drug Prescribing." *The New England Journal of Medicine* 317(4):252.

[21]The study was conducted by the sales department of American Home Products Corporation. The whole program was run by the marketing department. Using Script Tract, an information base on physician's prescribing habits,

the firm targeted physicians who were high prescribers of beta blockers to receive the promotion.

[22]These figures are from the "Final Report" of the company, i.e., the glossy seven-page brochure distributed to participating physicians.

[23]The figures were supplied by Ayerst to the Massachusetts Attorney General's Office and reported to me by Marek L. Laas, Assistant Attorney General, Medicaid Fraud Control Unit, who negotiated a settlement of the case.

[24]The drug was on the formulary for the Massachusetts Medicaid Program, which gave the Massachusetts Attorney General's Office jurisdiction to bring suit under the state's Medicaid False Claims Act, M.G.L. ch. 118E, Section 21B. After a grand jury subpoena, an out-of-court settlement was reached on May 25, 1989. No action was taken against any of the participating physicians.

[25]*Fraud, Waste, and Abuse in the Medicare Pacemaker Industry: An Information Paper.* (Committee Print). Special Committee on Aging, United States Senate, 97th Congress, 2nd Session, September 1982. (See especially pp. 40-52.)

Fraud, Waste, and Abuse in the Medicare Pacemaker Industry. Hearings before the Special Committee on Aging, United States Senate, 99th Congress, 1st Session, September 10, 1982.

Pacemakers Revisited: A Saga of Benign Neglect: Hearing before the Special Committee on Aging, United Sates Senate, 99th Congress, 1st Session, May 10, 1985. (Serial No. 99-4.) (Senate Hearings 99-608.)

The 1982 hearings included testimony from attorneys bringing suits for malpractice, physicians as expert witnesses, former pacemaker company officials, patients, salesman, and transcripts of taped interviews. See the testimony of Mr. Greg Wasley, an attorney who represents patients in lawsuits against physicians who have improperly implanted pacemakers, pp. 16-19, 1982 hearings; Mrs. Edna Alderman, a woman who was subject to a needless pacemaker implant; Mr. Howard F. Hoffman, former director of sales for Telectronics; Richard Stanley, who worked for four pacemaker manufacturers (three of which as director of marketing).

Investigations by other government agencies supported these findings. See 1978 Federal Trade Commission investigation of Intermedics.

[26]See *Pacemakers Revisited: A Saga of Benign Neglect*, statement of William Stollhans. 1985. pp. 94-96 (payments of $250 to $450), and *Fraud, Waste and Abuse in the Medicare Pacemaker Industry*, 1982, statement of Senator John Heinz, 1982. p. 2 (payments of $150 to $200), quoting a California salesman for company number 14; *Fraud, Waste and Abuse in the Medicare Pacemaker Industry: An Information Paper*, 1982. p. 43. (payments of $150).

[27]See *Pacemakers Revisited: A Saga of Benign Neglect*, 1985, statement of William Stollhans, pp. 94-96.

Fraud, Waste, and Abuse in the Medicare Pacemaker Industry. 1982. (See especially pp. 40-52.)

[28]Another kind of dubious payment was supposedly made to compensate physicians for "unreimbursed" medical expenses. Since Medicare pays all expenses except a deductible, in most cases such compensation guarantees the physician payment of the patient's portion and amounts to a $300 to $500 rebate to physicians.

[29]Devices called *programmers* set the pacemaker rate. These devices cost $200 to $300 and retail for $2,000 to $3,000. Analyzers are used to test the placement of the electrodes and to gauge how much stimulation is needed. They cost $2,000 to $3,500 retail. Transtelephonic transmitters are used to send an electrocardiogram over a telephone. Their retail cost is $200 to $300. Receivers are used by physicians to transform and print the telephone signals of patients' electrocardiograms. Their retail cost is $2,500 to $3,000. Miniclinics are portable devices used to monitor the performance of pacemakers. They are sold for $300 to $400. Source: 1982 Committee on Aging, *Information Paper*, p. 47.

This equipment is given to physicians to get them to use the pacemakers. Said one salesman, "All of our equipment is offered totally free of charge. . . . What we want, what we would like is if the doctor likes our pacemaker, we want him to refer our name, or to use our pacemaker as much as possible." 1982 Committee on Aging, *Information Paper*, p. 47.

[30]The following summary is based on testimony presented in the trial transcript and other legal papers. The jury and court did not make specific findings of fact. But Dr. Balasco did not present any evidence to contradict the testimony at the trial, and the government presented canceled checks and testimony from employees of the firms as to the purpose of the payments. See *United States of America v. Felix M. Balasco*. United States District Court for the District of Rhode Island. Trial transcript. CR NO. 85-059. January 8-10, 13-17, 1986.

Felix Balasco was found guilty of extortion in violation of Title 18 U.S.C., Section 1951 (a); Medicare fraud, in violation of Title 42, U.S.C., Section 1395nn(b)(1)(B); and conspiracy, in violation of Title 18, U.S.C., Section 371. He was sentenced to 10 years in prison and fined $70,000. See CR 85-059 Judgment and Probation/Commitment Order April 4, 1986, signed by Judge Raymond J. Pettine.

The Medicare charge for which he was convicted was soliciting payments of $4,400 from Bio-Med Technologies, an agent for Pacesetter, and $10,000 from Telectronics for implanting its pacemakers.

[31]See, e.g., *Felix M. Balasco*. 1986. Trial transcript. Testimony of Roger Anderson. January 14, pp. 74, 82, 102-105.

The government introduced as evidence bank deposit slips to Dr. Balasco's account for the sums of money paid by the firms. Trial transcript. January 14, 1986, pp. 68-71.

[32]*Felix M. Balasco*. 1986. Trial transcript. Testimony of Wendy Fisher. (See especially pp. 6, 25, 29).

[33]*Felix M. Balasco*. 1986. Trial transcript. Testimony of John Oliver. pp. 24-27.

[34]*Felix M. Balasco*. 1986. Trial transcript. Testimony of Robert F. Bunch. p. 88. The cost of the trip was nearly $4,800. (Robert Bunch was regional and later national sales manager of Teletronics.)

[35]*Felix M. Balasco*. 1986. Trial transcript. Testimony of Robert F. Bunch. pp. 113-114, Testimony of James Duncan. p. 86.

[36]*Felix M. Balasco*. 1986. Trial transcript. Testimony of Wendy Fisher. pp. 29-30.

[37]*Felix M. Balasco*. 1986. Trial transcript. Testimony of Thomas Cohen. Testimony of Barry Forwand. January 9, p. 123.

[38]*Felix M. Balasco*. 1986. Trial transcript. Testimony of John Oliver. January 9, p. 108.

[39]Inspector General's Office. 1986. *Medicare Cataract Implant Surgery*. (March). Office of Analysis and Inspections, Office of the Inspector General. 1988. *Medicare Certified Ambulatory Surgical Centers: Cataract Surgery Costs and Related Issues*. Washington, D.C: Department of Health and Human Services, OIA-09-88-00490.

Kickbacks in Cataract Surgery: Hearing before the Special Committee on Aging, United States Senate, 100th Congress, 2nd Session, Philadelphia, May 23, 1988 (Serial No. 100-22).

Cataract Surgery: Fraud, Waste, and Abuse: Hearing before the Subcommittee on Health and Long-Term Care of the Select Committee on Aging, House of Representatives, 99th Congress, 1st Session, July 19, 1985, Committee Publication No. 99-531.

[40]Comment 86; December 18, 1987 letter of Hunter R. Stokes, M.D., secretary for governmental relations, American Academy of Ophthalmology. See Section IIA, p. 13.

[41]*Kickbacks in Cataract Surgery*, statement of Bryan Mitchell, Deputy Inspector General, Department of Health and Human Services. 1988. pp. 34-37.

A draft of the report is included as an appendix to the testimony, pp. 280-289. Nearly half of the highest-paid ophthalmologists referred patients to optometrists for postoperative care, but only 10% of ophthalmologists in the mid-income range made such referrals. Ophthalmologists who referred postoperative care received 32% of their referrals from optometrists, while ophthalmologists who did not received only 7% of their referrals from optometrists.

[42]Comment 117; December 18, 1989 letter of Stephen A. Obstbaum, M.D., president, American Society for Cataract and Refractive Surgery. Obstbaum says that this practice occurs frequently and should be prohibited.

[43]*Cataract Surgery: Fraud, Waste, and Abuse*. 1985. p. 15.

[44]*Cataract Surgery: Fraud, Waste, and Abuse*: Subcommittee on Health and Long-term Care of the Select Committee on Aging, House of Representatives, 99th Congress, 1st Session, Pepper, Claude. 1985.

Cataract Surgery: Fraud, Waste, and Abuse, statement of Gordon Smith. Member, board of directors, Association of Eye and Ear Hospitals, and executive director, Eye Foundation, Birmingham, Alabama, 1985. pp. 62-63.

These practices appear to continue. See Comment 63; December 16, 1987 letter of Joseph Mandato, president, Ioptex Research, Inc., and Comment 117; December 18, 1989 letter of Stephen A. Obstbaum, M.D., president, American Society for Cataract and Refractive Surgery.

[45]Comment 117; December 18, 1989 letter of Stephen A. Obstbaum, M.D., president, American Society for Cataract and Refractive Surgery.

[46]*Kickbacks in Cataract Surgery*. 1988. pp. 14-16.

[47]See, e.g., *Kickbacks in Cataract Surgery*. 1988.

[48]Comment 54; December 11, 1987 letter of U. J. Berzins, M.D., an ophthalmologist in private practice in Salem, Oregon, and a member of the State Board of Medical Examiners.

[49]The American Optometric Association acknowledges the existence of this practice but suggests that it should be excluded from prosecution under the Medicare kickback statute because "there is no exchange of monies or any form of remuneration between providers." Comment 64; December 17, 1987 letter of James W. Clark, Jr., director, Washington, D.C., office, American Optometric Association. The American Academy of Ophthalmology acknowledges the practice and suggests it should be prohibited. Comment 86; December 18, 1987 letter of Hunter R. Stokes, M.D., secretary for governmental relations, American Academy of Ophthalmology.

[50]Comment 86; December 18, 1987 letter of Hunter R. Stokes, M.D., secretary for governmental relations, American Academy of Ophthalmology. See Section I(E)(2).

[51]See, e.g., *Kickbacks in Cataract Surgery*, 1988. Statements of Glenn Pomerance, M.D., and Charles Wright, M.D., and Appendix 5, "Documents and Letters Illustrating Referral Arrangements." pp. 246-280 and related materials attached to Appendix 4, pp. 170-189, 224-245.

[52]*Kickbacks in Cataract Surgery*, 1988. Appendix 4, "Fraudulent and/or Abuse Practices by Ophthalmologists Participating in the Medicare Program." Submitted by Scott P. Bowers, M.D., and Walter Wright, M.D. pp. 133-246.

[53]There are no accurate figures on the extent of these practices. But the American Clinical Laboratory Association believes the practices are widespread. See *Submission of the American Clinical Laboratory Association in Support of Legislation to Remedy Problems Created by Primary Care Physician-Ownership of Laboratories*. June 1987.

[54]760 F.2d 68 (1983).

[55]604 F.2d 509 (7th Cir. 1979).

[56]Press release, June 16, 1988, U.S. Department of Justice, United States Attorney, Eastern District of Pennsylvania.

[57]*Fraud and Abuse in the Medicare and Medicaid Programs*. Subcommittee on Health, Committee on Ways and Means, and Subcommittee on Health and the Environment, Committee on Interstate and Foreign Commerce, U.S. House of Representatives, 95th Congress, 1st Session, Joint Committee Print. March 3, 1977. (WMCP:95-6.) (See especially pp. 398-426.) This report includes excerpts from recorded conversations in which kickbacks were offered, a breakdown of the problem by state, and an analysis of difficulties in detection and prosecution.

[58]*Fraud and Abuse in the Medicare and Medicaid Programs*. 1977. p. 399.

Another example of how these kickbacks are disguised comes from W. M. William Winstanly, M.D. He ran the King Drive Medical Center in Chicago and reported that he received $100,000 from Medicaid. His rent was $1,050 a month. United Medical Laboratory, a clinical lab, subleased a 7 x 10 foot room for $950 a month and paid him $130 a month to hire an employee to draw blood. A pharmacy subleased space in his clinic for $1,000 a month. A dentist paid him $800 a month and an optician $400 a month. p. 400.

[59]42 Code of Federal Regulations 424.60.

[60]"Referral for Profit." American Physical Therapy Association. p. 5. Board of Directors Report to 1982 House of Delegates on Physician/Physical Therapist Practice Arrangements. (RC 59-81 and RC 64-81.)

[61]*Walter Ford v. William Cabot*. Superior Court of Fulton County, Georgia. First Amendment to Complaint. Civil Action No. D-334. Filed July 14, 1983.

[62]Sometimes these ventures are organized as privately held corporations with physicians as shareholders. The change to a corporate form does not affect the incentive to make referrals. It can affect taxes, state regulation, and control of the organization and can limit liability.

[63]Interview with Helen Trilling, Hogan & Hartson, October 27, 1992.

[64]The example comes from a Federal Trade Commission, Bureau of Competition opinion letter, November 6, 1985, from Walter T. Winslow, acting director, to H. Fred Varn, executive director, Florida Board of Dentistry. Attached as an appendix to Comment 120; December 17, 1987, letter of David L. Rogers.

[65]Kusserow, Richard P. 1989. *Financial Arrangements between Physicians and Health Care Businesses: Report to Congress*. Washington, D.C.: Department of Health and Human Services. (OAI-12-88-01410.)

[66]*Issues Related to Physician "Self-Referrals"*: Hearings before the Subcommittee on Health and the Subcommittee on Oversight of the Committee on Ways and Means, House of Representatives, 101st Congress, 1st Session, on H.R. 939. Testimony of Richard P. Kusserow. March 2, June 1, 1989. (Serial No. 101-58.) pp. 124-144.

[67]*Issues Related to Physician "Self-Referrals."* 1989. p. 128.

[68]Mitchell, Jean M., and Elton Scott. 1992. "New Evidence on the Prevalence and Scope of Physician Joint Ventures." *Journal of the American Medical Association* 268 (1):80-84.

Mitchell, Jean M., and Elton Scott. 1992. "Evidence on Complex Structures of Physician Joint Ventures Under Existing Regulation." *Yale Journal of Regulation* 9 (2):489-520.

State of Florida Health Care Cost Containment Board and the Department of Economics and Department of Finance, Florida State University. 1991. *Joint Ventures Among Health Care Providers in Florida: Volumes I-III.* State of Florida Health Care Cost Containment Board.

[69]The share of physicians owning other facilities was smaller: 40% for physical therapy or rehabilitation centers, 20% for durable equipment suppliers, 13% for home health agencies, 12% for nursing homes, 5.3% for acute care hospitals.

[70]Mitchell, Jean M. and Elton Scott. 1992. Physician Ownership of Physical Therapy Services: Effects on Charges, Utilization, Profits, and Service Characteristics. *Journal of the American Medical Association* 268(15):2055-2059.

[71]Mitchell, Jean M. and Jonathan H. Sunshine. 1992. "Consequences of Physicians' Ownership of Healthcare Facilities-Joint Ventures in Radiation Therapy." *New England Journal of Medicine* 327(21):1497-1501.

[72]Undated circular of the Cooperative, p. 1.

[73]January 26, 1988 letter from Charles L. Robinette, Jr., M.D., chairman, Coordinating Committee, to colleagues.

[74]November 2, 1988 letter from National Physical Therapy Management, Inc., Houston, Texas.

[75]February 5, 1989 letter and circular by Philip K. Hensel, M.D., president, and Jerry B. Silver, Senior vice president, CP Rehab Corporation West, Newport Beach, California.

[76]November 11, 1985 letter from Duncan Services, Republic, Missouri, a firm that sells, leases, and services physical therapy equipment.

[77]From an undated "Physician Participation Package" as part of a solicitation of investment issued by American Pain and Stress Clinics.

[78]Kusserow, Richard P. 1989. *Financial Arrangements: Report to Congress.*

[79]The report notes that the actual effect is higher, since the group used to compare the patients of physician owners is "all patients." This group includes the patients of physician investors.

[80]Metric Medical Laboratories at one time imposed such requirements on physician limited partners. The partnership agreement included the following clause: "[I]n addition to death, retirement or withdrawal from active practice, utilization of another laboratory other than Metric Medical Laboratories, or establishment or expansion of in-house laboratories can be considered as grounds for immediate return of investment capital, at the market price at the time." Since the time of this agreement, Metric Medical Laboratories has bought out its physician owners.

See *In the Matter of Daniel A. Abessinio, D.O.,* Administrative Complaint filed before the Department of Licensing and Regulation of the Board of Osteopathic Medicine and Surgery on September 4, 1986.

[81]Physicians Diagnostic Associates of Huntsville, Ltd. October 22, 1985. Private placement memorandum. p. 3.

[82]Based on MRI of Elizabeth Associates, L.P., March 26, 1986. Confidential private placement memorandum. Additional information provided by Barry H. Ostrowsky, of the law firm Brach, Eichler, Rosenberg, Silver, Bernstein, Hammer & Gladstone (Roseland, N.J.).

[83]Dr. Molitor, as the general partner, has a 15% stake in the partnership and receives a corresponding share of its profits.

[84]The facility has produced even higher volumes than projected in the private placement memorandum. Interview with Barry H. Ostrowsky. November 8, 1989.

[85]The example comes from Comment 59; December 15, 1987 letter from Hospital Corporation of America Donelson Hospital, Donelson, Tennessee (near Nashville), Cornelius Serle, administrator.

[86]Lancaster Hospital. April 21, 1988. Private placement memorandum. "Investor Suitability Standards." pp. 23-24.

[87]Lancaster Hospital. 1988. p. 1.

[88]Strictly speaking, the hospital allows the physician investors to receive "advances" based on earnings. To the extent that earnings at the end of the year do not cover the advances received, the investors are supposed to repay funds advanced.

[89]The prospectus does not state these facts explicitly. But a review of the contracts and financial information makes it clear.

The return to investors would be based on the incremental net revenue (INR). Investors would receive 1% of any INR less than $1,771,000; 1.25% of the INR greater than $1,771,000 but less than $2,155,000; and 1.50% of the INR greater than $2,155,000.

The INR equals the net operating revenue minus the baseline amount, which is set at $2,860,000. In 1987 the net operating revenue for the surgical center and the gastrointestinal unit was $3,950,228. Thus, for that year, the INR was $3,950,228 - $2,860,000 = $1,090,228; 1% of $1,090,228 is $10,902.

The prospectus states that no fewer than 9 and no more than 35 investors are sought. If 35 physicians invested $10,000, the hospital would raise $350,000 in capital. Assuming that in the first year of operation the INR was the same as that of the year before the joint venture started, the hospital would pay out $10,902 X 35 = $381,570.

In a telephone conversation on October 13, 1989, Steve Courtier, the hospital administrator, told me that the surgery and gastrointestinal unit was never established. However, the hospital has established two other joint ventures with physicians: one is a CT scanner unit, and the other is an outpatient surgery center. Mr. Courier declined to release information about the organization of these joint ventures.

[90]National Medical Enterprise. March 17, 1989. Prospectus for 200 Class A Limited Partnership units.

NME owns or leases 38 acute care hospitals, 66 psychiatric hospitals, 25 rehabilitation hospitals, and 366 long-term care facilities. Information provided by NME. 1989. *Prospectus.*

[91]NME. 1989. *Prospectus.* p. 18.

[92]NME. 1989. *Prospectus.* p. 7.

[93]NME. 1989. *Prospectus.* p. 12. Additional information on past and projected patient census is provided in Exhibit D, Financial Forecast of NME Hospitals, Inc. pp. 7, 15.

[94]NME would sell the facility (but not the land) to the limited partners and lease it back from them. The rent was set to amortize the debt assumed by the partnership and provide a fixed return of $1,200 per $15,000 invested. NME. 1989. *Prospectus.* p. 11.

[95]This income was called *contingent rent revenue* and is based on hospital revenues that exceed a specified baseline amount. NME. 1989. *Prospectus.* Appendix E, Financial Forecast of NME Hospitals, Inc. pp. 4, 12. Investment Summary, p. 5.

[96]A total of $500,000 would be used to pay for the expenses of the public offering.

[97]NME. 1989. *Prospectus.* p. 9.

[98]Perry, Linda. 1989. "Physician Ownership May Give Hospitals a Shot in the Arm." *Modern Health Care* (June 30):25-34.

[99]Source: Advisory Board Company. 1990. *Competitive Strategy:10+ Long Term Strategic Positions for Hospitals.* CEO Series Vol. 2, p. 72. The Advisory Board uses a pseudonym. But it lists its source for the data as *HealthWeek* (April 25, 1988), which should list the name of the hospital.

[100]Advisory Board Company. 1990. Vol. 2, p. 80.

"Doctors Invest, Hospital Profits Healthy." *Los Angeles Times*, October 2, 1988.

Naughton, Diane H. 1989. "MD Ownership of Hospitals: Is It Healthy?" *Health Care Competition Week* 6(36):4-7.

[101]Freudenheim, Milt. 1991. "Cashing in on Health Care's Troubles." *New York Times* (July 21):Section 3, pp. 1, 6.

Tamsho, Robert. 1992. "Columbia Hospital is Expanding, One Market at a Time." *The Wall Street Journal.* (December 4):B4

[102]Comment 107; December 18, 1987 letter of John Horty, president, National Council of Community Hospitals. p. 7.

[103]Hospitals have lost business in response to the growth of agencies providing home health care and infusion therapy. In response, some hospitals are developing their own subsidiaries and joint ventures to provide home care. For examples, Massachusetts General Hospital and New England Medical Center have formed a joint venture that owns a home health care agency.

Some hospitals have had their discharge planners recommend the affiliated home health care venture, and this has prompted competitors to file antitrust lawsuits. Key issues in these suits include what options are available to patients, who makes the choice of home health providers, and the role of hospital affiliate personnel in promoting agencies. See, e.g., *Key Enterprises of Delaware, Inc. v. Venice Hospital*, 919 F. 2d 1550 (11th Cir. 1990).

[104]Some hospitals are developing joint ventures with home health care agencies, too. There are even greater problems when hospitals and physicians are co-venturers in home health care, e.g., Tri-State Home Therapeutics. Physicians can decrease hospital costs by discharging Medicare patients early. At the same time, they can increase revenue for the home health care provider and them-selves because a sicker patient will need more days of home health care. If physicians have a financial interest in the hospital and the home health care provider, their conflicts of interest are multiplied.

[105]Information drawn from Tri-State Home Therapeutics, Inc., and Ohio Corporation. July 15, 1987. Confidential private placement memorandum.

[106]Tri-State Home Therapeutics. 1987. "IV DESCRIPTION OF THE BUSINESS, No. 8 *Shareholder Loans*." pp. 12-13.

[107]The prospectus obscures this fact. One part states the financial requirements to be a potential qualified investor. However, another provision gives T^2 exclusive choice of who to sell shares to from among potential qualified investors. Although the prospectus does not explicitly say that only physicians would be investors, the Development Agreement, included as an appendix, states that the contract is between T^2 Medical Management and "the undersigned physicians, all residents of the Cincinnati, Ohio area." Tri-State Home Therapeutics. 1987. Appendix F Development Agreement, p. 1.

[108]Tri-State Home Therapeutics. 1987. "IV DESCRIPTION OF THE BUSINESS, No. 3 *Marketing Plan*." p. 11.

"[P]hysicians who invest in the Corporation, as owners of the Corporation, will most likely be better informed regarding the services being provided by the Corporation and may be more inclined to refer patients to the Corporation." p. 4.

[109]Tri-State Home Therapeutics. 1987. "VIII RISK FACTORS, No. 5 *Competition*." p. 23.

Once physicians became investors, they could not sell their shares to others without corporate approval. This tied physicians to the corporation and prevented them from selling their shares to investors who cannot refer patients. See Tri-State Home Therapeutics. 1987. "VIII RISK FACTORS, No. 11 *Restrictions on Transferability of Shares*," p. 24. Tri-State has the right to first refusal in the event that investors want to sell their shares. "IX THE SHAREHOLDERS AGREEMENT, No. 11, *Right of First Refusal*." p. 29.

[110]Tri-State Home Therapeutics. 1987. "VIII RISK FACTORS, No. 12 *Ethical Considerations*." p. 25.

[111]Information on T^2 draws on the following. Sternberg, Steve. 1992. "Rx for Profit: Doctors Get Rich by Sending Patients to Firms in Which They Own an Economic Stake." *Atlanta Constitution* (December 13):1, A8,9.

T² Medical, Inc. Common Stock *Prospectus*, May 11, 1988.

[112]*Physician Ownership in Pharmacies and Drug Companies*. 1964. Subcommittee on the Judiciary. Hearings before the Subcommittee on Antitrust and Monopoly, 88th Congress, 2nd Session, pursuant to S. Res. 262. Washington, D.C.: U.S. Government Printing Office.

The Medical Restraint of Trade Act. 1967. Subcommittee on the Judiciary. Hearings before the Subcommittee on Antitrust and Monopoly, 90th Congress, 1st Session, pursuant to S. Res. 26 on S. 260. Washington, D.C.: U.S. Government Printing Office.

[113]Uken, Carol. 1992. "Long Island, R.I.s picket physician-owned pharmacies." *Drug Topics*. 136(19):110, 112.

"Interview with James Henning, President, Medical Associates of America, December 16, 1992."

[114]Daumier print, original text: "Diable! ne plaisantez pas avec cette maladie! .... Croyez moi, buvez de l'eau, beaucoup d'eau. Frottez vous les os des jambes et revenez me voir souvent, ça ne vous ruinera pas mes consultations sont gratuites.... Vous me devez 20 F pour ces deux bouteilles (On reprend le verre pour 10 centimes)."

[115]*Dispensing of Drugs*. Hearings before the Subcommittee on Health and the Environment of the Committee on Energy and Commerce, House of Representatives, 100th Congress, 1st Session, on H.R. 2093. April 22, 1987. Testimony of Nancy W. Dickey, M.D., American Medical Association. (Serial No. 100-36.) p. 15.

[116]A report by the Department of Health and Human Services, Office of the Inspector General, states that 31 states have minimal or no regulations on physicians dispensing drugs, 13 have only modest restrictions, and 7 have strict regulations. Office of the Inspector General. 1988. *Physician Drug Dispensing: An Overview of State Regulation*. Washington, D.C.: Department of Health and Human Services.

[117]*Physician Drug Dispensing*. 1988. Three-fourths of the officials surveyed indicated that they believed that 5% or less of their state's physicians dispensed drugs. One-half of those surveyed believed the practice was growing.

[118]Haney, Daniel Q., and Fred Bayles. "Patients, Money Promised to Doctors Selling Drugs." Associated Press, June 4, 1991.

[119] Ikegami, Naoki. 1991. "Japanese Health Care: Low Cost, Regulated Fees." *Health Affairs* 10(3):87-109, at 90.

Iglehart, John K. 1988. "Health Policy Report: Japan's Medical System: Part Two." *The New England Journal of Medicine* 319(17):166-1172.

[120]Source: Center for the Study of Drug Development, Database on Marketed Drugs. Tufts University: Medford, MA.

[121]Pharmaceutical Manufacturers Association. 1991. *Annual Survey Report: U.S. Pharmaceutical Industry—1989-1991*. Washington, D.C. The statistics are adjusted for inflation.

[122]*Dispensing of Drugs.* 1987. Source of examples from Congressman Ron Wyden and attributed to Dr. Harrison Rogers, past president, AMA. p. 1.

[123]Advertisement of the Pharmaceutical Corporation of America, quoted in "Drug Repackagers on the Make." 1987. *National Association of Retail Druggists Journal* (March):18, note 7.

[124]Information supplied from the Income Prospectus and "Patients' Diets Which Make Doctors Fat." 1989. *Public Citizen Research Group Health Letter* 5(6):12.

[125]Hemenway, David, Alice Killen, Suzanne B. Cashman, Cindy Lou Parks, and William J. Bicknell. 1990. "Physicians' Responses to Financial Incentives: Evidence from a For-Profit Ambulatory Care Center."*New England Journal of Medicine* 322(15):1059-1063.

Hillman, Bruce J., Catherine A. Joseph, Michael R. Mabry, Jonathan H. Sunshine, Stephen D. Kennedy, and Monica Noether. 1990. "Frequency and Costs of Diagnostic Imaging in Office Practice—A Comparison of Self-Referring and Radiologist-Referring Physicians." *New England Journal of Medicine* 323(23):1604-1608.

[126]Kusserow, Richard P. 1990. *Ensuring Appropriate Use of Laboratory Services: A Monograph.* Office of the Inspector General. Department of Health and Human Services. Washington, D.C.: OEI-05-89-89150.

McIllrath, Sharon. 1991. "Coalition Fights Plan to Roll Lab Fees into Visit Payments." *American Medical News* (February 11):29.

[127]Kusserow, Richard P. 1990. *Ensuring Appropriate Use.*

[128]The American Pharmaceutical Association estimates that most pharmacies stock 3,000 prescription items, while most physicians who dispense stock fewer than 50 drugs. *Dispensing of Drugs.* 1987. Testimony of Mr. Larry Braden. p. 84.

[129]In 1986 disciplinary actions for inappropriate prescribing of drugs accounted for nearly one-half of all state licensing board disciplinary actions. See Office of the Inspector General. June 1986. *Medical Licensure and Discipline: An Overview.* Boston: Department of Health and Human Services. (Control Number P-01-86-00064.) p. 13.

[130]Comment 80; December 17, 1987 letter of Nancy A. Wynstra, senior vice-president and general counsel, Allegheny Health Services, Inc., Pittsburgh.

[131]Health Care Advisory Board. 1989. *Physician Bonding: Volume II: Perfecting the Physician Network.* See "Tactic # 5 Hospital-Owned Primary Care Networks." pp. 77-106.

The Health Care Advisory Board bases its recommendations on case studies. Although it often cites financial data, the names of the parties are changed to keep their identities confidential.

[132]Grayson, Mary A. 1989. "Breaking the Medical Gridlock."*Hospitals* (February 20):32-37.

[133]Health Care Advisory Board. 1989. See "Tactic #5 Hospital-Owned Primary Care Networks." p. 80.

[134]Health Care Advisory Board. 1989. "Tactic #5." p. 82.

[135]Health Care Advisory Board. 1989. "Tactic #5." p. 89.

[136]Health Care Advisory Board. 1989. "Tactic #5." p. 96.

However, the Health Care Advisory Board says that hospitals can make these practices profitable and recommends paying physicians a percentage of the practice revenues they generate rather than the profits. This method of compensating physicians gives an incentive to provide increased outpatient services as well as increased patient admissions. It thus vitiates one of the possible benefits of a hospital-owned primary care practice: the elimination of fee-for-service incentives to increase services by using salary for compensation.

[137]Jackson and Coker. 1990. Flyer: *Physician's Marketing and Management.*

[138]Jackson and Coker. 1988. *Physician Recruiting Trends.*

[139]Jackson and Coker press release announcing the results of a nationwide survey of 114 hospitals. December 2, 1987.

[140]Jackson and Coker. 1988. *Physician Recruiting Trends.*

[141]Health Care Advisory Board. 1989. See "Tactic #8, Redoubled Recruitment, Conclusion #111." p. 138.

One such arrangement is described in an IRS private ruling letter, March 15, 1990. The hospital offered a physician $150,000 over 4 years.

[142]Jackson and Coker. "Memorandum: Possible Jeopardy of Tax Exemption Due to Physician Recruiting Incentives." October 13, 1986.

[143]Telephone interview with Mark Bryant, Jackson and Coker. December 14, 1989.

[144]Telephone interview with Randall W. Gott, director of research and training, Jackson and Coker, February 20, 1991.

[145]These programs are not limited to physicians on the hospital's medical staff. Woeppel, Charles E. 1990. "Building Physician Loyalty." *Health Care Executive Briefings* 3(2):1-3.

[146]Comment 80; December 17, 1987 letter of Nancy A. Wynstra, senior vice-president and general counsel, Allegheny Health Services, Inc., Pittsburgh. See paragraph 7.

[147]Woeppel, Charles E. 1990. "Building Physician Loyalty."

[148]Jackson and Coker. 1989. *Physician Recruiting Trends.*

[149]Health Care Advisory Board. 1987. *Physician Bonding, Volume I: Overview of Strategies Coast to Coast.*

[150]Health Care Advisory Board. 1987. pp. 141-146.

[151]Health Care Advisory Board. 1987. "Case Study #12 Rocky Point Medical Center." p. 209.

[152]These practices are hard to document. However, the American Hospital Association suggests that health care organizations often have formal or informal cross-referral arrangements, and practitioners have noted the trend as well. See Comment 101; December 18, 1987 letter of Jack W. Owen, executive

vice-president, American Hospital Association; Comment 28; December 1, 1987 letter of Michael S. Morishima, M.D.

[153]"Admissions Take Off." A flyer of The Coker Group.

[154]Telephone interview with Charles E. Woeppel, vice-president of Jackson and Coker. February 20, 1990.

[155]Health Care Advisory Board. 1989. See "Tactic #3 Massive Contract Management." p. 63.

[156]Health Care Advisory Board. 1989. See "Tactic #3, Conclusion #32." p. 66.

[157]The scenarios are based on the depositions—pretrial testimony provided under oath— of Lee Roy Joyner, M.D., Robin Lane, M.D., and John Colton, president of HCA, and on the trial transcript. The suit is *Monroe Medical Clinic and Dr. Henry E. Jones v. Hospital Corporation of America, HCA Health Services of Louisiana, Inc. a/k/a HCA of North Monroe Community Hospital, and Arlen Reynolds.* C.A. 87-851 and C.A. 87-4178, 4th District Court, Ouachita Parish, Monroe, LA. The complaint was filed on March 5, 1987. The court entered judgment on September 13, 1991.

Joyner is not a party to the suit and left the North Louisiana Clinic. He resigned over a disagreement with the policies of the North Monroe Community Hospital administrator, Dr. Robin Lake.

[158]The trial testimony on the unfair business practices was contested. As an indication of the alleged practices, testimony at trial indicated that when Dr. Jones objected to the hospital's practices, the hospital retaliated. Some patients said that the emergency room referred them to new doctors for follow-up care, rather than to Dr. Jones, their usual physician. The hospital also lured two physicians away from Dr. Jones's office, including his brother, and subsidized their competing practice next door. North Monroe Hospital also made payments to several other physicians. One physician was paid nearly $100,000 a year for a part-time position in charge of the hospital quality assurance program while maintaining an active private practice that generated patient admissions.

For an account of the trial and the multiple complex financial transactions, see the series of articles by Valerie Crain in *The Monroe News-Star* on August 11, 14-17, 20-25, and 27-31, 1991.

For a skillful narrative of the story from the perspective of the physicians who objected to these practices, written before the trial, see Bogdanich, Walt. "Candy from Strangers," in *The Great White Lie: How America's Hospitals Betray Our Trust and Endanger Our Lives.* New York: Simon and Schuster. The lawsuit case was also reported in *Health Policy Week* (1989) 18(31):1-3.

[159]Dr. Robin Lake's testimony includes some contradictory points. He says that the payment was to be $30,000 a month for three years, which equals $1,080,000. But later he says that the payment was to be $960,000. The money was divided equally among the eight physicians. If HCA paid $960,000, the subsidy amounted to $3,333 a month per physician, i.e., $40,000 a year per physician.

Deposition of Robin Lake, M.D. pp. 18-21.

[160]*Monroe Medical Clinic v. H.C.A.* Joyner deposition. p. 22.

[161]*Monroe Medical Clinic v. H.C.A.* Joyner deposition. p. 23.

[162]*Monroe Medical Clinic v. H.C.A.* Joyner deposition. p. 24.

[163]*Monroe Medical Clinic v. H.C.A.* Joyner deposition. pp. 60-63.

[164]*Monroe Medical Clinic v. H.C.A.* Joyner deposition. p. 40.

[165]*Monroe Medical Clinic v. H.C.A.* Joyner deposition. pp. 46-47.

[166]*Monroe Medical Clinic v. H.C.A.* Joyner deposition. p. 48.

[167]*Monroe Medical Clinic, Inc. v. H.C.A., et al.* Civil Action No. 87-851. Judgment filed September 13, 1991.

[168]Joyner's testimony explains:

> Q: *Did they expect you to up admissions in periods when admissions were low?*
>
> A: I think they knew that if you had your practice there and you were on the take, that you were going to do that, so they didn't have to really say that.
>
> Q: *Was it your opinion that they expected it?*
>
> A: Yes. I knew they expected it.

(*Monroe Medical Clinic v. H.C.A.* Joyner deposition. pp. 72-73.)

[169]Crain, Valerie. 1991. "Hospital Official: Payments Halted for Business Reasons," quoting testimony of Dr. David Raines. *The Monroe News Star* (August 22):1, 2A.

[170]*Monroe Medical Clinic v. Hospital Corporation of America,* CA No. 87-851, 4th Judicial District, Louisiana, before Judge Michael Ingram. Testimony of Dr. Marshall Leary, August 23, 1992, p. 1458.

[171]*Advertising, Marketing and Promotional Practices of the Pharmaceutical Industry*: Hearings before the Committee on Labor and Human Resources, U.S. Senate, 101st Congress, 2nd Session, December 11 and 12, 1990.

Senator Kennedy, who chaired the hearings, was interested primarily in the cost of these marketing practices. He claimed that the sums spent on these practices raised the price of prescription drugs. The hearings led other government agencies to investigate the practice. See, e.g., Kusserow, Richard P. 1991. *Promotion of Prescription Drugs Through Payments and Gifts.* Washington, D.C.: Office of the Inspector General, Department of Health and Human Services.

[172]Memorandum of Michael M. Simpson, Congressional Research Service, December 9, 1990. Mr. Simpson analyzed data provided by 16 pharmaceutical firms on their marketing practices for the Senate Labor and Human Resources Committee in 1988 and compared them to data obtained from surveys conducted in 1974, 1975, and 1976.

[173]The data for previous years were adjusted for inflation. The $40 million figure is in 1988 dollars.

In 1974, 20 firms were surveyed. Some of these firms had merged, which accounts for the differences in the number of firms surveyed each year.

[174]Another problem with the data is that they represent practices for one year only. Typically, marketing programs and spending follow cycles due to the introduction of new products and market competition. The Senate committee does not know whether this year represents a typical or deviant year for spending and practices.

[175]*Examination of the Pharmaceutical Industry 1973-74*: Hearing before the Subcommittee on Health of the Committee on Labor and Public Welfare, United States Senate, 93rd Congress on Section 3441 and Section 966. Part 3, Statement of Spencer T. King, Towson, M.D., former sales representative of Pfizer, Inc., March 8, 1974. p. 754.

[176]*Examination of the Pharmaceutical Industry 1973-74*. Statement of Spencer T. King. 1974. p. 755.

[177]*Examination of the Pharmaceutical Industry 1973-74*. Statement of Spencer T. King. 1974. p. 746.

[178]*Examination of the Pharmaceutical Industry 1973-74*. Statement of Senator Kennedy. 1974. pp. 1273-1274.

[179]*Examination of the Pharmaceutical Industry 1973-74*. Statement of Roger J. Bulger, M.D. 1974. p. 1276.

[180]Waud, Douglas R. 1992. "Pharmaceutical Promotions—A Free Lunch." *New England Journal of Medicine* 327(5):351-353.

[181]*Examination of the Pharmaceutical Industry 1973-74*. Testimony of Morton D. Bogdonoff, M.D. 1974. p. 1361.

[182]*Examination of the Pharmaceutical Industry 1973-74*. Testimony of Morton D. Bogdonoff, M.D. 1974. p. 1348.

[183]Page, Leigh. 1992. "Are Goody Grab Bag Days Over? Dermatologists Eye New Ethics." *American Medical News* (February 3):3, 30, 31.

[184]Kusserow, Richard P. 1992. *Promotion Through Payments and Gifts: Physicians' Perspectives*. Washington, D.C.: Office of the Inspector General, Department of Health and Human Services. OIE-01-90-00481.

[185]The best sources for describing the range of these gifts are the companies that give them. Industry observers have said that they carefully target particular gifts to specified physicians and monitor their effect on physician prescribing and industry sale of products. However, firms are reluctant to discuss their practices. The examples used here are thus based on interviews with physicians, the television show *Frontline*, "Prescriptions for Profit," published literature, and Senate hearings in 1974 and 1990. These examples are illustrative of the range of gifts that firms have used over a period of years. Firms vary the gifts they give, depending on marketing fashion and consumer tastes.

[186]Eli Lilly was the main supplier of stethoscopes to medical students.

[187]Stross, Jeff K. 1987. "Influential Sources and Clinical Systems." *Journal of General Internal Medicine* 2(3):155-159.

[188]These were provided by firms that sold drugs to treat arthritic patients.

[189]Upjohn Company gives out review texts.

[190]Ciba-Geigy is known for its symposia, which consist of anatomical drawings. These were provided on a periodic basis. The whole series has now been collected and sold as an atlas, and is considered the standard work in the field. Transparencies of anatomical drawings are given to faculty members for use in making presentations, upon their request.

[191]Wilkes, Michael S., and Miriam Shuchman. 1989. "Pitching Doctors." *The New York Times Sunday Magazine* (November 12):88, 91, 126, 128-129.

[192]*Examination of the Pharmaceutical Industry 1973-74.* Statement of Donald Van Roden. p. 208.

[193]One manufacturer distributed dashboard sun shields bearing the phrase "Once Daily, Feldene First," an advertisement for piroxicam. See Schiedermayer David L., and W. Paul McKinney. 1988. "The Feldene Connection: Drug Dealing in the Doctor's Parking Lot?" *The New England Journal of Medicine* 319(19):1291-1292.

[194]*Advertising, Marketing and Promotional Practices of the Pharmaceutical Industry.* 1990. Some examples provided from the testimony of John C. Nelson, M.D.

[195]Residents at the Case Western University Hospital of Cleveland were treated to a cruise on Lake Erie. In the 1974 Senate hearings, many witnesses said that firms featured steak dinners.

[196]Chren, Margaret, C. Seth Landefeld, and Thomas Murray. 1989. "Doctors, Drug Companies, and Gifts." *Journal of the American Medical Association* 262(24):3448-3451. Westwood Pharmaceutical provided a check for $156 to senior residents.

[197]Example of Dr. Mary-Margaret Chren, Assistant Professor, Department of Dermatology, Case Western Reserve University.

[198]*Advertising, Marketing and Promotional Practices of the Pharmaceutical Industry.* 1990. Testimony of Nicole Lurie, M.D.

[199]Example of Dr. Mary-Margaret Chren.

[200]Example provided by Susan Tolle, M.D., Oregon Health Services, director of the Ethics Center, University of Oregon in Portland.

[201]For example, in January 1989, Dexell, Inc., invited dermatologists to attend a dinner and meeting at the Stouffer Inn in Cleveland on "Topical Antifungals and Topical Antibiotics" and offered $100 for attendance. From a company flyer.

Other firms that have paid physicians $100 to attend a dinner at which their products are discussed include Burroughs Wellcome, Ciba-Geigy, and Dexell, Inc. *Advertising, Marketing and Promotional Practices of the Pharmaceutical Industry.* 1990. Testimony of Sidney Wolf.

[202]Huston, Phillips. 1989. "Those Promotional Dinners: Food for Thought." *Medical Marketing & Media* (October 20):78-90, at 78. (Quoting Greg Boron, vice-president, Thomas S. Boron, Inc.)

[203]Huston, Phillips. 1989. "Those Promotional Dinners." p. 90.

[204]McGregor, Maurice. 1988. "Pharmaceutical 'Generosity' and the Medical Profession." *The Annals of the Royal College of Physicians and Surgeons of Canada* 21(5):289.

Goldfinger, Stephen E. 1987. "Sounding Board: A Matter of Influence." *The New England Journal of Medicine* 316(22):1408-1409.

Wilkie, Clare E., R. W. Fakes, Thomas C. O'Dowd, Roger Whibley, Ian Lenox-Smith, and J. M. Clifford. 1986. "Doctors and the Drug Industry." *British Medical Journal* 293(6529):1170-1171.

Rochmis, P.G. 1982. "Seminars for Physicians." *Journal of the American Medical Association* 248(13):1580-1581.

In an interview with *Frontline* at the November 1988 Ciba-Geigy conference devoted to the drug Valtarin, Fred McDuffie, M.D., former director of the American Asthmatic Foundation, said that it is understood that information critical of the product will not be presented at these meetings. Elie Arlie and Joe Rosenblum. 1988. "Prescriptions for Profit." *Frontline* (March 28).

[205]Some examples drawn from *Advertising, Marketing and Promotional Practices of the Pharmaceutical Industry.* 1990. The hearings listed a number of firms that had such programs. These included Hoffman-LaRoche, Wyeth-Ayerst Labs, Burroughs-Wellcome, and Ciba-Geigy. Testimony indicated that many other companies follow the practice.

[206]AMA Council on Ethical and Judicial Affairs. 1990. *Gifts to Physicians from Industry.* (Report: G I-90). (December 4):1.

[207]*Advertising, Marketing and Promotional Practices of the Pharmaceutical Industry.* 1990. Testimony of John C. Nelson, M.D. Dr. Nelson is an obstetrician and gynecologist in private practice associated with the University of Utah College of Medicine. He was a charter member of the Medicare Prospective Payment Assessment Commission.

Dr. Nelson was concerned because the cost of the patch is more than that of traditional therapy and delivers a lower dose, supposedly to reduce side effects. But he says it may not be clinically effective because of the low dose and states that there are insufficient data to determine if it is effective.

See also Nelson, John C. 1990. "A Snorkel, a 5-iron, and a Pen." *Journal of the American Medical Association* 264(6):742.

[208]"A Candid Conversation with a Pacemaker Salesman." 1982. *Committee on Aging Information Paper* and the other two 1982 pacemaker reports.

[209]Comment 85; December 17, 1987 letter and memorandum of James B. Powell, M.D., president, Roche Biomedical Laboratories, Inc. The comment is a complaint about the practices of competitors.

[210]*William Cabot.* 1983. First Amendment to Complaint. paragraph 14, p. 2.

[211]Ford would also receive any profits resulting from the sale of equipment.

[212]*William Cabot.* 1983. First Amendment to Complaint. paragraph 14, p. 2. Complaint Paragraph 14, Exhibit A, Paragraphs 9-10, Articles of Limited Partnership, Smyrna Physical Therapy Center.

[213]The partnership agreement also helped shield the income from taxes by placing part of it in the names of their children.

[214]In 1982, the Official Code of Georgia was amended to make it illegal for physical therapists to split fees, including payment through a limited partnership arrangement. When Ford learned this, he told Cabot and his colleagues that he could no longer continue the financial arrangement. Cabot immediately ceased referring patients and encouraged other physicians in the area to do likewise; Ford's private practice dried up. The cessation of referrals after the new law prevented Ford from paying Cabot suggests that Cabot and his referring colleagues were primarily motivated by personal profit in making referrals.

[215]Comment 70; December 17, 1987 letter of Joanne B. Erde for the Florida law firm of Mershon, Sawyer, Johnson, Dunwody & Cole.

[216]Comment 70; December 17, 1987 letter of Joanne B. Erde for the Florida law firm of Mershon, Sawyer, Johnson, Dunwody & Cole. p. 3. Example B.

[217]Erde wrote that under her fourth variation, "It is unlikely that any patients other than the patients of each physician joint venturer will utilize that physician's joint venture." Since the referring physician or physician group pays only for services provided to its own physicians, and since they share profits generated from providing these services, the link between referral and profits is nearly indistinguishable from a kickback.

[218]Comment 78; December 17, 1987 letter of Robert D. Masher, Nossaman, Guther, Knox, & Eliot, Los Angeles. The comment does not indicate whether such an arrangement was put into effect or was merely proposed.

[219]See the discussion of the Furth trial in the section on kickbacks from hospitals.

[220]*Russell Furth*. Trial transcript. 1986. vol. 2, p. 201; vol. 3, pp. 3–6; vol. 4, pp. 65, 66; vol. 2, p. 48.

The tool to be utilized for invitation or continued participation on the advisory committee will be numbers of admission consistent with quality care. If admissions fall below the anticipated number, then they will be removed from the committee. Their replacement will be any other physician on staff eligible who has a justifiable high admission rate. (Twelve to fifteen) admissions per month will be considered the bench-mark number when assessing activity. Government's Exhibit No. 7. Minutes of advisory meeting. June 5, 1985.

The $1,000 payment, when prorated to 12 patients, is $83 a patient; when prorated to 15 patients, it is $66 a patient.

[221]*Russell Furth*. Trial transcript. vol. 4, pp. 103–104.

Furth: ... I'm helping Murphy and Goodie with their rent, not their full rent, but part of it, and, ah, I didn't compensate Goodie last month, because she kind of died.

McShane: You mean admissions were down.

Furth: Well, they were last month. (laughing)

...

Furth: [S]he asked me if she could be on the advisory committee.

McShane: Oh, I see.

Furth: And I said there's a problem. Said I am (inaudible) and the physicians over at the clinic know that you are getting compensation for rent.

McShane: Oh, okay.

Furth: None of the other doctors over there are.

McShane: I see.

Furth: So if I put—if you're on the committee, you're getting more than everybody else is.

McShane: Sure.

Furth: For the same—

McShane: The same activity.

Furth: Yeah.

Chapter 4

[1]Comment 129; December 17, 1987 letter of Jim Codo, a medical laboratory salesperson.

[2]Pauly, Mark V. 1979. "The Ethics and Economics of Kickbacks and Fee Splitting." *The Bell Journal of Economics and Management Science* 10(1):344-352.

Pauly also suggests that in the face of bans on fee splitting and kickbacks, physicians may use other forms of vertical integration (multispecialty group practices) or ownership of specialty facilities to achieve similar results. p. 349.

[3]The kickback needs to be equal to or greater than the rewards from the general practitioner providing the medical care. A similar rationale is used to justify referral fees among lawyers.

[4]However, there are indirect incentives to make referrals. Tort law requires physicians to refer to specialists when that is the standard practice. Failure to do so can result in malpractice liability.

[5]At one time, Metric Medical Laboratories imposed such requirements on physician limited partners. The partnership agreement included the following clause: "[I]n addition to death, retirement or withdrawal from active practice, utilization of another laboratory other than Metric Medical Laboratories, or establishment or expansion of in-house laboratories can be considered as ground for immediate return of investment capital, at the market price at the time." See *In the Matter of Daniel A. Abessinio, D.O.* Administrative Complaint filed before the Department of Licensing and Regulation of the Board of Osteopathic Medi-

cine and Surgery on September 4, 1986. Since then, Metric Medical Laboratories has bought out its physician owners.

[6]Information drawn from the February 11, 1987, and November 11, 1988, prospectuses for the PCS Limited Partnership.

[7]The first 140 partnerships were sold for $9,500. The remainder are planned to be sold for $11,000.

[8]Some of these factors were mentioned as evidence that this kind of venture would not be considered a kickback under the Medicare fraud and abuse statute in an opinion letter filed with the SEC by the lawyer representing PCS. December 30, 1986, letter from Lynn Shapiro Snyder of the law firm Epstein, Becker, Brosody & Green, P.C., to Mr. James L. Flore, president, PCS. The letter was filed as an appendix with the firm's SEC Registration Statement.

[9]The financial forecast included in the February 11, 1987, prospectus assumes that the partners will be 90% of the customers for the forecasted period (December 31, 1988, through December 31, 1992). (Appendix D, "Forecasted Financial Statements," p. 9.) However, the forecast in the November 11, 1988, prospectus assumed that 75% of the business would come from limited partners. (Appendix D "Forecasted Financial Statements," p. 18.) The first forecast also assumes that these physicians will use the labs for 85% of their tests. The second forecast says only that physicians will use the lab for the majority of their tests.

Although PCS sold shares to the general public, the general partners reserved the right to reject any subscriber even if he or she met all the qualifications (November 11, 1988, *Prospectus*, p. 68). This allowed PCS to control the ratio of physicians and other providers to non-referring investors.

[10]The November 11, 1988, prospectus assumes that partnerships will be sold to 504 physicians or providers (10 units per month over a period of 50 months; see p. D.14). Of the first 147 units sold, 50 were sold to one hospital. It is unclear how many of the remaining units were sold to physicians.

Legislation restricting physician self-referral to clinical laboratories for Medicare patients forced PCS to restructure. In September 1991, the limited partners unanimously agreed to sell their ownership interest to the general partner who in turned sold this interest to Manor Health Care, Inc., a firm with extensive holdings in nursing homes. The company is now owed 51% by Manor Care, Inc., 49% by James Flore, the president. The expectation is that Manor Care nursing homes will provide an important source of referrals. Telephone interview with James Flore, December 8, 1992.

[11]Morreim, E. Haavi. 1989. "Conflicts of Interest: Profits and Problems in Physician Referrals." *Journal of the American Medical Association* 262(3):390-394.

Morreim, E. Haavi. 1990. "Physician Investment and Self-referral: Philosophical Analysis of a Contentious Debate." *Journal of Medicine and Philosophy* 15(4):425-448.

[12]It is true that most physician owners invest relatively moderate sums, usually about $10,000. But they still can lose these funds, and presumably they invested them to earn money.

[13]Mitchell, Jean M., and Elton Scott. 1992. "New Evidence on the Prevalence and Scope of Physician Joint Ventures." *Journal of the American Medical Association* 268(1):80-84.

[14]See Abood, Richard R. 1989. "Physician Dispensing: Issues of Law, Legislation and Social Policy." *American Journal of Law and Medicine* 14(4):307-352. Abood notes that pharmacists can serve as a check on physicians and ensure that they have not made errors.

[15]For a review of the pros and cons of physician dispensing discussed in relation to the physician's role as a patient advocate, see Relman, Arnold. 1987. "Doctors and the Dispensing of Drugs." *The New England Journal of Medicine* 317(5):311-312.

[16]*Dispensing of Drugs*: Hearings before the Subcommittee on Health and the Environment of the Committee on Energy and Commerce, House of Representatives, 100th Congress, 1st Session, on H.R. 2093. See the testimony of Daniel Oliver and Jeffrey Zuckerman, FTC. April 22, 1987. (Serial No. 100-36.) pp. 8-11. This reflects the position of Reagan appointees, who developed a new and radical view of market competition. In 1970, Casper Weinberger, as head of the FTC, supported legislation to restrict physician dispensing on the grounds that it was unfair competition and might allow monopoly pricing or overprescribing.

See *Regulation of Trade in Drugs*: Hearings before the Consumer Subcommittee of the Committee on Commerce, U.S. Senate, 91st Congress, 2nd session. June 1970, p. 13.   Brownman, Stephens, and Bangert. *Physician Merchandising* (April 23, 1979). FTC Memorandum No. CH80007.

[17]*Dispensing of Drugs*. 1987. See, the statements of Charles M. West, executive vice-president, National Association of Retail Druggists. pp. 53-83.

See the Report of the Pennsylvania Department of Aging on the Costs of Its Pharmaceutical Assistance Contract for the Elderly. Quoted in "Drug Repackagers on the Make." 1987. *National Association of Retail Druggists Journal* 109:20, note 7.

Andritz, Mary H., and Matthew P. Rogan. 1988. "Drug Dispensing by Physicians: Promoter's Claims Examined." *Pediatrics* 82(3):504-509.

The Virginia Pharmaceutical Association performed a study that revealed that the price physicians paid for drugs was nearly always higher than the average wholesale price of the drugs and often higher than the retail price paid by patients. See "Statement to the Virginia Board of Medicine from the Pharmacists of Virginia Concerning the Dispensing of Medications by Physicians," in *Physician Dispensing for Profit*. Alexandria: National Association of Retail Druggists. 1987.

[18]Hoffer, George E. 1975. "Physician-Ownership in Pharmacies and Drug Repackagers." *Inquiry* 12(March):26-36.

Similar results were found for physician owners of pharmaceutical companies. Myers, Maven John. 1966. *Prescribing Habits of Physicians Who Own Pharmaceutical Companies*. Doctoral dissertation, University of Wisconsin. Meyers also found evidence that physicians who owned pharmacies misprescribed drugs.

[19]The Consumer Federation of America supported the bill introduced by Representative Wyden, which would have restricted physician dispensing of drugs.

[20]Glassman-Oliver consulting report on dispensing quoted in remarks of Thomas E. Menighan, American Pharmaceutical Association, at the AMA Annual State Legislation Meeting, Palm Springs, California, January 8, 1988.

[21]While scheduling may seem to be a minor concern, that depends on the perspective. There are cases when physicians have scheduled CAT and MRI scans at 2:00 a.m. at facilities in which they invest, while other independent facilities charged less and were available during the day. Most patients' interests are not served by such scheduling. The situation would be different if the patient faced a choice and was compensated for making the inconvenient choice.

[22]Titmuss, Richard Morris. 1971. *The Gift Relationship: From Human Blood to Social Policy.* New York: Vintage Books.

[23]Hughes, Evert. 1983. "Good Men, Dirty Work," in *The Gift*, Lewis Hyde, ed. New York: Random House.

Turner, Jonathan. 1982. *The Structure of Sociological Theory.* Homewood, Ill.: The Dorsey Press.

Ekeh, Peter. 1974. *Social Exchange Theory: The Two Traditions.* Cambridge: Harvard University Press.

Mauss, Marcell. 1967. *The Gift: Forms and Functions of Exchange in Archaic Societies.* (Ian Cunnison, trans.) New York: Norton.

Simmel, Georg. 1964. "Faithfulness and Gratitude," in *The Sociology of Georg Simmel.* (Kurt Wolff, trans.) Glencoe, Ill.: Free Press.

Blau, Peter M. 1964. "Social Exchange," in *Exchange and Power in Social Life.* New York: Wiley.

Homans, George. 1958. "Social Behavior as Exchange." *American Journal of Sociology* 63(6):597-606.

Many languages use the same word for bribe and gift. In many Asian countries *baksheesh* means gift, bribe, alms, and tip. In French *pot de vin* means tip and bribe.

[24]Chren, Margaret, C. Seth Landefeld, and Thomas Murray. 1989. "Doctors, Drug Companies, and Gifts." *Journal of the American Medical Association* 262(24):3448-3451.

Goldfinger, Stephen E. 1987. "A Matter of Influence." *The New England Journal of Medicine* 316(22):1408-1409.

[25]"What we usually call gratitude ... goes much beyond the ordinary form of thanks for gifts.... [G]ratitude actually consists, not in the return of a gift but in the consciousness that it cannot be returned, that there is something which places the receiver into a certain permanent position with respect to the give ..." Simmel, Georg. 1950. "Faithfulness and Gratitude." p. 392.

[26]Miller, Kenneth, William A. Gouveia, Michael Barza, et al. 1985. "Undesirable Marketing Practice in the Pharmaceutical Industry." *The New England Journal of Medicine* 313(1):54.

[27]42 U.S.C. Secs 1320a-7b.

[28]Fisher, Susan Heilbronner. 1991. "The Economic Wisdom of Regulating Pharmaceutical 'Freebies.'" *Duke Law Journal* 1991(1):206-239.

[29]Wilkes, Michael S., Bruce H. Doblin, and Martin Shapiro. 1992. "Pharmaceutical Advertisements in Leading Medical Journals: Experts' Assessments." *Annals of Internal Medicine* 116(11):912-919.

[30]Personal communication with Dr. Michael S. Wilkes, October 21, 1992.

[31]*Advertising, Marketing and Promotional Practices of the Pharmaceutical Industry*: Hearings before the Committee on Labor and Human Resources, U.S. Senate, 101st Congress, 2nd Session, Testimony of Frederick Fenster, M.D. December 11 and 12, 1990.

[32]Avorn, Jerry, Milton Chen, and Robert Hartley. 1982. "Scientific versus Commercial Sources of Influence on the Prescribing Behavior of Physicians." *The American Journal of Medicine* 73(1):4-8.

[33]*Advertising, Marketing and Promotional Practices in the Pharmaceutical Industry*. Testimony of Frederick Fenster. 1990.

[34]Bowman, Marjorie A. 1986. "The Impact of Drug Company Funding on the Content of Continuing Medical Education." *Mobius* 6(1):66-69.

[35]The author notes that the sponsors had a role in choosing the instructor and suggests that they were apt to choose physicians who were favorably disposed to their product. But the issue of choice is not so simple. By sponsoring physicians to make presentations, pharmaceutical companies can help influence their judgment—if not in a specific case, perhaps over time.

[36]The author used a form of content analysis, and reviewers made assessments of the frequency of the language used and the characterization of the drugs. Initially, two reviewers assessed the content of transcribed tapes independently. The materials were reviewed again by three pairs of students who were unfamiliar with the purpose of the project or the sponsor of the course.

[37]Bowman, Marjorie A., and David L. Pearle. 1988. "Changes in Drug Prescribing Patterns Related to Commercial Company Funding of Continuing Medical Education." *Journal of Continuing Education in the Health Professions* 8(1):13-20.

[38]*Advertising, Marketing and Promotional Practices of the Pharmaceutical Industry*. Testimony of Nicole Lurie. 1990.

Lurie, Nicole, Eugene C. Rich, Deborah E. Simpson, Jeff Meyer, David L. Schiedermayer, Jesse L. Goodman, and W. Paul McKinney. 1990. "Pharmaceutical Representatives in Academic Medical Centers: Interactions with Faculty and House Staff." *Journal of General Internal Medicine* 5(3):240-243.

[39]Shama, Avraham, and Jack K. Thompson. 1989. "Gifts Build Goodwill and Market Share." *Journal of Retail Banking* 11(2):55-59.

[40]Hite, Robert E., and Joseph A. Bellizzi. 1987. "Salespeople's Use of Entertainment and Gifts." *Industrial Marketing Management* 16(3):179-285.

[41]For an analysis of efforts to hold physicians and other providers accountable through such programs as well as other means, see Gray, Bradford. 1991. *The Profit Motive and Patient Care: The Changing Accountability of Doctors and Hospitals.* Cambridge: Harvard University Press.

For a history and description of utilization review programs, see Gray, Bradford H., and Marilyn J. Fields, eds. 1989. *Controlling Costs and Changing Patient Care: The Role of Utilization Management.* Washington, D.C.: National Academy Press.

[42]The idea of utilization review was first discussed in print in 1954. See Carter, Fred. 1954. "The Utilization Committee." *The Modern Hospital* 83(3):64.

[43]PSRO Law enacted in 1972 as P.L. 92-603.

[44]Congressional Budget Office. 1979. *The Effects of PSROs on Health Care Costs: Current Findings and Future Evaluations.* Washington, D.C.: Congressional Budget Office.

Professional Standards Review Organization 1979 Program Evaluation. 1979. Washington, D.C.: U.S. Department of Health and Human Services, Health Care Financing Administration.

Dobson, Allen, Joanne G. Greer, Ronald A. Carlson, et al. 1978. "PSROs: Their Current Status and Their Impact to Date." *Inquiry* 15(2):113-128.

[45]Marmor, Theodore R., and James A. Morone. 1980. "Representing Consumers' Interests: Imbalanced Markets, Health Planning and HSAs." *Milbank Memorial Fund Quarterly* 58(1):125-165.

[46]Physicians' conflicts of interest are now being built into the evaluation of PROs. To review the performance of PROs, the federal government established a Super-PRO that sampled and reassessed cases reviewed by PROs. There was disagreement in about 10% of the cases. These reviews were to serve an educational function. They did not affect the initial PRO decisions. But efforts are now underway to use the Super-PRO to assess PROs formally and determine whether their contract will be renewed. Disagreements between the PRO and Super-PRO concerning the quality of care, the appropriateness of the level of medical care provided, and local medical practice can be appealed. The Health Care Financing Administration has contracted with the AMA to conduct the final reviews that resolve disputes between the PRO and Super-PRO. McIllrath, Sharon. 1990. "AMA Takes on Role as Mediator Between PROs, SuperPRO." *American Medical News* (November 23/30):1, 33.

Under the plan, the AMA would recruit local physicians to conduct the reviews on a volunteer basis. It would allow PRO reviewers to be these reviewers, so long as they had not earned more than 15% of their income from the PRO they were reviewing. In addition, no physician would be a consultant if he or she had a conflict of interest stemming from having a relationship with the patient or physician whose case is reviewed, or if the physicians had been involved in reviewing the case previously.

This appeal process reintroduces the physicians' conflicts of interest into patient care determinations. Reviewers are physicians in practice who act as consultant reviewers on the side, not as a full-time occupation. These physicians often will have colleagues in the organizations they review with whom they will have to deal after their PRO work. Some will be reviewing their own hospital and PRO. It can be expected that physicians' main loyalty will lie with their main colleagues, hospitals, and PROs for whom they work more frequently rather than with the appeal board.

The conflict-of-interest provisions established to counter this bias are ineffective. First, it is up to the physician consultants themselves to decide whether or not they have a conflict of interest. There is no mechanism to supervise them. Like other AMA voluntary policies on conflicts of interest, these are unenforceable, and physicians are no more likely to comply with them than with other voluntary policies, especially because they will be the judges of last resort, from whom there is no appeal. Second, the guidelines are weak, so that even if physicians comply with them, reviewers will have significant conflicts of interest. The rule against PRO reviewers not being allowed to review any PRO from which they derive more than 15% of their income is weak. Physicians who work for a PRO have a financial and organizational commitment to that organization, which compromises their judgment and loyalty as reviewers, even if they earn less than 15% of their income from the PRO. Furthermore, since most reviewers for PROs work only part-time, it is unlikely that this rule will bar many physicians.

[47]Feldstein, Paul J., Thomas M. Wickizer, and John R.C. Wheeler. 1988. "Private Cost Containment: The Effects of Utilization Review Programs on Health Care Use and Expenditure." *The New England Journal of Medicine* 318(20):1310-1314.

[48]However, certain PROs also review quality of care in HMOs. In addition, the Health Care Financing Administration is now conducting two experiments to evaluate the use of review in outpatient care in physicians' private offices. Medicare may well extend such review programs to outpatient care in the future.

[49]Vibbert, Spenser. 1989. "Is Utilization Review Paying Off?" *Business & Health* 7(2):20-26, at 24.

[50]Kusserow, Richard P. 1990. *Ensuring Appropriate Use of Laboratory Services: A Monograph*. Washington, D.C.: Office of the Inspector General. Department of Health and Human Services. OEI-05-89-89150.

[51]This trend may be particularly pronounced for clinical or diagnostic tests because utilization review programs rarely review outpatient care. Furthermore, physicians often perceive that ordering diagnostic tests will protect them in the event that they are sued for malpractice.

[52]The exception may be in insurance programs that offer a closed panel of physicians and providers. Here the patient explicitly trades free choice when purchasing the insurance in return for other benefits such as lower copayments, more comprehensive coverage, or convenience. But even within closed panel programs, primary care physicians have a choice of specialists and providers to whom they may refer patients. Within this context, patients have a right to expect that physicians will use the patients' interest as the basis for choosing the specialist or provider.

[53]*Sarchett v. Blue Shield of California*, 43 Cal. 3d 1, 233 Cal. Rptr. 76, 729 P. 2d 267 (1987).

Wickline v. California 192 Cal. App. 3d 1630, 239 Cal. Rptr. 810 (1986).

[54]*Schware v. Board of Bar Examiners*, 353 U.S. 232. (1957).

The specific powers of licensing boards varies, depending on state statutes.

[55]*Schware v. Board of Bar Examiners*.

[56]See Reaves, Randolph P. 1984. *The Law of Professional Licensing and Certification*. Charlotte, N.C.: Publications for Professionals.

Morris, William Otis. 1984. *Revocation of Professional Licenses by Governmental Agencies*. Charlottesville, Va.: The Michie Company.

[57]The paucity of concern for physicians' conflicts of interests by state licensing boards can be gauged by examining the cases and issues discussed in two leading books on professional licensing:

Morris, William Otis. 1984. *Revocation of Professional Licenses by Governmental Agencies*.

Reaves, Randolph P. 1984. *The Law of Professional Licensing and Certification*.

[58]Telephone interview with Mr. Dale Breaden, associate executive vice-president, Federation of State Medical Licensing Boards.

[59]Kusserow, Richard, P. August 1990. *State Medical Boards and Medical Discipline*. Washington, D.C.: Office of the Inspector General. Department of Health and Human Services. OEI-01-89-00560.

[60]Ortega, Bob. 1992. "Gypsy Medicine: State Medical Boards let Doctors Who Move Escape Any Discipline." *Wall Street Journal* (November 11):1, A5.

Physician Discipline: Can State Boards Protect the Public?: Hearing before the Subcommittee on Regulation, Business Opportunities and Energy, of the Committee on Small Business, House of Representatives, 101st Congress, 2nd Session. June 8, 1990. (Serial No. 101-65.)

Kusserow, Richard P. 1990. *State Medical Boards*.

Gianelli, Diane M. 1990. "IG Report Suggests Medical Boards Don't Discipline Enough Doctors." *American Medical News* (June 15):1, 29.

"State Medical Board Doctor Disciplinary Actions: 1987." 1989. *The Public Citizen Health Research Group* 5(11):1-4.

Kusserow, Richard P., Elisabeth A. Handley, and Mark R. Yessian. 1987. "An Overview of State Medical Discipline." *Journal of the American Medical Association* 257(6):820-824.

Brinkley, Joel. 1986. "State Medical Boards Discipline Record Number of Doctors in 1985." *The New York Times* (November 9):1, 26.

Relman, Arnold S. 1985. "Professional Regulation and the State Medical Boards." *The New England Journal of Medicine* 312(12):784-785.

Feinstein, Richard J. 1985. "The Ethics of Professional Regulation." *The New England Journal of Medicine* 312(12):801-804.

[61]Kusserow, Richard P. 1990. *State Medical Boards*.

[62]Kusserow, Richard P. 1990. *State Medical Boards*. p. 9.

[63]P.L. 101-58, 1990.

[64]Delmar, Diana. 1990. "State Boards Laud Federal Bill to Aid Doctor Disciplining." *Physicians' Financial News* (September 30):1, 16.

[65]Office of the Inspector General. 1989. *Financial Arrangements Between Physicians and Health Care Business: State Laws and Regulations: A Management Advisory Report*. Washington, D.C.: Department of Health and Human Services. OAI-12-88-01412. Since the report, Texas has enacted legislation prohibiting fee-splitting.

[66]Arizona Revised Statutes Annotated, Sec. 13-3713.

California Business & Professional Code.

[67]Virginia Code, Sec. 54-278.

[68]Alabama Code, Sec. 22-1-11.

[69]New York General Law, Sec. 801.

[70]Office of the Inspector General. 1989. *Management Advisory Report*. p. 6.

[71]My analysis is based on recent legislation and two reports.

McDermott, Will, and Emery. Survey of Physician Self-Referral/Physician Ownership Statutes and Regulations. August 20, 1991.

Office of the Inspector General. 1989. *Financial Arrangements Between Physicians and Health Care Business: State Laws and Regulations: A Management Advisory Report*. Washington, D.C.: Department of Health and Human Services. OAI-12-88-01412.

[72]Florida (with certain exceptions) prohibits self-referral to clinical laboratories, physical therapy, radiation therapy, diagnostic imaging, and comprehensive rehabilitative services. Self-referral is permitted for other ser-vices so long as ownership is disclosed. (Patient Self-Referral Act of 1992; Florida 1992 Regular Session, Chapter 92-178.) However, there are exceptions for demonstrated need in communities, and for self-referral to publicly traded companies. Illinois prohibits health care workers from referring patients for medical services to entities outside of offices or group practices (Health Care Workers Self-Referral Act 1992, H.B. 4163). Michigan law prohibits physicians from directing or requiring an individual to purchase services from any facility in which the physician has a financial interest (Michigan Statutes Annotated Section 14.5). Minnesota law directs the Commissioner of Health to adopt rules that restrict financial or payment relations that involve self-referral and requires the state to follow federal Medicare guidelines until state regulations are promulgated (H.F.

2800, April 1992). Missouri law prohibits physicians from referring patients to medical facilities or suppliers in which they invest (Mo. Rev. Stat. Section 334.100.[2], [19], [21]). Montana law prohibits physicians from owning an interest in pharmaceutical firms except for shares of publicly traded stock (Montana Code Section 37-2-102). Nevada prohibits physicians from referring patients to laboratories in which they invest unless the lab operates solely to provide services to the physician's own patients (Nevada Revenue Statute Section 630.305.7). Nevada law also precludes physicians from owning more than 10% of the stock of any pharmacy (Nev. Rev. Stat. 630.305.3). New Jersey, with numerous exceptions, prohibits physicians from referring to facil-ities in which they own a financial interest except in publicly traded companies (N.J. Rev. Stat. Section 45:9-22.5). Exceptions include self-referral to bioanalytic laboratories, pharmacies, home health care agencies, nursing homes, radiology, and physical therapy. New York prohibits self-referral in clinical laboratory services, x-rays, or imaging services (S.9028, July 1992, Amending Article 2 of the Public Health Law 2-D.)

[73]Illinois Health Care Workers Self-Referral Act 1992, H.B. 4163 (becomes effective January, 1993). New Jersey Statutes Annotated Section 45:9-22.5. Michigan Statutes Annotated, Section 14.15 (1101) (Callahan 1985).

[74]California Business and Professional Code, Section 4080.5(a) (West Supp. 1989).

Pennsylvania Statutes Annotated, Title 63, Section 390-5(a)(9) (Purdon 1961).

[75]Colorado Administrative Code, Section 1.00.15 (1985).

[76]*Inland Empire Optical, Inc.*, 76 Wash. 2d. 407 (1969).

[77]See Burns, L., and D. Mancino, eds. 1987. *Joint Ventures Between Hospitals and Physicians: A Competitive Strategy for the Health Care Marketplace.* Homewood, Ill.: Dow Jones-Irwin. p. 101, note 102.

[78]Arizona Medical Practice Act. Arizona Revised Statutes Annotated, Section 32-1401 (12) (u) (ff).

California Business and Professional Code, Section 654 (1)-(2).

Connecticut General Statute Section 20-7 a(b).

Delaware Board of Medical Practices (Rules and Regulations) Section 15 (24 Delaware C. Section 1173 (b) (3)) and Sec. 15 (k).

Florida Statutes, Section 458.327 (c); 458.331; 455.25.

Illinois Health Care Workers Self-Referral Act 1992, H.B. 4163.

Maryland Code Annotated, Health Occ., Sec 1-206.

Massachusetts General Laws Annotated, Chapter 112, Section 1, Section 12AA; Chapter 440, Section 21, Section 23P 1/2.

Minnesota Statutes Annotated, Section 147.091, Subsection 1, (P).

New York July 1992; S. 9028 Amending Article 2 of the Public Health Law 2-D.

Nevada Revised Statutes, Section 630.305 (6).

New Jersey Statutes Annotated Section 45:9-22.5.

35 Pennsylvania Consolidated Statutes, Section 449.22 (1988-66 P.L. 403, Section 2).

Rhode Island General Laws, Section 5-37-22.

Tennessee Physicians Conflict of Interest Disclosure Act of 1991, effective January 1, 1992.

Virginia Code, Section 54-278.3

Washington Revised Code, Section 19.68.010.

West Virginia Medical Practices Act, West Virginia Code, Section 30-3-14 (c)(7).

[79] Arizona, California, Maryland, Missouri, Minnesota, Nevada, New Jersey, Rhode Island, Washington, Virginia, and West Virginia.

[80] Until 1992, Florida required disclosure only when the physician owned more than 10% of the facility, while Virginia requires disclosure of "any financial interest." Massachusetts only requires disclosure to patients for physical therapy. California physicians must disclose their ownership to referred patients if they hold over a 5% interest. California Business and Professional Code, Section 654.2 (West Supp. 1986).

[81] Office of the Inspector General. 1989. *Management Advisory Report*.

[82] Michigan Statutes Annotated, Section 14.15 (1101) (Callahan 1985).

[83] *Lester v. Kelley*, Case no. 79-189821-CZ; State of Michigan Circuit Court, County of Oakland, October 6, 1982.

[84] Opinion of the Michigan Attorney General 5498 (1979).

[85] *Samuel Indenbaum, M.D., and Felix J. Liddell, M.D. v. Michigan Board of Medicine and Michigan Department of Licensing and Regulation*. Case No. 89-376715-AA, Circuit Court for the County of Oakland. May 7, 1990.

[86] *Indenbaum v. Michigan Board of Medicine*, No. 129223 August 6, 1992, (Unpublished Opinion).

[87] Michigan Office of the Attorney General. Personal communication.

[88] Kusserow, Richard P. 1989. *Report to Congress*.

[89] Massachusetts, Montana, Texas, and Utah disallow physician dispensing except in emergencies, when pharmacy services are unavailable, or when the physician is providing for the patient's immediate needs. Arizona either disallows physician dispensing altogether or allows it only in emergencies. Office of the Inspector General. 1989. *Physician Drug Dispensing: An Overview of State Regulations*. Washington, D.C.: Department of Health and Human Services.

[90] See *Dispensing Drugs*, testimony of Daniel Oliver and Jeffrey Zuckerman. 1987 hearings.

[91] *Physician Drug Dispensing*. 1989.

[92] Office of the Inspector General. June 1986. *Medical Licensure and Discipline: An Overview*. Washington, D.C.: Department of Health and Human Services.

[93] *Physicians' Ownership in Pharmacies and Drug Companies*: Hearings before the Subcommittee on Antitrust and Monopoly of the Committee on the Judi-

ciary, U.S. Senate, 88th Congress, 2nd Session on S. 262. August 4, 5, 6, 11, 12, and 14, 1964. Washington, D.C.: U.S. Government Printing Office.

The Medical Restraint of Trade Act: Hearings before the Subcommittee on Antitrust and Monopoly of the Committee on the Judiciary, U.S. Senate, 90th Congress, 1st Session on S. 260. Parts 1 and 2. January 24, 25, 26, 30, 31; February 1, 6, 7, 9, 23, February 24; March 1 and 3, 1967.

Senator Phil Hart introduced legislation and conducted hearings in 1970 (S.1575). *Regulation of Trade in Drugs.* 1970.

Rep. Ron Wyden (D.-Oregon) introduced H.R. 2093 on April 9, 1987 and held hearings. *Dispensing of Drugs.* 1987, pp. 13-36. Rep. Ron Wyden introduced a similar bill (H.R. 2168) in 1988.

The bills introduced by Representative Wyden in 1987 and 1988 would have amended the Federal Food, Drug and Cosmetic Act to prohibit practitioners from dispensing certain drugs. The bill made exceptions for dispensing in emergencies, when there was no pharmacy within 15 miles of the physician's office, and in certain rural areas and Indian health clinics.

[94]*Dispensing of Drugs.* 1987. See testimony of Nancy W. Dicey. pp. 13-36.

[95]Report of the Council on Ethical and Judicial Affairs. *Conflict of Interest.* Report A (I-86). Chicago: AMA, p. 5.

AMA. 1992. *Current Opinions of the Council on Ethical and Judicial Affairs.* "Opinion 8.06." Chicago: AMA.

[96]Title 20 (Social Service Block Grants) and Title 5 (Maternal and Child Health Block Grants) of the Social Security Act.

[97]Another avenue of federal regulation is through health care provided by the Department of Defense under the Civilian Health and Medical Program of the Uniformed Services (CHAMPUS). The Department of Defense Appropriates Act, 1991, P.L. 101-511 Section 8044, limits payments to doctors for inpatient mental health when the doctor refers patients to facilities in which they had a financial interest. Proposed regulations would amend 32 CFR 199(g)(73).

[98]House of Representatives Report No. 393, 95th Congress, 1st Session, reprinted in 1977 *U.S. Code Congressional & Administrative News.* p. 3039.

[99]Violation of the statute constitutes a felony, with punishment including up to $25,000 in fines and a prison term of up to ten years.

[100]*United States v. Zacher,* 586 F.2d 912 (2nd Cir. 1978); *United States v. Porter,* 591 F.2d 1048 (5th Cir. 1979).

[101]*United States v. Hancock,* 604 F. 2d 999 (7th Cir. 1979); *United States v. Weingarden,* 468 F. Supp. 410 (E.D. Mich. 1979); *United States v. Tapert,* 625 F.2d 111 (6th Cir. 1980); *United States v. Ruttenberg,* 625 F.2d 173 (7th Cir. 1980); *United States v. Greber,* 760 F.2d 68 (3rd Cir. 1985); *United States v. Kats,* 871 F.2d 105 (6th Cir. 1989); *United States v. Bay State Ambulance and Hospital Rental Services, Inc.,* 874 F.2d 20 (1st Cir. 1989). Final Decision on Review of Administrative Law Judge Decision. *The Inspector General v. the Hanlester Network et al.* Department of

Health and Human Services; Departmental Appeals Board; Appellate Division; Doc. Nos. C-186 through C-192, C-208, C-213. Doc. No. 1275. Reported in Commerce Clearing House Medicare and Medicaid Guide. Par. 39,566. Decision on Remand of the Administrative Law Judge. *The Inspector General v. The Hanlester Network et al.* Department of Health and Human Services; Departmental Appeals Board; Civil Remedies Division; Doc. No. C-448. Doc. No. CR 181. Reported in Commerce Clearing House Medicare and Medicaid Guide, par. 40,064.

The current statutory language is quite broad and prohibits soliciting, offering, receiving, or paying, directly or indirectly, any remuneration in return for making a referral or ordering any service or item. It excludes only price discounts that are disclosed and reflected in charges made by providers and payments by employers to employees for provision of covered services.

[102]Very few kickback cases were prosecuted prior to the 1977 amendments. When asked why, U.S. Attorneys and State Attorneys have reported that "kickbacks [cases] were among the most complicated and difficult to prove." It is even harder to prove that physicians provided unnecessary services in return for payment, unless the overutilization is "grossly unreasonable." *Fraud and Abuse in the Medicare and Medicaid Programs.* Subcommittee on Health, Committee on Ways and Means, and Subcommittee on Health and the Environment, Committee on Interstate and Foreign Commerce, U.S. House of Representatives, 95th Congress, 1st Session, Joint Committee Print. March 3, 1977. (WMCP:95-6.) pp. 14, 402.

Although the fraud and abuse statute was amended to prohibit still other questionable additional conduct and facilitate prosecution, these same difficulties in prosecution persist. Richard Kusserow, the Health and Human Services Inspector General, reiterated recently that the kickback law is inadequate "to prevent outright kickbacks and bribes which are offered or paid to induce the referral of Medicare business." October 31, 1989 letter of Richard Kusserow to Rep. Pete Stark.

The Justice Department and the Department of Health and Human Services do not keep statistics on indictments and prosecutions for particular offenses.

[103]Relman, Arnold S. 1980. "The New Medical-Industrial Complex." *The New England Journal of Medicine* 303(17):963-970.

[104]Ruffenach, Glenn. 1992. "Medical Firms' Stocks Plunge on Probe News." *Wall Street Journal* (June 26):B4.

[105]"FBI Increasing Health Fraud Criminal Investigations Capability Over 30% with the reassignment of 50 counter intelligence agents to specialized health care investigative units." Werble, Cole and David Blue, eds. 1992. *F-D-C Reports Health News Daily* 4(23)(February 4).

[106]1992 West Law 253545 (E.D.Texas).

[107]Sternberg, Steve. 1992. "Doctor's Hospital Pact Sparks Federal Inquiry." *Atlanta Constitution* (November 19):1, A17.

Recruitment Agreement Between Cobb County Kennestone Hospital Authority and George J. Kanes, M.D., May 15, 1992.

[108]Final Decision on Review of Administrative Law Judge Decision. *The Hanlester Network et al.* Doc. Nos. C-186 through C-192, C-208, C-213. Doc. No. 1275.

Decision on Remand of the Administrative Law Judge. *The Hanlester Network et al.* Doc. No. C-448. Dec. No. CR 181.

See also Crane, Thomas S. 1992. "The Problem of Physician Self-Referral Under the Medicare and Medicaid AntiKickback Statute: The Hanlester Network Case and the Safe Harbor Regulation." *Journal of the American Medical Association* 268(1):85-91.

[109]Final Decision on Review of Administrative Law Judge Decision. *The Hanlester Network et al.*, p. 36, note 22.

[110]No prosecutorial action was brought against physician investors who received the payments in the *Hanlester* case even though the statute forbids both paying and receiving. This may be due to the lack of resources for prosecution. It may be more time-consuming and costly to investigate and prosecute many individuals who receive kickbacks than a single or small group of payers. It is also possible that prosecutors believe that judges and juries would be more sympathetic to physicians than to managers, businesspeople, or firms.

[111]Medicare and State Health Care Programs Fraud and Abuse; OIG AntiKickback Regulations. 56 *Federal Register* 35952.01, July 29, 1991. These rules amend 42 Code of Federal Regulations part 1001 by adding a new subpart E, "Permissive Exclusions." Sections 1001.951-1001.953.

The process was started by a notice of proposed rule making regarding "payment practices which, although potentially capable of inducing referrals of business covered by the Medicare program, are not to be considered kickbacks." 52 *Federal Register* 38794 (October 19, 1987). Comments were solicited. The Department of Health and Human Services published a proposed rule in 53 *Federal Register* 51856 on December 23, 1988. It withdrew the proposed rule in 53 *Federal Register* 52448 on December 28, 1988, in order to allow the Office of Management and Budget to review it. A final proposed rule was issued on January 23, 1989. 54 *Federal Registrar* 3088-3095 (January 23, 1989).

[112]Perry, Linda. 1989. "'Safe Harbor' Rules Harsher Than Expected." *Modern Healthcare* 19(49):40.

In reporting on the draft rules, the journal noted that resource constraints will stop the government from challenging joint ventures unless they are clearly illegal and added: "As a result, a joint venture probably won't be challenged if it meets all of the criteria outlined in the safe-harbor regulations except the 50% rule." (The draft final rule set the upper limit for investors at 50%, but the final rule changed this to 40%.)

[113]My summary combined some of the rules. The regulations and explanation total 35 pages of small print. My summary outlines the main features but necessarily simplifies.

[114]These include provisions barring businesses from giving investors who can refer patients different investment terms from other investors; giving physicians better terms based on a record of making a large number of referrals in the past or being likely to make a large number of referrals in the future; and provisions preventing businesses from loaning funds to referring investors in order to make the investment.

[115]The office announced it would propose safe harbors for investments in rural areas, investments in ambulatory surgery centers, investment in group practices composed exclusively of active investors, practitioner recruitment, subsidies for obstetrical malpractice insurance, referral deals for subspecialty service, cooperative hospital service organizations, purchase of group practices by hospitals, rural hospital purchase of physician practices as part of recruitment programs, and transactions between subsidiaries of the same firm. Yongstrom, Nina. 1992. *Health Care Financial Relationships* 1(7):2.

[116]The discussion is based on the draft safe harbors dated October 1, 1989

[117]However, the agreement cannot condition the recruitment income subsidy and other benefits on the physician referring patients or require that the physician have privileges exclusively at that hospital.

[118]The enabling legislation for this restriction was the Omnibus Reconciliation Act of 1980, P.L. 96-499, 94 Stat 2599, 42 U.S.C. Section 1395n(a)(2)(1988). Interim final rules were published in the *Federal Register* on October, 1982, and confirmed on June 30, 1986, in 51 *Federal Register* 23541; codified in 42 C.F.R. Section 424.22(d), 42 C.F.R. Section 105.1633

[119]October 31, 1989 letter of Richard P. Kusserow to Rep. Pete Stark.

[120]Medicare Catastrophic Coverage Act of 1988. P.L. 100-360, Section 203(c)(1)(F) (Section 1834 of the Social Security Act). Reprinted in 1988 *U.S. Code Congress & Administrative News* (102 Stat.) 722.

The statute included four exceptions: (a) when physician ownership in the health care facility is in publicly traded stock purchased on the same terms as available to the public; (b) when physician ownership is in a sole rural provider; (c) when the physician receives reasonable compensation for services he or she provides but not compensation for patient care, and the fees cannot vary with the volume of referrals; and (d) when falling within exceptions promulgated by the Department of Health and Human Services.

[121]Ethics in Patient Referral Act, H.R. 939 (1989).

[122]Exceptions were made for sole providers in rural areas, for ownership of publicly traded stock, and for services in group practices and HMOs.

[123]Also opposing the legislation were the American Academy of Neurology, the American College of Rheumatology, and the American Academy of Family Physicians.

[124]Omnibus Reconciliation Act of 1989, P.L. 101-239, Title 6. Section 6204 Adding Section 1877 to the Title 18 of the Social Security Act.

Iglehart, John K. 1989. "The Debate Over Physician Ownership of Health Care Facilities." *The New England Journal of Medicine* 321(3):198-204.

Iglehart, John K. 1990. "Congress Moves to Regulate Self-Referral and Physicians' Ownership of Clinical Laboratories." *The New England Journal of Medicine* 322(23):1682-1687.

[125]These limitations are subject to certain caveats.

[126]Intentional subterfuges to get around these arrangements (such as cross-referrals) are subject to even higher fines up to $100,000.

[127]Omnibus Reconciliation Act of 1990, Section 4164(b) Amending Sections 1124, and 4201(e) of Title XI of the Social Security Act.

Proposed regulations specify reporting requirements. "Medicare Program; Physician Ownership of, and Referrals to, Health Care Entities That Furnish Clinical Laboratory Services." 57 *Federal Register* 8588 (March 11, 1992). Congress has mandated a study of ownership of hospitals and other medical facilities by referring physicians. When this information becomes available, it may well provide the basis for further legislation.

[128]The President's Comprehensive Health Reform Program. February 6, 1992. p. 68.

Three other bills limiting physician self-referral were introduced in 1992. Reps. John Kasich and Rick Santorum introduced H.R. 5142; Rep. Robert Michel introduced H.R. 5325; and Brock Adams introduced S. 3186, the Ethics in Referral and Billing Act of 1992.

[129]There are several other requirements for tax-exempt status, but these are not relevant to physician conflict-of-interest policy.

[130]Such payments include those made to hospital-physician joint ventures, to physician-recruitment programs, to physicians for purchasing their practice, and to other physician bonding programs.

Mackelvie, Charles, and Mary Lynn McGuire. 1990. "Fraud, Abuse and Inurement: The Growing Impact on Provider-Physician Relations." *Journal of Health and Hospital Law* 23(1):1-9.

Sullivan, T. J., and V. Moore. 1990. "A Critical Look at Recent Developments in Tax Exempt Hospitals." *Journal of Health and Hospital Law* 23(3):65-83, 80.

[131]Internal Revenue Service, *General Counsel Memorandum* 39,498 (January 28, 1986).

Bromberg, Robert S. 1988. "Hospital-Physician Arrangements: A New Threat to Exemption." *Southwest Winds* (Newsletter of the Southwestern Ohio Chapter of the Healthcare Financial Management Association) (August-September):1, 4-8.

Bromberg, Robert S. 1988. "The Effect of Incentive Compensation Arrangements for Physicians and Executives on Hospital Exemption Hospital-Physician Arrangements." *Kentucky Hospitals* (Summer):38-41.

[132]IRS. *General Council Memorandum* 39862: Hospital Physician Joint Ventures. November 21, 1991.

Peregrine, Michael W., and Bernadette M. Broccolo. 1991. "Health Care Joint Ventures After GCM 39862: The Chief Counsel's Boarding-House Reach." *The Exempt Organization Tax Review* 4(10):1309-1319.

The IRS plans to issue another General Council Memorandum on physician recruitment payments. Personal Communication with T. J. Sullivan, senior attorney, Employee Benefits and Exempt Organizations, IRS.

[133]Clayton Act, 38 Stat. 730, as amended, 15 U.S.C.A. Sections 12-27.

Federal Trade Commission Act, 38 Stat. 717, as amended, 15 U.S.C.A. Sections 41-58.

Sherman Act, 26 Stat. 209, as amended, 15 U.S.C.

[134]*Goldfarb v. Virginia State Bar*, 421 U.S. 773 (1975).

Arizona v. Maricopa County Medical Society, 457 U.S. 332 (1982).

[135]*American Medical Association v. Federal Trade Commission*, 638 F. 2d 443 (2nd Cir. 1980), *aff'd. Mem.* 455 U.S. 676 (1982).

[136]*Jefferson Parish Hospital v. Hyde*, 466 U.S. 2 (1984).

[137]*Health First v. Bronson Methodist Hospital*, (CCH) Para. 69,200 (W.D. Mi. 1990).

Key Enterprises of Delaware v. Venice Hospital. 919 F 2d 1550 (11th Cir. 1990).

[138]Senator Hart also investigated physician dispensing of other medical products such as eyeglasses.

[139]Medical Restraint of Trade Act. 1967.

Physician Ownership in Pharmacies. 1964. p. 243.

[140]Comments of the FTC Concerning the Development of Regulations Pursuant to the Medicare and Medicaid AntiKickback Statute, December 18, 1987 (LRR-17-NI).

[141]The same physician-owner incentives for self-referral that lie at the heart of the conflict-of-interest issue may give rise to antitrust concerns: the potential in some cases for creating or enhancing market power in markets for the ancillary goods or services, resulting in higher prices and lower-quality health care to consumers and monopoly profits to some health care suppliers.

Arguit, Kevin. 1992. *A New Concern in Health Care Antitrust Enforcement: Acquisition and Exercise of Market Power by Physicians Ancillary Joint Ventures* (Remarks Before the National Health Lawyers Association, January 30.) Arguit suggested that such arrangements might violate Section 2 of the Sherman Act, Section 5 of the Federal Trade Commission Act, or Sections 1 or 7 of the Clayton Act.

[142]Witt, A. 1991. "Drug Company Supported Activities in Scientific or Educational Contexts: Draft Concept Paper."

[143]*Examination of the Pharmaceutical Industry: 1973-1974:* Hearings before the Subcommittee on Health of the Committee on Labor and Public Welfare, United States Senate, 93rd Congress, 1st and 2nd Sessions, Part 3, March 8, 12, 13; Part 4, May 3, 1974.

[144]Memorandum of Michael M. Simpson, Congressional Research Service, December 9, 1990. Mr. Simpson analyzed data provided by 16 pharmaceutical firms on their marketing practices to the Senate Labor and Human Resources Committee in 1988 and compared them to data obtained from surveys conducted in 1974, 1975, and 1976. In nearly every case, there was a slight drop in promotional practices following the 1974 hearings and a major resurgence afterward.

The firms providing data were Abbott, American Cyanamid-Lederie, Bristol-Meyers, Burroughs-Wellcome, Ciba-Geigy, Hoffman-LaRoche, Johnson & Johnson, Eli Lilly, Merck Sharp & Dohme, Merrell Dow, Norwich, Pfizer, Searle, Smith Kline, Syntex, Upjohn, Warner Lambert, and Wyeth-Ayerst.

[145]S. 1831, 1977 Amendments to the Food, Drug and Cosmetics Act, Introduced July 11, 1977.

[146]*Advertising, Marketing and Promotional Practices of the Pharmaceutical Industry.* 1990.

[147]Council on Ethical and Judicial Affairs. 1990. "Gifts to Physicians." *Journal of the American Medical Association* 265(4):501. The opinion is dated December 3, 1990, a week before the hearings and long after the AMA was asked to testify. The Judicial Council also adopted a report on December 4, 1990. "Gifts to Physicians from Industry." Report:G (I-90). The opinion was published and made known to members in the January 23/30 issue of the *Journal of the Ameri-can Medical Association.* However, *American Medical News* covered the hearings and noted in its December 14 issue that the Council on Ethical and Judicial Af-fairs had adopted a new opinion and the House of Delegates had adopted a report. See Merz, Beverly. 1990. "AMA Issues Rules on Drug Firm Gifts." *American Medical News* (December 14):1, 33.

[148]The AMA policy did not address conferences sponsored by private firms or the practice of firms giving sample drugs and other products to physicians for use by patients.

[149]The Senate hearing revealed instances of firms maintaining high drug prices once justified by high production costs, even after production costs dropped substantially. The reason was that the firms' managements believed the market would bear the price. When these decisions were made, there was no discussion of benefits to patients. See the discussion of Abbott Laboratories' pricing of TRH, testimony of David Jones, former executive director of public and professional affairs of Ciba-Geigy and vice president of public affairs for Abbott Laboratories. December 11, 1990. *Advertising, Marketing and Promotional Practices in the Pharmaceutical Industry.*

[150]Council on Ethical and Judicial Affairs. October 9, 1991. *Annotated Guidelines on Gifts to Physicians from Industry.* Chicago: AMA.

[151]Kusserow, Richard P. 1992. *Promotion of Prescription Drugs Through Payments and Gifts: Physicians' Perspectives.* Washington, D.C.: Office of the Inspector General, Department of Health and Human Services. OIE-01-90-00481.

The survey asked physicians to report on gifts and payments received between fall 1991 and fall 1992. The AMA guidelines were announced in December 1991. Some of the practices reported might have stopped in 1992. However, the American Medical News reports that many of these practices persist. Page, Leigh. 1992. "Are Goody Grab Bag Days Over? Dermatologists Eye New Ethics." *American Medical News* (February 3):3, 30, 31.

[152]Page, Leigh. 1992. "Are Goody Grab Bag Days Over?" pp. 3, 30, 31.

[153]Infectious Diseases Society of America. 1984. "Statement on Ethical Conduct in Research by the Infectious Diseases Society of North America." *Journal of Infectious Diseases* 150:(5)792-793.

[154]American Surgical Association, *Minutes of the One Hundred and Seventh Meeting*, April 21, 1987. p. lxxxvi.

[155]American College of Physicians. 1990. "Physicians and the Pharmaceutical Industry." *Annals of Internal Medicine* 112(8):624-626.

Chapter 5

[1]Brennan, Troyen A. 1991. *Just Doctoring: Medical Ethics in the Liberal State*. Berkeley: University of California Press. p. 71.

[2]Incentives to reduce care also counter another distortion in medical markets, namely, insurance. This removes financial barriers to access for insured people and eliminates any incentive they have to use resources frugally. A still more fundamental distortion is uncertainty, which makes patients depend on physicians and skews decisions. Arrow, Kenneth. 1963. "Uncertainty and the Welfare Economics of Medical Care." *American Economic Review* 53(2):941-973.

[3]There is an exception: approximately 15%, or 37 million Americans, have no health insurance.

[4]This is called a *prospective payment system*, which pays hospitals using DRGs. In fact, the system is more complex. If the cost of treatment greatly exceeds the DRG payment, Medicare will pay one-half of the extra cost. The payment is adjusted for hospital region, teaching status, and other criteria.

[5]For a sample of views of proponents of such incentives, see the following articles:

Hall, Mark A. 1988. "Institutional Control of Physician Behavior: Legal Barriers to Health Care Cost Containment." *University of Pennsylvania Law Review* 137(2):431-536.

Egdahl, Richard H., and Cynthia H. Taft. 1986. "Financial Incentives to Physicians." *The New England Journal of Medicine* 315(1):59-61.

Rabkin, Mitchell T. 1983. "Control of Health Care Costs: Targeting and Coordinating the Economic Incentives." *The New England Journal of Medicine* 309(16):982-984.

[6]For a summary of evidence of underuse of medical services and the effect on quality of care, see Lohr, Kathleen N. 1990. "Quality Problems and the Burdens of Harm: Evidence of Underuse," in *Medicare: A Strategy for Quality Assurance*, Kathleen N. Lohr, ed. Washington, D.C.: National Academy Press. Ch. 7.

[7]Stone, Alan A. 1985. "Law's Influence on Medicine and Medical Ethics." *The New England Journal of Medicine* 312(5):309-312.

[8]It might be argued that salaried practice does not make physicians neutral with respect to providing medical services because the risk of malpractice liability provides incentives for physicians to practice defensive medicine, i.e., to perform minimally useful diagnostic tests merely to document the basis for their clinical decisions. Financial incentives to reduce diagnostic tests, it can be argued, are necessary to counter this tendency. However, this approach to discouraging defensive medicine is roundabout and not particularly effective. A more direct approach would be for institutional providers to pay the cost of malpractice insurance.

[9]For a thoughtful discussion of the undesirable consequences of using incentives to promote desirable behavior in another context, see Kelman, Steven. 1981. *What Price Incentives?: Economists and the Environment*. Boston: Auburn House.

[10]*Health Maintenance Organization* is a legislative term used to describe pre-paid group practices qualifying for certain federal benefits. In common usage, it often refers to prepaid group practice generally, and includes so-called Competitive Medical Plans and many other similar arrangements.

[11]See Brown, Larry. 1983. *Politics and Health Care Organizations: HMOs as Federal Policy*. Washington, D.C.: The Brookings Institute.

[12]More recently, HMOs have developed three organizational tiers which increase the ways in which financial risk can be apportioned. See Hillman, Alan L., W. Pete Welch, and Mark V. Pauly. 1992. "Contractual Arrangements Between HMOs and Primary Care Physicians: Three Tiered HMOs and Risk Pools." *Medical Care* 3(2):136-148.

[13]Some analysts now suggest that differences in institutional structure are less significant than the different financial incentives and styles of management different HMOs use. See Welch, W. Pete, Alan L. Hillman, and Mark V. Pauly. 1990. "Toward New Typologies for HMOs." *The Milbank Quarterly* 68(2):221-243.

[14]There are numerous definitions of managed care. A few prominent ones are as follows:

"A coordinating and rationing strategy designed to make the unique role of the primary care provider the key to cost control." Freund, Deborah, and Robert

E. Hurley. 1987. "Managed Care in Medicaid: Selected Issues in Program Origins, Design, and Research." *Annual Review of Public Health* 8:137-163.

"[A] health care plan that attempts to influence physician practice in contrast to traditional indemnity insurance that pays the health bills for services specified in the health benefit." Egdahl, Richard H. 1988. "Managed Care in the U.S." Pew Seminar on Managed Care, Boston University Health Policy Institute. January 29, 1988.

"Management of resources used by physicians in the care of patients, driven by financial considerations." Rabkin, Michael. Pew Seminar on Managed Care, Boston University Health Policy Institute. April 8, 1988.

[15]Even within fee-for-service practice there are various styles. See Wennberg, John E., and A. Gittelshon. 1973. "Small Area Variations in Health Care Delivery." *Science* 183(117):1102-1108.

Nevertheless, fee-for-service encourages overuse of services. For a summary of evidence of overuse of medical services, see Institute of Medicine. 1990. *Medicare: A Strategy for Quality Assurance.* Ch. 7.

[16]Hillman, Alan L. 1987. "Financial Incentives for Physicians in HMOs: Is There a Conflict of Interest?" *The New England Journal of Medicine* 317(27):1743-1748.

Hillman, Alan L., Mark V. Pauly, and Joseph J. Kerstein. 1989. "How Do Financial Incentives Affect Physicians' Clinical Decisions and the Financial Performance of Health Maintenance Organizations?" *The New England Journal of Medicine* 321(2):86-92.

[17]I use the term *profitable* to cover both profit in for-profit HMOs and a "surplus" in non-profit HMOs.

[18]Hillman, Alan L. 1987. "Financial Incentives."

Welch, W. Pete, Alan L. Hillman, and Mark V. Pauly. 1990. "Financial Incentives."

[19]Gold, Marsha, and Ingrid Reeves. 1987. "Preliminary Results of the GHAA-BC/BS Survey of Physician Incentives in Health Maintenance Organizations (HMOs)." *Research Briefs* (1):1-15.

Typically, bonuses are explicitly linked to the volume of services used. Sometimes, however, bonuses are based on HMO profits. Profit sharing provides the same incentives for physicians as bonuses based on the volume of services used since the main costs to an HMO are the medical services they provide.

[20]Sullivan, Lewis. 1990. *Incentive Arrangements Offered by Health Maintenance Organizations and Competitive Medical Plans to Physicians.* Washington D.C.: Department of Health and Human Services. PB 90-20263/AS and PB 90-202649/AS. Vol. II. Appendix I: May 18, 1988. ICF Report submitted to Office of the Assistant Secretary for Planning and Evaluation, Department of Health and Human Services. Ch. III-2.

[21]Gold, Marsha, and Ingrid Reeves. 1987. "Preliminary Results."

For a thoughtful discussion of incentives and recent trends see, Hillman, Alan L. 1991. "Managing the Physician: Rules Versus Incentives." *Health Affairs* (10(4):138–146.

[22]For example, the California Primary Care Management Medicaid program gives physicians the option of bearing the risk for diagnostic tests, X-rays, and drugs. See Welch, W. Pete, Alan L. Hillman, and Mark V. Pauly. 1989. *Toward a Typology of HMOs Reflecting Financial Incentives to Physicians.* Washington, D.C.: The Urban Institute.

[23]See Welch, W. Pete. 1989. *Giving Physicians Incentives to Contain Costs Under Medicare: Lessons from Medicaid.* Washington D.C.: The Urban Institute. Working Paper 3872-01. See the case study of Kitsap, Washington HIO.

[24]General Accounting Office. 1988. *Medicare: Physician Incentive Payments by Prepaid Health Plans Could Lower Quality of Care.* Washington, D.C.: Department of Health and Human Services. HRD-89-29.

[25]Moore, Stephen H., D. P. Martin, and W. C. Richardson. 1983. "Does the Primary-Care Gatekeeper Control the Costs of Health Care? Lessons from the SAFECO Experience." *The New England Journal of Medicine* 309(22):1400-1404.

Lavin, John H. 1980. "When Primary Doctors Run the Whole Show." *Medical Economics* (December 22):25-42.

Moore, Stephen. 1979. "Cost Containment Through Risk-Sharing by Primary-Care Physicians." *The New England Journal of Medicine* 300(24):1359-1362

[26]Based on information provided in Kahn, Lawrence. 1988. *Medical Developments* 3(2) and Bluechoice documents.

[27]Primary care physicians can also receive income from providing services not covered in the capitation agreement on a fee-for-service basis and by sharing savings from managing home care cases.

[28]These figures assume a practice of 1,850 primary care patients.

[29]Berenson, Robert A. 1987. "Hidden Compromises in Paying Physicians." *Business and Health* (July):18-22.

[30]Berenson, Robert A. 1987. "Financial Confessions of a Sawbones: In a Doctor's Wallet." *The New Republic* (May 18):11-13.

[31]Berenson, Robert A. 1987. "Financial Confessions."

[32]Kolata, Gina. 1988. "Being Thorough Can Be Costly—To the Doctor." New York Times (March 20):Sec. 4, p. 6.

[33]Hillman, Alan A., Pauly, Mark V., and Kerstein, Joseph J. 1989. "Financial Incentives."

[34]Hillman, Alan L., Mark V. Pauly, Keith Kermann, and Caroline Rohr Martinek. 1991. "HMO Managers' Views on Financial Incentives and Quality." *Health Affairs* 10(4):206-219.

[35]Haney, Daniel Q., and Fred Bayles. 1991. "HMO Doctors Can Earn More for Doing Less." Associated Press (November 19).

[36]Millenson, Michael L. 1987. "Health Care Debate Rages: Cost-Paring: Good Business or Bad Medicine?" *Chicago Tribune* (June 14):1, 3-5.

[37]Millenson, Michael L. 1987. "Health Care Debate."

[38]Some economists say that people are influenced most by marginal gains or losses from particular decisions. However, others say that money, like anything else, has decreasing marginal utility and will be less desirable as the supply increases. There is a growing literature that suggests that physicians work to achieve a target income. If this is so, they will be less susceptible to incentives as they approach or exceed this income level.

For a discussion of the target income hypothesis, see Cromwell, Jerry, and Janet B. Mitchell. 1986. "Physician-Induced Demand for Surgery." *Journal of Health Economics* 5(4):293-313.

Reinhardt, Uwe W. 1985. "The Theory of Physician-Induced Demand: Reflections After a Decade." *Journal of Health Economics* 4(2):87-93.

Rossiter, Louis F., and Gail R. Wilensky. 1983. "A Reexamination of the Use of Physician Services: The Role of Physician-Induced Demand." *Inquiry* 20(2):162-172.

Wilensky, Gail R., and Louis F. Rossiter. 1983. "The Relative Importance of Physician-Induced Demand in the Demand for Medical Care." *Health and Society* 61(2):252-277.

Fuchs, Victor R. 1978. "The Supply of Surgeons and the Demand for Operations." *Journal of Human Resources* 13 (Supplement):35-56.

Sloan, Frank A., and Roger Feldman. 1978. "Competition Among Physicians," in *Competition in the Health Care Sector: Past, Present, and Future*, Warren Greenberg, ed. Germantown, Aspen Systems.

[39]Hillman, Alan L., W. Pete Welch, and Mark V. Pauly. 1992. "Contractual Arrangements Between HMOs and Primary Care Physicians: Three Tiered HMOs and Risk Pools." *Medical Care* 3(2):136-148.

[40]For a description of prospective payment using DRGs, see Vladeck, Bruce C. 1984. "Medicare Hospital Payment by Diagnosis-Related Groups." *Annals of Internal Medicine* 100(4):576-591.

[41]Harris, Jeffrey E. 1977. "The Internal Organization of the Hospital: Some Economic Implications." *Bell Journal of Economics* 8(2):467-482.

[42]Koska, Mary T. 1990. "Physician Practices Go Under the Microscope." *Hospitals* (February 20):32-37.

[43]Tierney, William M., Michael E. Miller, and Clement J. McDonald. 1990. "The Effect on Test Ordering of Informing Physicians of the Charges for Outpatient Diagnostic Tests." *The New England Journal of Medicine* 322(21):1499-1504.

[44]See the series of articles by Fred Bayles and Daniel Haney, of the Associated Press, entitled "Doctors for Sale." These articles deal with the carrots and sticks that hospitals use to get physicians to admit patients and practice in a manner that promotes hospitals' financial well-being. Released October 14, 1990: "Hospitals Give Doctors Money, Freebies for Patients." Released October 15, 1990: "Money for Patients: One Hospital's Story."

[45]Hollywood Community Hospital. April 25, 1985 letter from Patrick Petre, Assistant Administrator to hospital doctors.

[46]General Accounting Office. 1988. *Physician Incentives.*

[47]Paracelsus stopped its physician incentive plan following a 1985 investigation by the Department of Justice for Medicare fraud. Other hospitals with similar incentive plans have followed suit. Although the initial impetus for the Paracelsus investigation was the incentive plan, the Justice Department also investigated billing and other practices. As part of a settlement of all potential claims, PHC agreed to pay $4.45 million in reimbursement, fines, and interest and to provide $100,000 in medical services to indigent persons living in Orange County. Department of Health and Human Services. Office of the Inspector General. *Fact Sheet on the Paracelsus Investigation.*

General Accounting Office. 1988. *Physician Incentives.*

Kreche, Kathryn A. 1986. "Abusing the Patient: Medicare Fraud and Abuse and Hospital-Physician Incentive Plans." *University of Michigan Journal of Law Reform* 20(1):279-304.

The Paracelsus case was also instrumental in prompting Congress to pass legislation limiting risk-sharing in HMOs.

[48]Interstudy proposed the idea, and it has received considerable attention. However, it has rarely been used.

[49]Richards, Glenn. 1984. "How Do Joint Ventures Affect Relations with Physicians?" *Hospitals* 58(23):68-74.

[50]Richards, Glenn. 1984. "Joint Ventures."

[51]Dechene, James C. 1987. "Physician Incentive Programs: Are They Legal?" *HealthSpan* 4(1):3-9.

[52]Perry, Linda. 1989. "Physician Ownership May Give Hospitals a Shot in the Arm." *Modern Healthcare* (June 30):25-34.

[53]Often these arrangements involve a complicated series of ownership and leasing arrangements between the hospital and physicians.

[54]For a review of recent developments and the legal issues, see Hall, Mark A. 1988. "Institutional Control."

See also Hershey, Nathan. 1986. "Applying Utilization Review Findings in Medical Staff Appointment and Reappointment Decisions." *Quality Assurance and Utilization Review* 1(4):109-110.

[55]Eller, John J., and Sanford V. Teplitzky. 1986. "Considering Economic Factors in Hospital Privilege Decisions." *HealthSpan* 3 (August-September):11-14.

Ellwood, Paul M., Jr. "When MDs Meet DRGs." *Hospitals* 57(24):62-66.

Glandon, Gerald L., and Michael A. Morrisey. 1986. "Redefining the Hospital-Physician Relationship Under Prospective Payment." *Inquiry* 23(2):166-175.

For a study of one hospital's changed by-laws to account for physician costs, see Cantrell, Leonard E., and Jeffrey A. Frick. 1986. "Physician Efficiency and

Reimbursement: A Case Study." *Hospital and Health Services Administration* (November-December):43.

"Economic Credentialing Is Fine—For Tightrope Walkers." 1990. *Hospital Peer Review* 15(4):49-51.

[56]Blum, John D. 1991. "Economic Credentialing: A New Twist in Hospital Physician Appraisal Processes." *Journal of Legal Medicine* 12(4):427-475.

Koska, Mary. 1991. "Hospital CEOs Divided on Use of Economic Credentialing." *Hospitals* 65(6):42, 44, 46, 48.

[57]Hospitals frequently will maintain a referral service for patients who seek a physician for outpatient medical care. Some hospitals have excluded "high-cost" physicians from their referral programs (i.e., those who order many tests and procedures), so that hospital revenues under Medicare's DRG reimbursement system are less than the costs of treating patients.

Franz, Julie. 1984. "Clipping Doctors from Referral Program Spurs Them to Clip Costs." *Modern Healthcare* (April):116, 118.

Chapter 6

[1]Stone, Alan A. 1985. "Law's Influence on Medicine and Medical Ethics." *The New England Journal of Medicine* 312(5):309-12.

[2]Geist, Robert W. 1974. "Incentive Bonuses in Prepayment Plans." *The New England Journal of Medicine* 291(24):1306-1308, at 1307.

[3]Schneyer, Theodore J. 1976. "Informed Consent and the Danger of Bias in the Formation of Medical Disclosure Practices."*Wisconsin Law Review* 1976(2): 124-170.

[4]The relation between hospitals, physicians, and patients resembles that of courts, criminal defense lawyers, and clients. Marc Galanter says that criminal defense lawyers are "repeat players" who have a vested interest in the system that may compromise their loyalty to clients, who interact with the justice system only occasionally. Galanter, Marc. 1974. "Why the 'Haves' Come Out Ahead: Speculations on the Limits of Legal Change." *Law and Society Review* 9(1):95-160.

[5]Annas, George J. 1988. *Judging Medicine*. Clifton, N.J.: Humana Press. See "The Hospital: A Human Rights Wasteland." pp. 4-26.

[6]However, more sober proponents acknowledge that not much is known about the effects of such incentive arrangements or about other crucial variables that affect the costs of caring for patients. See, e.g., Physician Payment Review

Commission. 1989. *Annual Report to Congress.* "Risk-Sharing Arrangements in Prepaid Health Plans, Washington. D.C." Ch. 15.

[7]The most common examples of such programs are Medicare's Professional Standards Review Program, private utilization review programs, and quality assurance programs. I discuss these later in the chapter in the section titled "The Limitations of Professional Review Organizations and Quality Assurance Programs."

[8]Sullivan, Lewis. 1990. *Incentive Arrangements Offered by Health Maintenance Organizations and Competitive Medical Plans to Physicians.* Washington D.C.: Department of Health and Human Services. PB 90-20263/AS and PB 90-202649/AS, Vol. II, Appendix I. May 18, 1988. ICF Report submitted to the Office of the Assistant Secretary for Planning and Evaluation, Department of Health and Human Services. Ch. IV.

[9]The first HMOs were staff model HMOs that employed physicians on salary. They often reduced hospitalization by 30%. Luft, Harold S. 1981. *Health Maintenance Organizations: Dimensions of Performance.* New York: Wiley

[10]See, e.g., Physician Payment Review Commission. *Annual Report.* 1989. "Risk-Sharing Arrangements in Prepaid Health Plans." Ch. 15. The report's recommendations include the following:

> HCFA should require prepaid health plans to limit the total risk assumed by individual physicians or small groups through some form of reinsurance or "stop loss" provisions, and it should require them to rely primarily on incentives to groups of physicians rather than to individual physicians.

See also the testimony of Karen Davis, Commissioner, Physician Payment Review Commission. *Fiscal Year 1990 Budget Issues Relating to Physician Incentive Payments by Prepaid Health Plans.* Hearings Before the Subcommittee on Health of the Committee on Ways and Means, House of Representatives, 101st Congress, 1st Session. April 25, 1989. (Serial No. 101-30.)

[11]Some writers have commented on this problem. Dr. Stephen Moore acknowledges the need to reduce the risk physicians bear in order to prevent undue pressure on physicians when they have a few very ill patients. In such situations, doctors can do everything reasonably possible within the realm of accepted medical practice to eliminate waste yet still lose money. Here risk sharing can promote improper behavior. Yet Moore attributes the failure of the SAFECO HMO to its providing incentives that were too weak. Moore, Stephen H., D.P. Martin, and W.C. Richardson. 1983. "Does the Primary-Care Gatekeeper Control the Costs of Health Care? Lessons From the SAFECO Experience." *The New England Journal of Medicine* 309(22):1400-1404.

[12]U.S. Healthcare, a national HMO, and Av-Med, a Florida-based HMO, have devised such programs. For a summary of the U.S. Healthcare program written by its employees, see Schlackman, Neil. 1989. "Integrating Quality Assessment and Physician Incentive Payment." *Quality Review Bulletin* (August):

234-237; Stocker, Michael A. 1989. "Quality Assurance in an IPA." *HMO Practice* 3(5):183-187.

U.S. Healthcare has revised the incentive formula it uses three times and is likely to do so again in the future.

For a discussion of the Av-Med program by its medical director, see Beloff, Jerome "Case Study/Av-Med Health Plan of Florida: The Physician Incentive Bonus Plan Based on Quality of Care." Ch. 13 in Boland, Peter. 1991. *Making Managed Health Care Work*. New York: McGraw-Hill.

[13]The incentive payments are only part of U.S. Healthcare's quality assurance program. My criticisms are directed not to the whole program, only to the idea that incentives for their quality measures can appropriately counter incentives to reduce services.

There is little public information about the effectiveness of the U.S. Healthcare program. U.S. Healthcare has published a brief description of the program (see the preceding note). It hired a consulting firm to evaluate the program and has released a four-page executive summary of the 100-page report. The summary portrays the program very favorably. However, the report itself is not public. U.S. Healthcare acknowledges that the consultants also suggested a number of changes, including improvement of the review of medical records by using more comprehensive criteria, more objective measures, and better-trained reviewers. See Schlackman, Neil. 1991. "Integrating Quality Assessment and Physician Incentive Payment." p. 236.

[14]Goffman, Erving. 1952. "On Cooling the Mark Out." *Psychiatry* 15(3):451-463.

[15]One study found that patient satisfaction was correlated with quality of care. Stewart, A. L., Sheldon Greenfield, R. D. Hays, et al. 1989. "Functional Status and Well-Being of Patients With Chronic Conditions: Results From the Medical Outcomes Study." *Journal of the American Medical Association* 262(7):907-913.

[16]*U.S. Healthcare's Quality Mission Statement*. 1992. (Unpublished photocopy). Telephone interview with Neil Schlackman, *U.S. Healthcare*, June 1992.

[17]For a discussion of fiduciary obligations, see Chapter 7.

[18]Halper, Thomas. 1989. *The Misfortune of Others: End-Stage Renal Disease in the United Kingdom*. New York: Cambridge University Press.

[19]However, there appear to be biases that prompt doctors to provide fewer services based on class, race and gender.

Wenneker, Mark B., William Rogers, and Sheldon Greenfield. 1992. "Income and Racial Differences in Utilization and Satisfaction for Patients in Doctor's Offices; The Results from the Medical Outcomes Study." (Unpublished manuscript.)

[20]When physicians receive incentives to reduce services, they become what Dr. Geist calls "Self-serving denial-of-care agents for the benefit of the 'buyer' of care seeking 'cost-control' of the 'health-care industry.'" Geist, Robert W. 1974. "Incentive Bonuses." p. 1307.

²¹Daniels, Norman. 1986. "Why Saying No to Patients in the United States Is So Hard: Cost Containment, Justice, and Provider Autonomy." *The New England Journal of Medicine* 314(24):1381-1383.

²²See, e.g., *Fiscal Year 1990 Budget Issues Relating to Physician Incentive Payments by Prepaid Health Plans*, Testimony of Harris Berman. 1989. p. 32.

²³For an account of how peer review and quality assurance programs can help promote accountability to patients, see Gray, Bradford H. 1991. *The Profit Motive and Patient Care: The Changing Accountability of Doctors and Hospitals.* Cambridge: Harvard University Press.

²⁴PRO Law: Enacted as P.L. 92-603 in 1972. Certificate of Need Law: Section 1122 of the 1972 Amendments to the Social Security Act, P.L. 92-603.

²⁵Blumstein, James F., and Frank A. Sloan. 1978. "Health Planning and Regulation Through Certificate of Need: An Overview." *Utah Law Review* 1978(1):3-37.

Professional Standards Review Organization 1979 Program Evaluation. 1979. Washington, D.C.: U.S. Department of Health and Human Services, Health Care Financing Administration.

Salkever, David S., and Thomas W. Bice. 1976. *Impact of State Certificate of Need Laws on Health Care Costs and Utilization.* National Center for Health Services Research, Health Resources Administration. Department of Health, Education, and Welfare.

Salkever, David S., and Thomas W. Bice. 1976. "The Impact of Certificate-of-Need Controls on Hospital Investment." *The Milbank Quarterly* 54(2):185-214.

²⁶Providers have indirect financial incentives to produce high-quality care because this affects the commitment of the public and physicians. But it is difficult for experts, let alone the public, to gauge quality. Moreover, developing a reputation for quality requires a long-term commitment. Most medical administrators are under greater pressure to attend to short-term profits rather than build a long-term reputation. Therefore, more direct financial incentives will have a stronger effect than indirect incentives to develop a reputation for quality.

Insurers that do not detect underservice risk paying more later if it leads to more costly medical problems. But many medical problems can be neglected or untreated without leading to greater expense. Some untreated medical problems may lead to death, which may decrease medical care expenses. Others may be tolerated by patients even though they lead to a lower quality of life.

There is also a difference between the cost of not detecting underservice for an individual patient and for groups. Underservice, when due to failure to perform tests, may lead to greater costs for an individual patient. But because the frequency of the problem may be low, it may be less costly for the insurer to pay the increased cost in a few cases than pay for the testing of all individuals who have symptoms that indicate that testing is appropriate.

[27]Lohr, Kathleen N., ed. 1990. *Medicare: A Strategy for Quality Assurance.* Washington, D.C.: National Academy Press. pp. 226-227.

Restuccia, Joseph D., Susan M. C. Payne, and Lenore V. Tracey. 1989. "A Framework for the Definition and Measurement of Underutilization." *Medical Care Review* 46(3):255-270, at 265.

[28]Restuccia, Joseph D., Susan M. C. Payne, and Lenore V. Tracey. 1989. "Definition and Measurement."

[29]Restuccia, Joseph D., Susan M. C. Payne, and Lenore V. Tracey. 1989. "Definition and Measurement."

[30]Although the United States is a leader in quality assurance programs, our technology is still underdeveloped and the nation currently lacks the capacity to achieve comprehensive and maximally effective quality assurance programs. Lohr, Kathleen N., and Steven A. Schroeder. 1990. "A Strategy for Quality Assurance in Medicare." *The New England Journal of Medicine* 322(10):707-712.

Lohr, Kathleen N. 1990. *Medicare.*

[31]Lohr, Kathleen N., and Steven A. Schroeder. 1990. "Quality Assurance." Lohr, Kathleen N. 1990. *Medicare.*

[32]Lohr, Kathleen N. 1990. *Medicare.* p. 170.

[33]Lohr, Kathleen N. 1990. *Medicare.*

Rubenstein, L. Z., L. V. Rubenstein, and K. R. Josephson. 1989. "Quality of Health Care for Older People in America." Paper prepared for the Institute of Medicine Study to Design a Strategy for Quality Review and Assurance in Medicare. Cited in Lohr, Kathleen N. 1990. *Medicare.* pp. 228-229. Rubenstein, et al., based this conclusion on a review of published literature. However, they suspect that these studies underestimate the problem.

[34]Gray, Bradford H., and Marilyn J. Fields, eds. 1989. *Controlling Costs and Changing Patient Care? The Role of Utilization Management.* Washington, D.C.: National Academy Press. Appendix E, Summaries of Committee Site Visits to Utilization Management Organizations, Organization 10, p. 270.

[35]The SuperPRO is an independent contractor hired to review the performance of PROs. PROMPTS-2 is a Health Care Financing Administration internal PRO monitoring protocol and tracking system used to monitor PROs' performance.

[36]GAO. May 1988. *Medicare: Improving Quality of Care Assessment and Assurance.* (GAO/PEMD-88-10). Washington, D.C.: Ch. 4.

Lohr, Kathleen N. 1990. *Medicare.* p. 181.

[37]GAO. May 1988. *Medicare.* Ch. 4.

[38]Lohr, Kathleen N. 1990. *Medicare.* p. 199.

[39]GAO. May 1988. *Medicare.* Ch. 4.

[40]GAO. May 1988. *Medicare.* Ch. 4.

[41]Senate Special Committee On Aging. 1987. *Medicare and HMOs: A First Look, With Disturbing Findings.* Minority Staff Report. (Senator Heinz, ranking member). (April 7). (See especially pp. 25-41.)

[42]Trauner, Joan B., and Sibyl Tilson. "Appendix B: Utilization Management and Quality Assurance in Health Maintenance Organizations: An Operational Assessment." In Gray, Bradford H., and Marilyn J. Field. 1989. *Controlling Costs.*

[43]Trauner, Joan B. and Sibyl Tilson. 1989. "Appendix B: Utilization Management."

[44]Joint Commission on Accreditation of Health Care Organizations. 1987. *Reports of the Findings of the Joint Commission's Quality Assurance Evaluation and Medical Records Audits of Health Maintenance Organizations in Ohio under the Medical Assistance Program.* Submitted to the Bureau of Alternative Delivery Systems, Ohio Department of Human Services. (December).

[45]Recently, investigative reports have again demonstrated that quality problems exist in HMOs. A series of newspaper articles in the fall of 1990 documented abuses in the Gold Plus Plan, owned by Humana, a major national health care provider. Bergal, Jenni, Nancy McVicar, and Fred Schulte. 1990. "Risky RX: The Gold Plus Plan for the Elderly." *Florida Sun Centennial.* Reprint of a four-part series (October 21-24). The articles led to congressional hearings in March 1991 before the Committee on Aging, which showed that it is far easier to design quality assurance systems that look good on paper than to make them work in practice.

[46]The HMO Act of 1973 and federal regulations provide the following:
Each health maintenance organization shall... (2) assume full financial risk ...except that a health maintenance organization may... (D) make arrangements with physicians or other health professionals . . . to assume all or part of the financial risk on a prospective basis for the provision of basic health services by the physicians or other health professionals . . . (Section 1301(c) HMO Act of 1973.) Each HMO... may... (4) make arrangements with physicians...to assume all or part of the financial risk . . . for the provision of basic health services by physicians or other health professionals . . . (42 C.F.R. 417.107 (b) (4).)
HMOs shall have effective procedures to monitor utilization and to control the cost of basic and supplemental health services and to achieve utilization goals, which may include mechanisms such as risk sharing, financial incentives or other provisions agreed to by providers. (42 C.R. R. 417.103(b).)
The Tax Equity and Fiscal Responsibility Act of 1982 (TEFRA) authorizes Medicare to enter into risk contracts with HMOs and Competitive Medical Plans and allows these organizations to pass on some portion of this risk to physicians.

(D) The entity assumes full financial risk . . . except that such entity may . . . (iv) make arrangements with physicians or other health professionals . . . to assume all or part of the financial risk on a prospective basis for the provision of basic health services by the physicians or other health professionals . . . (TEFRA, Section 1876 (b)(2)(D).)

[47]For example, Pennsylvania.

[48]Legislation introduced in Massachusetts in 1989 and 1990 would require HMOs and other health insurance providers to tell patients about any financial incentives that could influence physicians' treatment decisions. House bill 3342, 1990, An Act Relative to Public Disclosure by Health Insurers; Hearings Held, March 21, 1990. Reported favorably, April 25, 1990. For a news report, see Torry, Karen. 1989. "Mass Bill Would Require HMOs to Reveal Incentives." *American Medical News* (December 8):21.

Levinson, Douglas F. 1987. "Toward Full Disclosure of Referral Restrictions and Financial Incentives by Prepaid Health Plans." *The New England Journal of Medicine* 317(27):1729-1731.

[49]Section 9313(c), Omnibus Budget Reconciliation Act of 1986 (P.L. 99-509). 42 U.S.C. 1320a-7(b).

If a hospital, an eligible organization with a risk-sharing contract under section 1876, or an entity with a contract under section 1903(m) knowingly makes a payment, directly or indirectly, to a physician as an inducement to reduce or limit services provided . . . the hospital or organization shall be subject, in addition to any other penalties . . . , to a civil money penalty. . . .

[50]Competitive Medical Plans are like HMOs in that they are a form of pre-paid group practice. However, they do not meet federal qualification for HMOs, such as providing community-rated premiums and having open enrollment periods.

[51]Omnibus Reconciliation Act of 1990, Section 4204, Health Maintenance Organizations. "(a) Regulation of Incentive Payments to Physicians." This law became effective in 1992.

[52]"Requirements for Physician Incentive Plans in Prepaid Health Care Organizations." 1982. *Federal Register*, 57(240):59024-59041. December 14.

[53]Johnson, Julie. 1993. "Proposed Rules Would Protect Doctors Under Risk Contracts." *American Medical News* (January 18):7-8.

[54]Source: Managed Care Contract Report. March 1, 1992. Office of Prepaid Health Care, Health Care Financing Administration, Department of Health and Human Services. Washington, D.C.

There are approximately 34.7 million members covered by managed-care providers in the U.S. See Group Health Association of America. 1990. *National Directory of HMOs: 1990*. Washington, D.C.: Group Health Association of America.

Gold, Marsha. 1991. "Health Maintenance Organizations: Structure, Performance and Current Issues For Employee Health Benefits Design." *Journal of Occupational Medicine* 33(3):288-296.

[55]42 U.S.C. Section 1320 a-7a(b).

[56]Complaint, *Anthony Teti, Sr. v. U.S. Healthcare, Inc.*, C.A. 89-9808 U.S. District Court, Eastern District of Pennsylvania. (December 27, 1988.)

[57]At the time of the incident, U.S. Healthcare had a typical risk-sharing plan. It paid physicians by capitation, withheld 20% of the payment, and placed it in a referral fund. These funds were returned to physicians only if the allotted budget for specialty and hospital care was not exhausted; otherwise, they were used to cover the deficit. U.S. Healthcare now has a different compensation plan, described earlier in the chapter in the section titled "Financial Incentives That Help Patients." Some speculate that its new payment plan is a way to protect itself from liability. However, even the current payment arrangement provides incentives to restrict the volume of services.

[58]The trial court judge dismissed the lawsuit, saying that there was no basis for bringing a RICO claim. The plaintiffs appealed the dismissal, but their appeal was denied by the U.S. Court of Appeals for the 3rd Circuit by Judge Sloviter Order Numbers 89-2091/89-2092 (May 23, 1990). Following the appeal, the plaintiffs refiled the suit in state court.

[59]Stern, Joanne B. 1983. "Bad Faith Suits: Are They Applicable to Health Maintenance Organizations?" *West Virginia Law Review* 85(5):911-928.

[60]*Pilot Life Insurance Company v. Dedeaux*, 107 S.Ct. 1549 (1987).

The ERISA preemption does not apply to self-insured employers, individual purchasers of insurance, or employees covered by governmental insurance programs. This preemption may not be long-lived. In 1992 legislation was introduced in Congress that would eliminate the exception.

[61]Professor E. Haavi Morreim has suggested that suits for bad faith breach of contract against physicians are another way to hold physicians accountable to patients. Presumably courts could impose punitive damages on physicians who consciously act improperly, and this would deter physicians from misbehavior. Courts have not yet used this approach. Morreim, E. Haavi. 1990. "Physician Investment and Self-Referral: Philosophical Analysis of a Contentious Debate." *Journal of Medicine and Philosophy* 15(4):425-448.

[62]*Wickline v. State of California*, 192 Cal. App. 3rd 1630, 228 Cal. Reporter 661 (1986).

[63]*Pulvers v. Kaiser Foundation Health Plans*, 99 Cal. App. 3d 560, 160 Cal. Reporter 392 (1980).

[64]42 U.S.C. Sec. 300e (Section 1301).

[65]*Bush v. Dake*, C.A. No. 86-25767 Circuit Court, Saginaw County, Michigan.

[66]Group Health Services paid primary physicians on a per-capita basis and made them bear part of the financial risk of referring patients for specialty care of diagnostic tests.

[67]*Bush v. Dake*, Opinion of the Court on Motion for Partial Summary Disposition. April 27, 1989.

[68]*Kelly Anne Sweede v. CIGNA Health Plan of Delaware*, Third Amended Complaint. C.A. No 87C-SE-171-1-CV, Superior Court, New Castle County, Delaware. September 1988. Sweede named other physicians as defendants as well.

[69]This judicial decision was reported to me by the plaintiff's lawyer. Apparently it was issued from the bench and is recorded only in the trial transcript, not in a written judicial decision.

[70]See *Defendant CIGNA Healthplan of Delaware, Inc.'s Opening Brief in Support of Its Motion for Summary Judgment.* December 15, 1988. C.A. No. 87C-SE-171-1-CV. State of Delaware, New Castle County, Superior Court.

Plaintiff's Answering Brief in Opposition to CIGNA Healthplan of Delaware, Inc.'s Motion for Summary Judgment and Motions in Limine. January 9, 1989.

Defendant CIGNA Healthplan of Delaware, Inc.'s Reply Brief in Support of Its Motion for Summary Judgment. January 20, 1989.

The parties settled the suit out of court before the judge ruled on the motion to dismiss. CIGNA also makes this claim in its fourth affirmative defense to the second amended complaint.

[71]The risk-sharing plan paid primary care physicians by capitation but withheld 20% of the payment to cover the cost of medical care referrals and hospitalizations if they exceeded the budget. Withheld funds not used for referrals and hospitalization were distributed first to participating specialists, up to a total amount withheld, and then to primary care physicians. Primary care physicians could also receive a bonus if utilization of resources was below a target.

[72]*Boyd v. Albert Einstein Medical Center*, C.A. No. 4887, Court of Common Pleas, Civil Division, Philadelphia, Pennsylvania. July 1983.

Boyd v. Albert Einstein Medical Center, 547 A.2d 1229 (1988).

[73]*Boyd v. Albert Einstein Medical Center* (1988).

The plaintiffs claim that the treating physicians were ostensible agents of the HMO, thereby making the HMO legally responsible for their negligence. In response to the defendant's motion for summary judgment, the trial court dismissed the lawsuit, stating that there was no legal basis for holding the HMO responsible. But the appeals court reversed the lower court's dismissal, stating that the HMO might be responsible for the negligence of its physicians and that this could only be decided by a trial that determined the facts.

[74]*McClellan and Shotel v. HMO-PA*, 413 Pa. Super 128, 604 A.2d 1053 (1992).

[75]*McClellan and Shotel v. HMO-PA*, 413 Pa. Super 128, 604 A.2d 1053 fn 5 (1992).

[76]Civil Action number 4887.

[77]The law calls these *hold-harmless* or *indemnification clauses.* CIGNA required the IPA to indemnify it in the event that CIGNA was found liable for any negligence of physicians.

[78]One lawyer has advised HMOs to protect themselves by "having patients sign waivers indicating that they know their MDs are independent of the HMOs." He reportedly also advocated disclosing financial incentives to physicians. Harris, Meyer. 1988. "Lawyer: Suits Blaming HMO Controls for Malpractice May Have Jury Appeal." *American Medical News* (July 28):1, 10.

[79]Medical Practice Study Group, Harvard University. 1990. *Patients, Doctors, and Lawyers: Medical Injury, Malpractice Litigation, and Patient Compensation in New York.*

[80]Localio, A. Russell, Anne G. Lawthers, Troyen A. Brennnan, Nan M. Laird, Liesi E. Herbert, Lynn M. Peterson, Joseph P. Newhouse, Paul C. Weiler, and Howard H. Hiatt. 1991. "Relations Between Malpractice Claims and Adverse Events Due to Negligence." *The New England Journal of Medicine* 325(4):245-251.

[81]Medical Practice Study Group, Harvard University. 1990. *Patients, Doctors, and Lawyers.*

Chapter 7

[1]Alexander, M. Carr-Sanders, and P. A. Wilson. 1933. *The Professions.* Oxford: Clarendon Press p. 426.

[2]The legislation prohibiting physicians from engaging in self-referral, discussed in Chapter 4 may be a harbinger of greater legislation. The National Science Foundation has proposed a rule that would require financial disclosure and address conflicts of interest of individuals receiving research funds. See "Investigator Financial Disclosure Policy." 57 *Federal Register.* p. 31540-31541. July 16, 1992. The National Institutes of Health has announced its intent to promulgate a rule governing conflicts of interest. Reppert, Barton. 1992. "NICH Conflicts-of-Interest Regs Impending." *The Scientist* 6(20):1,8.

[3]Although the categories are not mutually exclusive, writers sometimes distinguish between wage labor, business, and professions. Wage laborers work for others and lack autonomy over their work. Individuals in business typically control their affairs and are expected to exploit market opportunities and pursue their self-interest. Professionals have obligations to act on behalf of their clients, even when this means forgoing business opportunities. Professionals are also supposed to have specialized knowledge and power, which distinguishes them from wage laborers and individuals in business. The relation between professionals and clients is one of authority, yet professionals are supposed to act for the benefit of clients. There are thus analogies between what the law defines as fiduciaries and the professions.

The clergy in the Middle Ages was probably the classic profession. Clergymen had specialized knowledge and power over the parishioner (their help was needed to get to heaven); and they were required to take a vow of poverty to help ensure that they did not act in their own interests. In modern times, people speak of medicine and law as classic professions.

For a sample of some recent literature on this subject see:

Friedson, Eliot. 1990. "The Centrality of Professionalism to Health Care." *Jurimetrics* 30(4):431-445.

Abott, Anderson Delane. 1988. *The System of Professions: An Essay on the Division of Expert Labor*. Chicago: Chicago University Press.

Friedson, Eliot. 1986. *Professional Powers*. Chicago: University of Chicago Press.

Haskell, Thomas L., ed. 1984. *The Authority of Experts*. Bloomington: Indiana University Press.

Geison, Gerald L., ed. 1983. *Professions and Professional Ideologies in America*. Chapel Hill: University of North Carolina.

Rottenberg, Simon. 1980. *Occupational Licensure and Regulation*. Washington, D.C.: American Enterprise Institute.

Larson, Margali Sarfatti. 1977. *The Rise of Professionalism: A Sociological Analysis*. Berkeley: University of California Press.

Blendstein, Burton J. 1976. *The Culture of Professionalism*. New York: W.W. Norton.

Johnson, Terence J. 1972. *Professions and Power*. London: MacMillan.

[4]Fried, Charles. 1976. "The Lawyer as Friend: The Moral Foundations of the Lawyer-Client Relation." *The Yale Law Journal* 85(8):1060-1089.

[5]My discussion of the concepts of *fiduciary* and *conflicts of interest* is based on the use of relevant principles in diverse areas of law, on secondary literature, and on analysis of fiduciary relationships. Fiduciary law is not a discrete area of law but a body of related principles that are applied in diverse contexts. Most writing on fiduciary law is limited to particular subjects. For example, there is an enormous literature on fiduciary principles in the law of trusts. See Scott, Austin Wakeman, and William Franklin Fratcher. 1987. *The Law of Trusts* (4th ed.). Boston: Little, Brown.

In-depth analysis of fiduciary law principles in general and comparative analysis of fiduciary law principles are underdeveloped. There are three main books:

Shepard, J.C. 1981. *The Law of Fiduciaries*. Toronto: Carswell.

Finn, P. D. 1977. *Fiduciary Obligations*. Sydney: Law Book.

Vinter, Ernest. 1955. *Treatise on the History and Law of Fiduciary Relationship and Resulting Trusts: Together with a Selection of Selected Cases*. (3rd ed.). Cambridge: Heffer.

There are also several articles. See, for example:

Cooter, Robert, and Bradley J. Freeman. 1991. "The Fiduciary Relationship, Its Economic Character and Legal Consequences." *New York University Law Review* 66(4):1045-1075.

Clark, Robert Charles. 1985. "Agency Costs versus Fiduciary Duties," in *Principles and Agents: The Structure of Business*, John W. Pratt and Richard Zeckhauser, eds. Boston: Harvard University Business School Press.

Frankel, Tamar. 1983. "Fiduciary Law." *California Law Review* 71(3):795-836.

Weinrib, Ernest J. 1975. "The Fiduciary Obligation." *University of Toronto Law Journal* 25:1-22.

Sealy, L.S. 1963. "Fiduciary Relationships." *Cambridge Law Journal*. pp. 119-140.

Sealy, L. S. 1962. "Fiduciary Relationships." *Cambridge Law Journal*, pp. 69-81.

Scott, Austin W. 1949. "The Fiduciary Principle." *California Law Review* 37(4):539-555.

[6]There have been other attempts to use a common term for the party on whose behalf the fiduciary acts. Sometimes writers use the term *beneficiary*. However, this term suggests that the party is receiving something, such as a gift, and this is not always the case. It also does not convey a central feature of the relationship, namely, that the party is *entitled* to expect certain things from the fiduciary. Tamar Frankel has coined the term *entrustor*, which conveys this sense with regard to the person on whose behalf the fiduciary acts. Frankel, Tamar. 1983. "Fiduciary Law." 800, fn. 17. But this term, too, has limitations. It suggests that the entrustor is giving power or authority to the trustee, which is not so in all situations. Sometimes a third party grants the authority or power to the fiduciary for the benefit of another. To meet some of these objections, I have coined the term *fiducie*. It does not suggest any particular kind of fiduciary relationship and clearly links the fiduciary to the party on whose behalf he or she acts.

[7]Although the concept of fiduciary in law originates in trust law in the Middle Ages, devices similar to trusts were also developed in Roman law and European civil law. Indeed, the idea of stewardship, which is similar, is found in the Bible. One noted scholar of trusts has compared the modern conceptions of fiduciaries to the parable of the unjust steward in the Gospel according to Saint Luke (chapter 16). Scott, Austin W. 1949. "The Fiduciary Principle." The parable uses the unjust steward's divided loyalties as an analogy for divided loyalties in serving both God and Mammon: ("No servant can serve two masters: for either he will hate the one, and love the other; or else he will hold to the one, and despise the other.").

[8]There are many reasons why a donor may want to give money or other property to an individual through a trust. The beneficiary may be a minor or legally incompetent (and not able to manage his or her affairs). Or a professional may be better able to invest the funds than the beneficiary. The settlor (the person who funds the trust) may want to transfer the property for restrictive purposes, such as the beneficiary's education, and a trust can ensure that the money is spent as indicated. If the donor bequeaths the money or other property through a will with the intent of having the beneficiary receive the money over several years, a trust can allow the trustee to control the distribution of funds as intended, whereas a direct gift would not.

Settlors may also want to divide their estates between several individuals, such as between their spouse and children, based on their needs. A trustee can be the neutral party who determines their relative needs. Trusts also allow flexibility in apportioning money. A fund can be invested, with interest flowing to one individual for a set period of time and the principal flowing to another at the expiration of that period. Trusts have also been used in business to achieve a number of purposes, including financing, issuing corporate bonds, real estate transactions, assignment for creditors, and liquidation of business affairs. See Isaacs, Nathan. 1929. "Trusteeship in Modern Business." *Harvard Law Review* 42(8):1048-1061.

Courts hold other property holders—bailees, executors, receivers, and guardians—to fiduciary standards. In all these relationships, one party holds or controls property for the benefit of others.

[9]Before the passage of the Rules Enabling Act in 1938, there were two parts of the Anglo-American judicial system: law and equity. Law was a highly formal and rigid system that did not adapt well to new circumstances. As a result, subjects would go to the King's chancellor to obtain a new remedy or some measure of justice that law could not provide. The chancellor's power was described as equity. Over time two distinct judicial systems emerged, each with its own courts, rules, and jurisdiction.

The creation of trusts was the product of these two systems. Title to property was controlled by law, but equity was allowed to control the use of property, thus bifurcating ownership interests between two different parties. For a discussion of the division of law and equity, see Maitland, F. W. (Revised by John Brunyate). 1936. *Equity*. London: Cambridge University Press. A summary of how the distinction lives on today is provided in Woodard, Calvin. 1986. "Progress and Poverty in American Law and Legal Education." *Syracuse Law Review* 37(3):795-850.

[10]*Restatement of Trusts (Second)*. 1959. St. Paul: American Law Institute. Section 179(1).

[11]*Restatement of Trusts (Second)*.

Enslen v. Allen, 160 Ala. 529, 49 So. 430 (1909).

[12]Scott, Austin Wakeman, and William Franklin Fratcher. 1987. *The Law of Trusts* (4th ed.). Boston: Little, Brown.

Scott, Austin Wakeman. 1967. *The Law of Trusts* (3rd ed.). Boston: Little, Brown. Vol. 2, Section 170.12, at 1326.

[13]Scott, Austin Wakeman. 1967. *Law of Trusts*. Vol. 3, Section 216, 216.3.

Scott, Austin Wakeman, and William Franklin Fratcher. 1987. *Law of Trusts*.

[14]Bogart, George C., and George T. Bogart. 1973. *Handbook of the Law of Trusts*, (5th ed.). St. Paul, Minn.: West. p. 343.

[15]*Garrett v. First Nat. Bank*, 233 Ala. 467, 172 So. 611 (1937).

[16]Scott, Austin Wakeman, and William Franklin Fratcher. 1987. *Law of Trusts*. Vol. 2A, Section 170.1, pp. 317-318.

[17]*In re. Kline*, 142 N.J.Eq. 20, 59 A.2d 14. (1948).

[18]*Continental Ill. Nat. Bank & Tr. Co. v. Kelley*, 333 Ill. App. 119, 76 N.E. 2d. 820 (1948).

[19]Another example is guardianship. Parents are the natural guardians of their children. They not only can hold property for the benefit of their children but also have the responsibility to educate, nurture, and care for them. If a child's natural parents are deceased or no longer willing or able to care for their child, courts will appoint another guardian. Guardians have discretion in fulfilling their obligations, but they are subject to supervision by courts. If a guardian acts in a manner contrary to the child's interest by neglecting or abusing the child, courts can remove the guardian and appoint a new one. Courts can also enjoin the child's guardian from acting in an abusive or neglectful manner. Parents and other guardians act like trustees and have authority to make decisions on behalf of their children for the benefit of the children. In this respect, parents also are fiduciaries, and courts have held them accountable to the high standards of conduct expected of fiduciaries. With respect to medical care, custody, and other things that are crucial to the well-being of children, guardians are expected to promote their wards' best interests.

[20]Agency involves several relationships, including master and servant, employer and employee, and proprietor and independent contractor. Agency can be general or for a limited purpose. *Restatement of Agency (Second)*. (1958).

For a discussion of the theoretical literature on principals and agents, see Buchanan, Allen. 1988. "Principal / Agent Theory and Decisionmaking in Health Care." *Bioethics* 2(4):317-333.

[21]*Restatement of Agency (Second)*. Section 13, comment a.

Hobson v. Eaton, 399 F.2d 781 (6th Cir. 1988).

[22]Seavey, Warren A. 1964. *Handbook of the Law of Agency*. (Section 147). St. Paul, Minn.: West.

Restatement of Agency (Second). Sections 387, 390. Section 390 reads: "Unless otherwise agreed, an agent is subject to a duty to his principal to act solely for the benefit of the principal in all matters connected with his agency."

Comment b. "The agent's duty is not only to act solely for the benefit of the principal but also to take no unfair advantage of his position in the use of information or things acquired by him because of the opportunities which his position affords... His duties of loyalty to the interest of his principal are the same as those of a trustee to his beneficiaries."

[23]*Restatement of Agency (Second)*. Sections 393-394, 389-392.

Nagle v. Todd 185 Md. 512, 45 A.2d 326 (1946).

[24]*Restatement of Agency (Second)*. Sections 395-396.

[25]*Restatement of Agency (Second)*. Section 387, Comment b.

[26]*Williams v. Queen Fisheries, Inc.*, 2 Wash. App. 691, 469 P.2d 583 (1970). *Restatement of Agency (Second)*. Section 387, Comment b.

[27]The Supreme Court has held that public employees may be dismissed "if they refuse to account for their performance of their public trust." *Uniformed Sanitation Men v. Commissioner of Sanitation*, 392 U.S. 280, 285 (1968).

[28]Ethics in Government Act of 1978, P.L. No. 95-521, 95th Congress, 2nd Session, 92 Stat., 1864, codified in relevant parts in 18 U.S. C. A. Section 207, as amended by P.L. 96-28, Sections 1 and 2, 96th Congress, 1st Session, 93 Stat. 76.

These statutes do not generally use the term *fiduciary*, although they set forth traditional fiduciary obligations. See Holmes, James E. 1961. "The Federal Conflicts of Interests Statutes and the Fiduciary Principle." *Vanderbilt Law Review* 14(4):1485-1509.

[29]*Meinhard v. Salmon*, 163 N.E. 545, 546 (N.Y.C.A.) (1928).

[30]*Restatement of Agency (Second)*. Section 1(1-3).

[31]Courts have applied fiduciary principles to three main groups: (a) *property holders*, such as trustees; (b) *representatives*, such as agents, partners, lawyers, elected officeholders, corporate officers and directors, and public officials; and (c) *advisers*, such as investment advisers, lawyers, and guardians. These three categories, which often overlap, are useful in suggesting the kinds of activities that courts have traditionally defined as fiduciaries. See Shepard, J. 1981. *Law of Fudicuiaries*. Ch. 2.

[32]It is not strictly accurate to make such generalizations without qualifiers. But my purpose here is to set forth the broad general standards to which fiduciaries are held, not to state a rule or qualifying test.

[33]However, parties can structure their relations so that they do not engage in activities that are currently subject to fiduciary law.

[34]Over time, courts have developed legal principles in several distinct areas of law and have applied these principles to new situations that appeared analogous. In addition, common law fiduciary principles have been the basis for new or more extensive obligations imposed by legislation. For example, Congress enacted the Investment Company Act and the Investment Advisers Act to remedy abuses in these fields. See Frankel, Tamar. 1978-80. *The Regulation of Money Managers: The Investment Company Act and the Investment Advisors Act*. Boston: Little, Brown.

[35]Many relationships have attributes of those recognized as fiduciary but are not themselves considered fiduciary relationships. For example, automobile mechanics give advice and have special expertise, and customers depend on their judgment and honesty; but auto mechanics are not considered fiduciaries. There are three reasons why activities such as these are not covered by fiduciary principles. First, and foremost, these activities are different in degree rather than in kind. Their importance and the degree of the purchaser's vulnerability are generally less than in fiduciary relationships. The market generally does an adequate job of holding the mechanics accountable. Second, courts and legislatures have been more willing to impose fiduciary standards on the classic

professions because of tradition, their independence, and self-regulation. Third, the decision to hold any class or individual to fiduciary standards is a social decision. If society, through the action of courts, legislatures, and other means, wishes to extend fiduciary obligations to auto mechanics or other groups, it can.

Even individuals performing roles that are not regulated explicitly as fiduciaries may be held to some similar obligations. Federal and many state consumer protection laws require sellers to make full disclosure of material facts to prospective purchasers and impose penalties for failure to do so and for making misrepresentations. These are similar to many disclosure obligations for brokers and others involved in the sale of securities regulated by the Securities Exchange Act of 1934 (29 United Sates Code, Section 1001 *et seq.*)

See, e.g., Federal Trade Commission Act, 15 U.S.C., Section 45, *et. seq.* Regulation of Business Practices and Consumer Protection Act, Massachusetts General Laws, Chapter 93-A.

Slaney v. Westwood Auto. 366 Mass 688, 705 (1975).

Bailey, Patricia P., and Michael Pertschuck. 1984. "The Law of Deception: The Past as Prologue." *American Law Review* 33(4):849-897.

Reich, Robert. 1979. "Towards a New Consumer Protection." *Pennsylvania Law Review.* 128(1):1-40.

[36]In recent years, many of the common law rules regarding fiduciaries have been codified in the United States Code. See Bogart, George C., and George T. Bogart. 1973. *Law of Trusts.* pp. 15-17 and extensive citations listed therein.

[37]One health law scholar has even asked whether fiduciary principles *should* constrain physicians' behavior. Miller, Frances H. 1983. "Secondary Income from Recommended Treatment: Should Fiduciary Principles Constrain Physician Behavior?" in *The New Health Care for Profit: Doctors and Hospitals in a Competitive Environment*, Bradford Gray, ed. Washington, D.C.: National Academy Press. pp. 153-170.

[38]*Miller v. Kennedy* 522 P.2d 852 (Wash. App. 1974).

Canterbury v. Spense, 464 F.2d 772 (D.C. App. 1972).

Cobbs v. Grant, 104 Cal. Rptr. 505 (1972).

Lockett v. Goodill 430 P.2d 589 (Wash. 1967).

Hammonds v. Aetna Casualty & Surety Co., 243 F. Supp. 793 (Ohio 1965)

[39]My discussion is limited to conflict-of-interest law for federal government employees. As of 1974, 43 states have adopted conflict-of-interest statutes. For an analysis of state laws, see Grant, James M. 1974. "Analysis of Financial Disclosure Laws of Public Officials." *Saint Louis University Law Journal* 18:641-661.

See also *Model State Conflict of Interest and Financial Disclosure Law.* 1979. New York: National Municipal League.

Council on Governmental Ethics Laws. 1979 Draft, Model Law.

For a discussion of the issues in Britain, see Williams, Sandra. 1985. *Conflicts of Interest: The Ethical Dilemma in Politics.* Aldershot: Gower.

[40]Swart, K. W. 1949. *Sale of Offices in the Seventeenth Century.* The Hague: Martinus Nijhoff.

[41]Filmer, Robert. 1949. *Patriarcha and Other Political Works by Robert Filmer.* Oxford: Oxford University Press. (Written in the 1630s and published in 1680 as *Patriarcha: Of the Natural Power of Kings.*)

[42]Locke, John. 1960. *Two Treatises on Government,* Peter Laslett, ed. Cambridge: Cambridge University Press. (Originally published in 1690.)

[43]Rogers, E. Mabry, and Stephen B. Young. 1975. "Public Office as a Public Trust: A Suggestion That Impeachment for High Crimes and Misdemeanors Implies a Fiduciary Standard." *The Georgetown Law Journal* 63(5):1025-1049.

The idea is not confined to contemporary society. In *The Republic of Plato,* the philosopher kings are guardians and receive only sustenance, in return for which they devote their entire attention to care of the state and themselves. *The Republic of Plato.* 1968. (Alan Bloom, trans.) New York: Basic Books. p. 543.

[44]Banfield, Edward C. 1975. "Corruption as a Feature of Governmental Organization." *Journal of Law and Economics* 18(3):587-605.

[45]Perkins, Roswell B. 1963. "The New Federal Conflict-of-Interest Law." *Harvard Law Review* 76(6):1113-1169, at 1117.

[46]My focus is on the main thrust of the statutes and the regulatory structures they create. I will state some qualifications in notes, but readers interested in the technical aspects of the statutes and the regulatory structure should consult the statutes and key studies listed below. In addition to regulations promulgated by the Office of Governmental Ethics which are generally applicable, agencies have established their own additional regulations.

Statutes

18 U.S.C. App. Section 101 *et. seq.*

5 U.S.C. Section 201 *et. seq.*

28 U.S.C. Section 591 *et. seq.*

P.L. 87-849 (1963); P.L. 95-521 (Ethics in Government Act of 1978); Ethics Reform Act of 1989, P.L. 101-194; 103 Stat. 1717; 5 U.S.C. App. 101 Note.

Regulations

5 CFR, 2634 Executive Personnel Financial Disclosure Requirements; Part 735 Agency Regulations Governing Ethical and Other Conduct and Responsibilities of Employees.

Limitations on Outside Employment and Prohibition of Honoraria; Confidential Reporting of Payment to Charities in Lieu of Honoraria, Part 2636; Standards of Ethical Conduct for Employees of the Executive Branch, 5 CFR 2635,August 7, 1992; Definition of Honoraria 5 CFR 601, January 8, 1992. P.L. 102-90, 1992 Legislative Branch Appropriations Act.

Presidential directives and agency regulations.

Executive Order No. 11222, Part II, Section 205; Part III, Section 3030, 30 *Federal Register.* 6469 (1965), as amended by Executive Order No. 11590, 36 *Federal Register* 7831, reprinted in 18 U.S.C. Section 201 (1976). Now superseded by "Principles of Ethical Conduct for Government Officers and Employees." Executive Order 12674. April 12, 1989. 54 *Federal Register* 15159-15162, as amended by Executive Order 1273, October 17, 1990, 55 *Federal Register* 42547-42550.

Studies

Roberts, Robert N. 1988. *White House Ethics: The History of the Politics of Conflict of Interest Regulation.* New York: Greenwood Press.

Vaughn, Robert A. 1979. *Conflict of Interest Regulation in the Federal Executive Branch.* Lexington, Mass.: Lexington Books.

Manning, Bayless. 1964. *Federal Conflict of Interest Law.* Cambridge: Harvard University Press.

Perkins, Roswell. 1963. "Conflict-of-Interest Law."

Association of the Bar of the City of New York. 1960. *Conflict of Interest and Federal Service.* Cambridge: Harvard University Press.

For a brief history and summary see, Amer, Mildred L. 1992. "Ethics in Government Reform of Laws and Regulations." *Congressional Research Service Issue Brief.* Washington, D.C: Congressional Research Service. Order Code IB89134.

[47]One writer on ethics codes of the U.S. Senate contrasts the corruption of individuals with arrangements that tempt otherwise honest ones. "The real danger we face does not come from a few greedy and corrupt individuals who manage to get into positions of power. It comes from our unwitting drift toward a system in which unethical behavior would be the sine qua non of political survival. In the past, ethics reform in the Congress has been directed toward individuals who corrupt the system. In the future, it must be directed toward a system that tends to corrupt individuals." Jennings, Bruce. 1981. "The Institutionalization of Ethics in the U.S. Senate." *The Hastings Center Report* 11(1) (Special Supplement):5-9, at 9.

[48]Perkins, Roswell. 1963. "Conflict-of-Interest Law." Perkins identifies five main provisions. See pp. 1117-1122.

Self-Dealing by a Public Official: "Public officials must disqualify themselves from participating in government action when a particular course of government action may significantly affect their personal economic interests." p. 1118.

Discretionary Transfer of Economic Value to a Public Official from a Private Source: "Public officials should not be allowed to accept transfers of economic value from private sources, even though no bribery is involved, if the transfer is at the discretion of the transferor as distinct from being pursuant to an enforceable contract or property right of the public official." p. 1119.

Assistance by Public Officials to Private Parties Dealing with Government: "[P]ublic officials should not in general be permitted to step out of their official roles to assist private entities or persons in their dealing with government." p. 1120.

Post-employment Assistance by Former Public Officials to Private Parties Dealing with Government: "[F]ormer public officials should not, within certain narrow limits of time and degree of connection with their former responsibilities, be

allowed to assist private entities or persons in their dealings with government."
p. 1121.

Private Gain Derived from Information Acquired in an Official Capacity: "Public officials should not be permitted to use for personal economic gain confidential information acquired in their official capacities." p. 1121.

[49]When the Attorney General receives information suggesting that a high-level executive branch official may have violated federal law, he is required to conduct a special preliminary inquiry. If there is sufficient evidence to merit a full investigation and if further investigation might reveal a personal, financial, or political conflict of interest by department officials, the Attorney General must request that the Court of Appeals for the District of Columbia appoint a special counsel to take charge of the case. When the court receives the Attorney General's request, it chooses the independent counsel and determines his or her jurisdiction (28 U.S.C., Section 593). The independent counsel is not subject to the control of the Department of Justice but has all the usual powers of Justice Department attorneys to investigate and, if necessary, prosecute officials.

[50]The language of Section 208 (a) is more precise. It refers to "he, his spouse, minor child, partner, organization in which he is serving as officer, director, trustee, partner or employee, or any person or organization with whom he is negotiating or has any arrangement concerning prospective employment."

The affiliations with organizations include nonprofit entities. The requirement of an employee to have knowledge of the financial interest allows the employee to own securities and other financial assets through a blind trust.

[51]18 U.S.C., Section 208 (b). The exemption must be given in advance of participation. The supervisor must find that the financial interest is so insubstantial as to be unlikely to affect the integrity of services that the government is likely to receive from the employee.

[52]18 U.S.C., Section 209(a) prohibits executive branch employees from receiving "any salary, or any contribution to or supplementation of salary, as compensation for his services as an officer or employee of the executive branch of the United States Government. . ."

[53]5 CFR Part 735.202; and agency rules promulgated pursuant to Executive Order 11222; 57 *Federal Register* 35006-35067. Standards of Ethical Conduct for Employees of the Executive Branch. Aug. 7, 1992.

[54]The Legislative Branch Appropriations Act of 1992, P.L. 102-90 (1992). There are provisions for waiving compliance with the monetary limit on gifts in limited circumstances.

[55]5 U.S.C. App. 7, Section 501 (a); 5 CFR, Part 2636.304. The restriction applies to noncareer employees af all three branches.

[56]5 U.S.C. App. 7 Section 501 (b).

[57]18 U.S.C., Section 207.

[58]18 U.S.C., Section 207 (b) and (f).

[59]18 U.S.C., Section 216.

[60]See presidential directives and agency regulations: Executive Order No. 11222, Part II, Section 205; Part III Section 3030, 30 Federal Register 6469 (1965), as amended by Executive Order No. 11590, 36 Federal Register 7831, reprinted in 18 U.S.C. Section 201 (1976); 5 CFR, Section 735, 204-5, 735-303 (1987).

[61]5 U.S.C. App. Section 101 *et. seq.* Reports must be retained by the government for six years and made available to the public.

[62]There are certain exemptions for small levels of income, personal hospitality, and small gifts from relatives. The precise requirements of what kinds of income must be listed, and how, are extremely detailed and take up a large part of the statute.

[63]The act requires officials to disclose any position of an officer, director, partner, proprietor, representative, employee, etc. 5 U.S.C., App. Sec 102 (a)(6)(A).

[64]In the executive branch, the Office of Government Ethics must approve the trust instrument and the trustee. The trustee must be independent of the employee, must be able to sell or transfer assets, and may not report details of the trust investments to the employee.

[65]Most of the problems found by GAO can be traced to the confidentiality of the current reporting system. Conflict-of-interest procedures are based totally on secretive, in-house review and enforcement. There is no public scrutiny of financial statements, of the procedures and justifications for granting exemptions, of the remedial actions prescribed to remedy conflicts, or of any other part of the process. All this has fostered neglect and outright abuse.
Common Cause. 1976. *Serving Two Masters: A Common Cause Study of Conflicts of Interest in the Executive Branch.* Washington, D.C.: Common Cause. pp. 15-16.

[66]28 U.S.C., Section 591 *et. seq.*

[67]Neely, Alfred S., IV. 1984. *Ethics-in-Government Laws: Are They Too "Ethical"?* Washington D.C.: American Enterprise Institute for Public Policy Research. pp. 1-58.
The theme is also developed in *Conflict of Interest and Federal Service.* 1960; Perkins, Roswell. 1963. *"Conflict-of-Interest Law."*
This is a peculiarly American issue. The United States has far more high-level employees who serve on a short-term basis than do Britain, France, and other countries with prestigious professional civil services.

[68]Manning, Bayless. 1964. *Federal Conflict of Interest Law.*
Knight, Frank H. 1961. "Some Comments on the Assumption Underlying the Conflict-of-Interest Concept." *University of Chicago Law School Conference on Conflict of Interest.* Conference Series No. 17. pp. 92-98.

[69]*National Treasury Union et al. v. United States.,* 788 F. Supp. 4 (D.D.C., 1992).

[70]Many gifts considered acceptable under the AMA's ethical guidelines are prohibited for physicians working in the federal government. Proposed regulations specifically note that a purchasing agent for a Veteran's Administration hospital may not routinely accept even a sandwich lunch from

a sales rep-resentative. Federal Register 56:3795, July 23, 1991. But the AMA says it is acceptable for physicians to accept modest meals from pharmaceutical industry representatives if they serve an educational function. Council on Ethical and Judicial Affairs. 1991. *Annotated Guidelines on Gifts to Physicians from Industry*. Chicago: American Medical Association.

[71]Weiss, Phillip. 1989. "Conduct Unbecoming?" *New York Times Sunday Magazine* (October 29):40, 68-71, 95.

Scientific Fraud. Hearings before the Subcommittee on Oversight and Investigations of the Committee on Energy and Commerce, House of Representatives, 100th Congress, 1st Session, May 4 and 9, 1989. Serial No. 101-64. Washington, D.C.: U.S. Government Printing Office.

[72]*S.E.C. v. Willis*, 777 F. Supp. 1165 (S.D.N.Y. 1991): 787 F. Supp. 58 (1992).

Lambert, Wade, and Edward Felsenthal. 1990. "Insider-Trading Rule Extends to Therapy Relationship." *The Wall Street Journal* (May 17):B10.

See also, Rodwin, Marc A. 1993. "Forum Commentary: Insider Information: A Legal and Ethical Analysis." *Ethics & Behavior* 3(1).

[73]Miller, Michael W. 1992. "Patients' Records Are Treasure Trove for Budding Industry." *The Wall Street Journal* (February 27):1, A6.

[74]This section focuses on laws and public policies. It does not discuss conflict-of-interest policies and codes of ethics of individual business organizations because these are private matters. Nevertheless, such policies abound. For a sample, see Southwestern Graduate School of Banking. 1980. *A Study of Corporate Ethical Policy Statements*. Dallas: Southwestern Graduate School of Banking Foundation. These policies typically protect corporations and other organizations from the conflicts of interest of employees. For example, policies often prevent employees who are responsible for purchasing materials for the firm from buying the materials from themselves, relatives, or business associates.

[75]My discussion of corporate law draws on the following:

Clark, Robert Charles. 1986. *Corporate Law*. Boston: Little, Brown.

American Bar Association. 1985. *Model Business Corporation Act Annotated* (2nd ed.). New York: Harcourt Brace Jovanovich.

Carey, William L., and Melvin Aron Eisenberg. 1980. *Cases and Material on Corporations* (5th ed.). Mineola, N.Y.: Foundation Press.

[76]Majority shareholders are also obligated to act in the corporation's interest.

[77]*Globe Woolen Co. v. Utica Gas & Electric Co.*, 121 N.E. 378 (N.Y. 1918).

[78]This summary of under what circumstances self-dealing is permitted is based on Delaware corporation law and the Model Business Corporation Act (MBCA). See Section 144, Delaware General Corporation Law, and Section 8.31 of the MBCA. These codes are models for many state laws. However, there is still considerable variety and confusion in the law on this point.

Corporations sometimes try to insulate self-dealing transactions through provisions in the articles of incorporation expressly authorizing it. Nevertheless, courts still have the power to void such transactions.

For a case illustrating the third circumstance, see *Flinger v. Lawrence*, 361 A.2d 218 (Del. 1976).

[79]Clark, Robert C. 1986. Section 5.4. pp. 182-189.

[80]Patients can get a second opinion from a physician.

[81]They are, however, quite good at making decisions involving value choices. Since many clinical choices involve a choice of values, it makes sense to promote the ideal of informed consent and patient participation in medical decision making.

[82]The Employment Retirement Income Security Act (ERISA) of 1974, P.L. 93-406 *et seq.* 129 U.S.C., Section 1001 *et. seq.*

[83]ERISA, Section 404.

[84]ERISA, Sections 409, 501.

[85]ERISA Sections 406-407 list prohibited transactions. Section 408 lists exemptions from prohibited transactions. Section 408 also empowers the Secretary of Labor to establish an exemptions procedure.

[86]ERISA, Sections 504 and 505.

[87]ERISA, Section 101-107.

[88]ERISA, Sections 202, 203, 302-306.

[89]The following are the main statutes and regulations: Securities Act of 1933, P.L. No. 22, 73rd Cong., 15 U.S.C. 77 *et seq.*; 1933 Act Rules, 17 C.F.R., Section 230 *et seq.*; Securities and Exchange Act of 1934; 1934 Act Rules, 17 C.F.R., Section 240; the Investment Company Act and the Investment Advisers Act of 1940. States also regulate the sale of securities.

The following are key secondary sources:

Ratner, David L. 1986. *Securities Regulation: Materials For a Basic Course*, (3rd ed.). St. Paul, Minn.: West.

Frankel, Tamar. 1978-80. *Regulation of Money Managers.*

Loss, Louis. 1961. *Securities Regulation* (2nd ed.). Boston: Little, Brown.

For an introduction, see Ratner, David L. 1978. *Securities Regulation in a Nutshell.* St. Paul, Minn.: West.

[90]Section 15(a), 1934 Act; Section 203, Investment Advisers Act of 1940.

[91]Section 20 of the 1934 Act, Section 15 of the 1934 Act; *Marbury Management v. Kohn*, 629 F.2d 705 (2nd Cir. 1980), establishes civil liability under common law.

Although I know of no studies comparing these fields, my impression is that the volume of suits and sums of money involved in lawsuits seeking tort and statutory damages in the securities field dwarfs the field of medical malpractice.

[92]Securities Act of 1933, P.L. No. 22, 73rd Congress, 15 U.S.C. 77 *et seq.* The 1934 Act, Sections 12, 13, 14, and 16, require disclosure for publicly traded companies and many other large companies.

Coffee, John C., Jr. 1984. "Market Failure and the Economic Case for a Mandatory Disclosure System." *Virginia Law Review* 70(4):717-753.

For an in-depth discussion of the policy debates about the SEC disclosure requirements, see Seligman, Joel. 1985. "The Corporate Disclosure Debate," in *The SEC and the Future of Finance*. New York: Prager. pp. 195-280.

Easterbrook, Frank H., and Daniel H. Fischel. 1984. "Mandatory Disclosure and the Protection of Investors." *Virginia Law Review* 70(4):669-715.

Securities Acts Amendments of 1964 extend disclosure requirements to many firms trading on OTC.

[93] 1933 Act, Section 5.

The 1934 Act, Section 12, requires registration with the SEC if the security is traded on a national securities exchange.

[94]Sections 7, and 10, Form A. Regulations S-K and S-X set forth requirements for disclosure of securities and financial statements.

The buyer often receives the prospectus after making the purchase. However, the requirement that sellers provide a prospectus probably helps deter oral misrepresentations.

[95] Securities Act of 1933, Section 11(e),(g), 12.

Escott v. Barchris Construction Corp., 283 F. Sup. 643 (S.D.N.Y. 1968).

[96]All parties that are potentially liable, except issuers, can avoid liability if they can prove either that they met prescribed standards of diligence in their work, did not know and did not have reason to know that the prospectus was misleading, or if they attempted to withdraw their approval of the prospectus and warn the SEC of the misleading statements. Securities Act of 1933, Sections 11, 12. Section 11(b).

[97]Investment Advisors Act, Sections 206(1)(2)(3);

University Management Corp., Adv-388 (1973);

Western Guarantee Management Corp., 34-8494 (1969).

SEC v. Capital Gains Research Bureau, 375 U.S.180 (1963).

[98]Section 17(d) and 17(e)(1) of the 1940 Act and antifraud provision of the Advisers Act. *SEC v. Capital Gains Research Bureau*, 375 U.S.180 (1963).

[99]Broker-dealers who fail to make such disclosure are liable for damages. *Zweig v. Hearst Corporation*, 594 F.2d 1261 (9th Cir. 1979). Rule 10(b)(5).

Arlene W. Hughes, 27 SEC 629 (1948).

[100]*Restatement of Agency (Second)*. Section 390.

Newkirk v. Hayden, Stone & Co., CCH [1964-1966 Trans. Binder] Fed. Sec. L. Rep. Par. 91,621 at 95,320 (S.D. Cal. 1965).

[101]*Restatement of Agency (Second)*. (1958). Sections 389, 390 comment c.

[102]SEC. June 20, 1936. *Report on the Feasibility and Advisability of the Complete Segregation of the Functions of Dealer and Broker*. Washington, D.C..
Opinion of the Director of Trading and Exchange Division. Adv-40 at 3, (1945).

[103]SEC Rule 15c1-7; *Horne v. Francis I. Dupont & Co.*, 428 F. Sup. 1271 (D.C.1977);

Shearson, Hammill & Co., 42 S.E.C. 811 (1965).

[104]*Charles Hughes & Co., Inc. v. SEC*, 139 F. 2d 434 (2nd Cir. 1943).

[105]*Merrill, Lynch.* SEC Ex. Act Rel. No. 14149.

Phillips v. Reynolds & Co., 294 F. Supp. 1249 (E.D. Pa. 1969).

[106]The adversarial ethic is most developed in litigation. However, the adversarial ethic and role applies in representing clients outside of litigation as well.

[107]Canon 6 of the 1908 Canons of Professional Responsibility states that "it is unprofessional to represent conflicting interests, except by express consent of all concerned given after a full disclosure of the facts." The Canon defines conflicting interests as occurring "when, in behalf of one client, it is [the lawyer's] duty to contend for that which duty to another client requires him to oppose."

[108]The Code of Professional Responsibility is divided into two main parts: Ethical Considerations (ECs), which set aspirational goals, and Disciplinary Rules (DRs), which are prescriptive and serve as a basis for taking disciplinary action.

In most jurisdictions, the Code of Professional Responsibility was adopted by the state supreme court, and thus takes precedence over all law except federal law and state constitutional law. Some states, however, have adopted the Code as guidelines. Federal courts have also widely adopted the Code as local rules. The *Model Rules* consist of 52 rules and comments explaining the rules. Some of the rules impose obligations and prohibitions, others delineate areas in which lawyers are not subject to discipline, and still others describe lawyers' roles.

[109]See Cratsley, John C. 1980. *Inherent Powers of the Courts.* Reno: National Judicial College, American Bar Association at the University of Nevada.

[110]*United Sewerage Agency v. Jelco, Inc.*, 646 F.2d, 1339, 1342, n.1 (9th Cir. 1981).

The 1969 Code of Professional Responsibility and the 1983 Model Rules of Professional Conduct state that violations of rules should not in themselves be a basis for liability. However, courts have looked to these codes as evidence of professional conduct. See *Woodruff v. Tomlin*, 616 F.2d 924, 936 (6th Cir.), cert. denied, 449 U.S. 888, 101 S.Ct. 246, 66 L. Ed. 2d 114 (1980).

[111]I use the term *codes of conduct* to refer collectively to the various codes adopted by courts as rules.

[112]Some courts speak of "irreconcilable conflicts." *In re Cohn*, 46 N.J. 202, 216 A.2d 1 (1969).

Other courts speak of "nonconsentable conflicts." *Valley Title Co. v. Superior Court*, 124 Cal. App. 3d 867, 177 Cal. Rptr. 643 (1981).

[113] "In the situations covered in DR 5-105(A) and (B), a lawyer may represent multiple clients if it is obvious that he can adequately represent the interests of each and if each consents to the representation after full disclosure of the possible effects of such representation on his independent professional

judgment on behalf of each." *(Code of Professional Responsibility.* 1969. Chicago: American Bar Association. DR 5-105(C).)

(a) A lawyer shall not represent a client if the representation of that client will be directly adverse to another client, unless:

(1) the lawyer reasonably believes the representation will not adversely affect the relationship with the other client; and

(2) each client consents after consultation.

(b) A lawyer shall not represent a client if the representation of that client may be materially limited by the lawyer's responsibilities to another client or to a third person, or by the lawyer's own interests, unless:

(1) the lawyer reasonably believes the representation will not be adversely affected; and

(b) the client consents after consultation. When representation of multiple clients in a single matter is undertaken, the consultation shall include explanation of the implications of the common representation and the advantages and risks involved. *Model Rules of Professional Conduct.* 1983. Chicago: American Bar Association. Rule 1.7. In the final analysis, courts decide whether a lawyer can adequately represent a client and whether it is reasonable to believe that representation will not be adversely affected. The individual lawyer's subjective intentions are not controlling. See Wolfram, Charles W. 1986. *Modern Legal Ethics.* St. Paul, Minn.: West. p. 341.

[114]Freedman, Monroe H. 1990. *Understanding Lawyers' Ethics.* New York: Matthew Bender.

Freedman, Monroe H. 1975. *Lawyers' Ethics in an Adversary System.* Indianapolis: Bobbs-Merrill.

Curtis, Charles. 1951. "The Ethics of Advocacy." *Stanford Law Review* 4 (December):3-23.

[115]Wolfram, Charles W. 1986. *Modern Legal Ethics.*

[116]*Code of Professional Responsibility.* 1969. Chicago: American Bar Association. D.R. 5-105 (D).

Model Rules of Professional Conduct. 1983. Rule 1.10.

[117]*Code of Professional Responsibility.* 1969. D.R. 5-105(D). "If a lawyer is required to decline employment or to withdraw from employment under a Disciplinary Rule, no partner or associate, or any other lawyer affiliated with him or his firm may accept or continue such employment" (as amended in 1974). Case law interprets this rule as allowing representation by affiliated lawyers if the conflict causing the initial lawyer to be disqualified can be cured by consent and the client consents. See, e.g., *In re Yarn Processing Patient Validity Litigation,* 530 F.2d 83 (9th Cir. 1976).

The Model Rules are less restrictive. *Model Rules of Professional Conduct.* 1983. Rule 1.10(a) prohibits lawyers associated in a firm from representing a client in four situations when any of the lawyers practicing alone would be prohibited from doing so: (a) representing the client will be adverse to another client; (b) the representation involves making a gift to lawyers in the firm or to one of their relatives; (c) the lawyer formerly represented a client with adverse interests in a substantially related matter; or (d) the lawyer would represent a client against a client the lawyer had represented as an intermediary.

Rule 1.10(b) prohibits lawyers leaving one firm and working for another from representing a client if there is a risk that they will use confidential information against the interests of the former client. But there is no presumption that all lawyers in the second firm are disqualified.

Rule 1.10(c) states that the client's consent can cure all imputed disqualifications.

[118]*Silver Chrysler Plymouth, Inc. v. Chrysler Motors Corporation*, 518 F. 2d 751 (2nd Cir. 1975).

[119]Wolfram, Charles W. 1986. *Modern Legal Ethics*. pp. 402–403.

[120]ABA Standards for Lawyer Disciplinary and Disability Proceedings, Section 3.4 (approved 1979).

[121]Wolfram, Charles W. 1986. *Modern Legal Ethics*. pp. 85–86.

[122]One indicator of the importance of conflicts of interest in legal ethics is the space devoted to the subject in the leading work on this subject. Charles Wolfram devotes over 250 pages to conflicts of interest in his 1,000-page treatise. However, this number underestimates the importance of conflicts of interest as part of the substantial ethical rules because another 250 pages of the treatise discusses the delivery of legal services and the judiciary, rather than substantive ethics. See, Wolfram, Charles, W. 1986. *Modern Legal Ethics*.

[123]This four-part categorization is my own. Most writers on legal ethics use multiple categories that define various kinds of conflicts of interest much more narrowly, such as simultaneous representation of clients with differing interests, representation of clients with differing interests successively, conflicts of interest involving former clients, problems of representing a corporate entity or the personal interest of the attorney, or conflicts of interest due to imputed disqualification. Other categories used include particular areas of practice such as criminal law, indemnity insurance, mediation, divorce, or representation of particular groups, such as the poor, government, buyers and sellers, or advocacy groups. Such categories are used, in part, to help guide lawyers to the rules applicable to particular situations they face. But they do not categorize conflicts of interest in an analytically interesting manner. See, e.g., Wolfram, Charles, W. 1986. *Modern Legal Ethics*.

Harvard Law Review. 1981. Special Issue: "Developments in the Law: Conflicts of Interest in the Legal Profession." 94(6):1247–1283.

[124]Lawyers' personal interests include not only financial interests but also other interests, such as political commitments. These too can create conflicts of interest, because they can compromise judgment or loyalty. My discussion focuses on financial conflicts.

For certain purposes, a lawyer's personal interests are deemed to include those of family members or associates. When a family member or close associate has a financial interest, it is considered as if it were the lawyer's.

[125]This is the one conflict of interest that is not explicitly addressed through rules regulating the conduct of lawyers. However, it is being addressed in the literature on lawyers' payments, and several authors have proposed reforms.

Kritzer, Herbert M., Austin Sarat, David M. Trubek, Kristin Bumiller, and Elizabeth McNichol. 1984. "Understanding Costs of Litigation: The Case of Hourly Fee Lawyers." *American Bar Foundation Research Journal* 1984(3):559-604.

Leubsdorf, John. 1981. "The Contingency Factor in Attorney Fees Awards." *Yale Law Journal* 90(3):473-513.

Clermont, Kevin M., and John D. Curriuan. 1978. "Improving on the Contingent Fee." *Cornell Law Review* 63(4):529-639.

[126]*Model Rules of Professional Conduct*. 1983. Rule 1.8(a)(2);

In re Kali, 124 Ariz. 592, 606 P.2d 808, 811 (1980).

In re Bartlett, 283 Or. 487, 584 P.2d 296 (1978). Cal.R. 5-101(2).

[127]*People v. Razatos*, 636 P.2d 666 (Colo. 1981).

Giovanazzi v. State Bar, 28 Cal. 3d 465, 169 Cal. Rptr. 581, 585, 619 P.2d 1005, 1009 (1980).

[128]Derrick Bell uses the term *constituents* to refer to civil rights advocates and leaders to whom lawyers representing plaintiffs in school desegregation lawsuits look for advice and approval. Bell, Derek. 1976. "Serving Two Masters: Integration Ideals and Client Interests in School Desegregation Litigation." *Yale Law Journal* 85(4):470-516.

[129]*Code of Professional Responsibility*. 1969. DR 5-107(B); DR 5-107(A); *Model Rules of Professional Conduct*. 1983. Rule 1.8(f).

[130]*Rogers v. Robson, Masters, Ryan, Brumund & Belom*, 81 Ill. 2d 201, 40 Ill. Dec. 816, 407 N.E. 2d 47 (1980).

"Guiding Principles" of the National Conference of Lawyers and Liability Insurers, in *Martindale-Hubbel Law Directory* 7:76M (1978); reprinted in *Federal Insurance Counsel Journal* 1970. 20:95.

[131]*National Association for the Advancement of Colored People v. Button*, 371 U.S. 415, 83 S. Ct. 328, 9 L. Ed. 2d 405 (1963).

[132]*I.B.M. Corp. v. Levin*, 579 F.2d 271 (3d Cir. 1978).

Grievance Committee v. Rottner, 15 2 Conn. 59, 203 A.2d 82 (1964).

[133]Rule 23 of the Federal Rules of Civil Procedure allows bringing lawsuits on behalf of a group of similarly situated plaintiffs, not all of whom need be identified. For a court to certify a class, the individuals must have common claims that can be adequately represented collectively.

[134]*Holoway v. Arkansas*, 435 U.S. 475 (1978).

Jedwabny v. Philadelphia Transportation Co., 390 Penn. 231, 135 A.2d 252 (1957).

[135]*Model Rules of Professional Conduct*. 1983. Rule 1.9(a).

T. C. Theatres, Inc. v. Warner Bros. Circuit Management Corp., 216 F. 2d 920 (2nd Cir. 1954).

[136]*Code of Professional Responsibility*. 1969. DR-7-106(B)(1).

Model Rules of Professional Conduct. 1983. Rule 3.3(a)(3).

In re Price, 429 N.E. 2d 961 (Ind 1982);

In re Drexler, 290 Minn. 542, 546 n.7, 188 N.W. 2d 436 (1971).

[137]*Federal Rules of Civil Procedure*. Rule 11.

The signature of an attorney or party constitutes a certificate by him that he has read the pleading; that to the best of his knowledge, information, and belief, formed after reasonable inquiry, it is well grounded in fact and is warranted by existing law or good faith argument for the extension, modification, or reversal of existing law; and that it is not interposed primarily for any improper purpose, such as to harass, to cause delay, or to increase the cost of litigation.

Model Rules of Professional Conduct. 1983. Rule 3.1.

[138]The Office of Governmental Ethics also scrutinizes the finances of *prospective* officials who have been nominated for executive appointments.

[139]For example, courts require that physicians obtain patients' informed consent prior to treatment, that physicians not abandon patients, and that physicians keep patient information confidential. These are traditional fiduciary obligations, but only a few of the many obligations that most fiduciaries must fulfill.

Humphers v. First Interstate Bank of Oregon, 696 P. 2d 527 (1985);

Alberts v. Devine, 395 Mass. 59 (1984);

Horn v. Patton, 287 So. Rep. 2d 824 (1974);

Ricks v. Budge, 64 P. 2d 208 (1937).

[140]An exception is the recent *Moore v. University of California*, 792 P. 2nd 479, 271 Cal. Rptr. 146, 51 Cal. 3rd 120 (1990). The Moore case, however, addressed financial conflicts of interest in research.

[141]Bogart, George C. and George T. Bogart. 1973. *Law of Trusts*. p. 343.

[142]Chapters 3 and 4 discuss gifts in more detail. Chren, Mary-Margaret, C. Seth Landefeld, and Thomas Murray. 1989. "Doctors, Drug Companies, and Gifts." *Journal of the American Medical Association* 262(24):3448-3451.

Jenike, M. A. 1990. "Relations between Physicians and Pharmaceutical Companies: Where to Draw the Line." *The New England Journal of Medicine* 322(8): 557.

[143]The federal Medicare program is now developing institutions to hold physicians to standards of technical performance and quality.

Relman, Arnold S. 1988. "Assessment and Accountability: The Third Revolution in Medical Care." *The New England Journal of Medicine* 319(18): 1220-1222.

Betz, Michael, and Lenahan O'Connell. 1983. "Changing Doctor-patient Relationships and the Rise in Concern for Accountability." *Social Problems* 31:84-95.

[144]Epstein, Arnold M. 1990. "The Outcomes Movement—Will It Get Us Where We Want to Go?" *The New England Journal of Medicine* 323(4):266-270.

Chapter 8

[1]Aristotle. *Nicomachean Ethics*. 1103b. Translated by Martin Ostwald. 1962. Indianapolis: Bobbs Merrill.

[2]Hirschman, Albert O. 1986. *Rival Views of Market Society and Other Recent Essays*. N.Y.: Viking Press, pp.145-6.

[3]American Medical Association. *Proceedings*. 1992. (June).

McCormick, Brian. 1992. "Referral Ban Softened: Frustrated Physicians OK Self-Referral if Doctors Disclose Ownership of Interests." *American Medical News* (July 6/13):1.

The Royal College of Physicians. 1986. "The Relationship Between Physicians and the Pharmaceutical Industry." *Journal of the Royal College of Physicians of London* 20(4):5-242.

Levinson, Douglas F. 1987. "Toward Full Disclosure of Referral Restrictions and Financial Incentives by Prepaid Health Plans." *The New England Journal of Medicine* 317(27):1729-1731.

Morreim, E. Haavi. 1989. "Conflicts of Interest: Profits and Problems in Physician Referrals." *Journal of the American Medical Association* 262(3):390-394.

Several states also require physicians to disclose financial conflicts of interest in referrals to patients.

[4]It is also possible that the AMA advocates disclosure as a means of staving off changes in medical organization, practice and finances that might reduce income or limit professional autonomy.

[5]My discussion of the limitations of disclosure draws heavily on the text of an article. See, Rodwin, Marc A. 1989. "Physicians' Conflicts of Interest: The Limitations of Disclosure." *The New England Journal of Medicine* 321(20):1205-1408.

[6]Appelbaum, Paul S., Charles W. Lidz, and Alan Meisel. 1987. *Informed Consent: Legal Theory and Clinical Practice*. New York: Oxford University Press.

Canterbury v. Spence, 464 F.2d 772 (D.C. Circuit. 1972).

Cobbs v. Grant, 502 P.2d 1 (Cal. 1972).

[7]Katz, Jay. 1984. *The Silent World of Doctor and Patient.* New York: The Free Press.

[8]Waitzkin, Howard. 1984. "Doctor-Patient Communication: Clinical Implications of Social Scientific Research." *Journal of the American Medical Association* 252(17):2441-2446.

President's Commission for the Study of Ethical Problems in Medicine and Biomedical Behavioral Research. 1982. *Making Health Care Decisions: the Ethical and Legal Implications of Informed Consent in the Patient-Practitioner Relationship: Empirical Studies of Informed Consent.* (Vol.3, appendices). p. 401.

[9]Schneyer, Theodore J. 1976. "Informed Consent and the Danger of Bias in the Formation of Medical Disclosure Practices."*Wisconsin Law Review* 1976(2):124-70.

[10]Faden, Ruth R., and Tom L. Beauchamp. 1986. *A History and Theory of Informed Consent.* New York: Oxford University Press. pp. 298-336.

McNeil, Barbara J., Stephen G. Pauker, Harold C. Sox, et al. 1982. "On the Elicitation of Preferences for Alternative Therapies." *The New England Journal of Medicine* 306(21):1259-1262.

[11]Lidz, Charles W., Alan Meisel, Eviatar Zerubavel, Mary Carter, Regina M. Sestak, and Loren H. Roth. 1983. *Informed Consent: A Study of Decisionmaking in Psychiatry.* New York: Guilford. pp. 128-129.

Korsch, Barbara M., and Negrete, Vida F. 1972. "Doctor-Patient Communication." *Scientific American* 227(6):66-74.

[12]Appelbaum, Paul S., Charles W. Lidz, and Alan Meisel. 1987. *Informed Consent.* p. 171.

[13]Appelbaum, Paul S., Charles W. Lidz, and Alan Meisel. 1987. *Informed Consent.*

Lidz, Charles W., Alan Meisel, Eviatar Zerubavel, Mary Carter, et al. 1983. *Informed Consent.* pp. 91-94.

Grundner, T.M. 1980. "On the Readability of Surgical Consent Forms." *The New England Journal of Medicine* 302(16):900-902.

[14]Appelbaum, Paul S., Charles W. Lidz, and Alan Meisel. 1987. *Informed Consent.* p. 166.

Beecher, Henry K. 1986. "Consent in Clinical Experimentation: Myth and Reality." *Journal of the American Medical Association* 195(24):124-125.

[15]Katz, Jay. 1977. "Informed Consent—A Fairy Tale? Law's Vision." *University of Pittsburgh Law Review* 39(2):137-174.

[16]Hillman, Bruce J., George T. Olson, Patricia E. Griffith, Jonathan H. Sunshine, Catherine A. Joseph, Stephen D. Kennedy, et al. 1992. "Physicians' Utilization and Changes for Outpatient Diagnostic Imaging in a Medicare Population." *Journal of the American Medical Association* 268(15):2050-2054.

Mitchell, Jean M. and Jonathan H. Sunshine. 1992. "Consequences of Physicians' Ownership of Healthcare Facilities-Joint Ventures in Radiation Therapy." *The New England Journal of Medicine* 327(21):1497-1501.

Mitchell, Jean M. and Elton Scott. 1992. "Evidence of Complex Structure of Physician Joint Ventures." *Yale Journal on Regulation* 9(3):489-520.

Mitchell, Jean M. and Elton Scott. 1992. "New Evidence on the Prevalence and Scope of Physician Joint Ventures."*Journal of the American Medical Association* 268(1):80-84.

Mitchell, Jean M. and Elton Scott. 1992. "Physician Ownership of Physical Therapy Services: Effects on Charges, Utilization, Profits, and Service Characteristics." *Journal of the American Medical Association* 268(15):2055-2059.

Swedlow, Alex, Gregory Johnson, Neil Smithline, Arnold Milstein. 1992. "Increased Costs and Rates of Use in the California Workers' Compensation System as a Result of Self-Referral by Physicians."*The New England Journal of Medicine* 327(21):1502-1506.

State of Florida Health Care Cost Containment Board and Department of Economics and Department of Finance, Florida State University. 1991. *Joint Ventures Among Health Care Providers in Florida: Volumes I—III.* Tallahassee, FL.

Hemmenway, David, Alice Killen, Suzanne B. Cashman, et al. 1990. "Physicians' Responses to Financial Incentives: Evidence From a For-Profit Ambulatory Care Center." *The New England Journal of Medicine* 322(15):1059-63.

Hillman, Bruce J., Catherine A. Joseph, Michael R. Mabry, Jonathan H. Sunshine, Stephen D. Kennedy, and Monica Noether. 1990. "Frequency and Costs of Diagnostic Imaging in Office Practice—A Comparison of Self-Referring and Radiologist-Referring Physicians."*The New England Journal of Medicine* 323(23):1604-1608.

Radecki, Stephen E., and James P. Steel. 1990. "Effect of On-Site Facilities on Use of Diagnostic Radiology by Non-Radiologists." *Investigative Radiology* 25(2):190-193.

Kusserow, Richard P. 1989. *Financial Arrangements Between Physicians and Health Care Businesses: Report to Congress.* Washington, D.C.: Office of Inspector General, Department of Health and Human Services. (DHHS Publication No. OA1-12-88-01410.)

Strasser, R.P., M.J. Bass, M. Brennan. 1987. "The Effect of an On-Site Radiology Facility on Radiologic Utilization in Family Practice." *Journal of Family Practice* 24(6):619-623.

Blue Cross and Blue Shield of Michigan, Medical Affairs Division. 1984. *A Comparison of Laboratory Utilization and Payout to Ownership.*

Department of Health and Human Services, Health Care Financing Administration, Division of Health Standards and Quality, Region V. 1983. *Diagnostic Clinical Laboratory Services in Region V.* (No. 2-05-2004-11).

U.S. Department of Health and Human Services, Health Care Financing Administration, Division of Health Standards and Quality, Region V. 1983. *Diagnostic Clinical Laboratory Services in Region V.* (No.2-05-2004-ll).

Medical Services Administration, State of Michigan. 1981. *Utilization of Medicaid Laboratory Services by Physicians With/Without Ownership Interest in*

Clinical Laboratories: A Comparative Analysis of Six Selected Laboratories. Michigan Department of Social Services, Medicaid Monitoring and Compliance Division.

Childs, Alfred A., and E. Diane Hunter. 1972. "Non-Medical Factors Influencing Use of Diagnostic X-ray by Physicians." *Medical Care* 10(4):323-335.

Childs, Alfred W., and D. W. Hunter. 1970. *Patterns of Primary Medical Care—Use of Diagnostic X-Ray by Physicians.* Berkeley: Institute of Business and Economic Research and the School of Public Health, University of California.

[17]Kusserow, Richard P. 1989. *Financial Arrangements.*

[18]For a discussion of physician use of resources in HMOs see, Luft, Harold S. 1984. *Health Maintenance Organizations: Dimensions of Performance.* New York: Wiley. Unfortunately, we do not yet have adequate means to measure underuse, and thus we are uncertain as to the consequences of these practices for the quality of care.

[19]Federal Trade Commission Act, 15 U.S.C., Sec. 41, *et. seq.*

Regulation of Business Practices and Consumer Protection Act, Mass. Gen. Laws, Ch. 93-A.

Bailey, Patricia B., and Pertschuk, Michael. 1984. "The Law of Deception: The Past As Prologue." *American Law Review* 33(4):849-897.

[20]*Slaney v. Westwood Auto.* 366 Mass. 688,705 (1975).

[21]Federal Food, Drug, and Cosmetic Act., 21 U.S.C. Secs. 201, 403.

United States v. Ninety-Five Barrels of ...Apple Cider Vinegar, 265 U.S. 438 (1924). 21 C.F.R. Secs 101.4, 101.22-35.

[22]Claxton, John D., Joseph N. Fry, and Bernard Portis. 1974. "A Taxonomy of Prepurchase Information Gathering." *Journal of Consumer Research* 1(December):35-42.

Newman, Joseph W., and Richard Staelin. 1971. "Multivariate Analysis of Differences in Buyer Decision Time." *Journal of Marketing Research* 8(May):192-8.

[23]Altman, Stuart H., and Marc A. Rodwin. 1988. "Halfway Competitive Markets and Ineffective Regulation: The American Health Care System." *Journal of Health Politics, Policy and Law* 13(2):323-339.

[24]Arrow, Kenneth J. 1963. "Uncertainty and the Welfare Economics of Medical Care." *American Economic Review* 53(2):941-73.

[25]The Boston Women's Health Book Collective. 1984. *The New Our Bodies, Ourselves.* New York: Simon & Schuster.

Malone, Thomas W. and Barbara Paul. 1991. "The Consumer Movement Takes Hold in Medical Care." *Health Affairs* 10:(4):268-281.

[26]Consumer Federation of America. 1989. *Public Opinion About Health Care Purchases: Cost, Ease of Shopping and Availability.*

[27]Reade, Julia M., and Richard M. Ratzan. 1989. "Access to Information—Physicians' Credentials and Where You Can't Find Them." *The New England Journal of Medicine* 321(7):466-8.

[28]In recent years the Health Care Financing Administration has published reports on hospital mortality and infection rates. These are not a good source for

consumer shopping. The reports are sold for hundreds of dollars and are not readily available. In addition, the data do not adequately account for the hospital case mix, the health status of patients treated, or other important variables. Yet this approach has been tried by state agencies, too. See Winslow, Ron. 1992. "Pennsylvania Heart Surgeons Rated by State." *Wall Street Journal* (November 20):B1, 5.

In 1990, *U.S. News and World Report* published a rating of hospitals. Rather than demonstrate the feasibility of providing helpful information to the public, the special issue is an example of the difficulty of doing so. "America's Best Hospitals." 1990. *U.S. News and World Report* (April 30):51-86. A novel approach to providing consumers with information was tried by *Boston Magazine* in 1990. It asked nurses in Boston to rate doctors they worked with and hospitals. Jahnke, Art. 1990. "The Doctors the Nurses Go To." *Boston Magazine* (October):77-83, 111-115.

[29]Kessler, David A. 1989. "The Federal Regulation of Food Labeling: Promoting Foods to Prevent Disease." *The New England Journal of Medicine* 321(11):717-25.

In the summer of 1991 the FDA proposed new labeling requirements that would require much stricter labeling of food. New nutritional labeling requirements will become effective in 1993. See Burros, Marian. 1991. "Coming to Stores Near You: New and Improved Labeling." *New York Times* (June 6):1. Burrows, Marian. 1992. "U.S. Will Require New Labels on Health on Packaged Food." *New York Times*. (December 3):1, A13.

[30]Koop, C. Everett. 1989. *Reducing Health Consequences of Smoking: 25 Years of Progress: A Report of the Surgeon General.* U.S. Department of Heath and Human Services. (DHHS Publication No. 89-8411.) pp. 478-481.

[31]In the past, disclosure of risks has clearly led courts to insulate firms from liability:

Humes v. Clinton, 792 P.2d 1032 (1990).

Wyeth Laboratories Inc. v. Fortenberry, 530 So. 2d 688 (Miss. 1988).

Cobb v. Syntex Laboratories, 444 So. 2d 203 (La. Ct. App. 1983).

Cipollone v. Liggette Group, Inc. 789 F.2d 181 (3rd Cir 1986).

In *Cipollone v. Liggette Group, Inc.*, 120L. Ed. 2d 407, 112 S. Ct. 2068, (1992), the Supreme Court ruled that disclosure of health risks in accordance with federal law does not preempt all civil suits against tobacco companies. Now, no easy generalizations are possible. The Supreme Court remanded the *Cipollone* case for a new trial. However, the lawyer for the Cippollone family voluntarily dismissed the lawsuit just under five months later, despite having won a $400,000-dollar verdict at the first trial before the case was appealed to the Supreme Court. Apparently the lawyers felt that the burden of proof the Supreme Court established was too high. See Strum, Charles. 1992. "Major Cigarette Suit Dropped by Cipollone Family After 10 Years." *New York Times* (Nov. 6):B 1, 5.

Annas, George. 1992. "Health Warnings, Smoking, and Cancer: The Cipollone Case." *The New England Journal of Medicine* 327(2):1604-1607.

[32]Public interest groups championed financial disclosure laws as a way to hold government accountable. See Common Cause. 1976. *Serving Two Masters: A Common Cause Study of Conflicts of Interest in the Executive Branch.* Washington D.C. Prior to laws requiring *public* disclosure, there was no way to insure government officials complied with disclosure requirements. In the report listed above, Common Cause marshaled evidence that the laws were not well enforced.

[33]Some corporate law scholars say this power of courts is insufficient and that the law should be changed to prohibit corporate self-dealing with limited exceptions which would be individually reviewed by the SEC. Clark, Robert Charles. 1986. *Corporate Law.* Boston: Little, Brown.

[34]Lawyers often speak of disclosure as *curing* a conflict of interest. This is merely a manner of speaking.

[35]*Model Rules of Professional Conduct.* 1983. Chicago: American Bar Association. Rules 1.7 (b), 1.13 (e), 1.9 (a), 2.2.

Code of Professional Responsibility. 1969. Chicago: American Bar Association. D.R. 5-105 (C).

Model Rules of Professional Conduct. 1983. Rules 1.7 (b), 1.13 (e), 1.9 (a), 2.2.

Wolfram, Charles W. 1986. *Modern Legal Ethics.* St. Paul: West Publishing. p. 345.

[36]Wolfram, Charles W. 1986. *Modern Legal Ethics.*

[37]Freedman, Monroe H. 1990. *Understanding Lawyers' Ethics.* New York: Matthew Bender.

Freedman, Monroe H. 1975. *Lawyers' Ethics in an Adversary System.* Indianapolis: Bobbs-Merrill.

Curtis, C. 1951. "The Ethics of Advocacy." *Stanford Law Review* 4 (December):3-23.

[38]*Code of Professional Responsibility.* 1969. D.R. 5-105 (D).

Model Rules of Professional Responsibility. 1983. Rule 1.10.

Wolfram, Charles W. 1986. *Modern Legal Ethics.* p.329.

[39]To avoid legal malpractice, experts advise lawyers to set up a conflict-of-interest screening system within their firms. Mallen, Ronald, and Jeffrey Smith. 1989. *Legal Malpractice* (3rd ed.). St. Paul: West Publishing. Section 2.5.

[40]45 CFR 46.

[41]Congress held hearings on conflicts of interest in research in 1988 and on September 15, 1989, the National Institutes of Health and the Alcohol, Drug Abuse and Mental Health Administration proposed conflict-of-interest guidelines for institutions receiving funds for biomedical or behavioral research. However, these were later withdrawn. Louis Sullivan, the Secretary of the Department of Health and Human Services, stated that he would issue regulations.

Subcommittee on Human Resources and Intergovernmental Relations of The House Committee on Government Operations. 100th Congress, 2nd Session. *Hearing: Federal Response to Misconduct in Science: Are Conflicts of Interest Hazardous to our Health?* Washington, D.C.: U.S. Government Printing Office. Sept. 29, 1988.

Request for comment on proposed guidelines for policies on conflict of interest developed by the National Institutes of Health and the Alcohol, Drug Abuse, and Mental Health Administration. NIH guide for grants and contracts. 1989. 18(32):1-5 (September 15).

[42]Reppert, Barton. 1992. "NIH Conflict-of-Interest Regs Impending." *The Scientist* 6(20):1,8.

[43]The Veteran's Administration Inspector General's investigation of Smith Kline & French and the PHARMCO project produced multiple reports which are available under the Freedom of Information Act.

The Senate also held hearings. See Subcommittee on Hospitals and Health Care, of the Committee on Veteran's Affairs, House of Representatives, 99th Congress, 1st Session, *Hearings: Possible Fraudulent Actions by VA Employees Involved in Drug Procurement or Research.*. Washington, D.C.: U.S. Government Printing Office. October 17, 1985. Serial No. 99-36.

The Veteran's Administration and Senate investigations were reported in the newspaper *U.S. Medicine* by Nancy Tomich, Terry Hemison and their colleagues. Relevant articles appeared in 1985 on August 15 (pp. 1, 15), September 1 (pp. 1, 14-15), September 15 (pp. 1, 8-9), October 1 (pp. 1, 10, 180), November 1 (pp. 1, 18), November 15 (pp. 1, 20-21), December 1 (pp. 1, 7), December 15 (pp. 1, 10-11), in 1986 in February (p. 3), in April (pp. 3, 27), November (pp. 3, 24, 25), December (pp. 1, 8, 9), and in 1987 on October 1 (pp. 1, 29-31).

[44]*Possible Fraudulent Actions by VA Employees Involved in Drug Procurement or Research.* 1985. Testimony of Mr. Audley Hendricks, Assistant General Counsel, Veteran's Administration. p. 20 .

[45]Sugarman, Jeremy and Madison Powers. 1991. "How the Doctor Got Gagged." *Journal of the American Medical Association* 266(23):3323-27.

Mariner, Wendy. 1992. "Mum's the Word: The Supreme Court and Family Planning." *American Journal of Public Health* 82(2):296-301.

[46]Field, Mark. 1953. "Structured Strain in the Role of the Soviet Physician." *American Journal of Sociology* 58(5):493-502.

[47]Walsh, Diana Chapman. 1988. *Corporate Physicians.* New Haven: Yale University Press.

Walsh, Diana Chapman. 1986. "Divided Loyalties in Medicine: the Ambivalence of Occupational Medical Practice." *Social Science and Medicine* 23(8): 789-96.

[48]Of course, the strength of the physicians' characters and their own moral sensibilities will affect how they respond to conflicts of interest. But for purposes of this discussion I am not addressing this issue, since conflict of interest policy cannot affect this directly.

[49]There may be indirect harm. The physician with a financial tie may not investigate alternative labs that produce better quality service. If the physician's lab has a higher than average error rate in its analysis, this could cause misdiagnosis and result in harm to the patient's health.

[50]Kusserow, Richard P. 1989. *Financial Arrangements.*

[51]Their arguments often apply to physician dispensing and kickbacks as well.

[52]There is strong evidence that physicians with incentives to refer patients in-house do so. Bruce Hillman has shown that doctors who refer patients for radiation therapy in their own offices used imaging exams 4 to 4.5 times more often than physicians who referred patients to radiologists in independent facilities with which they had no financial affiliation. Such doctors also charge significantly more than independent radiologists. As a result, mean imaging charges per episode of care were between 4.4 and 7.5 times higher for doctors who performed imaging in their own offices. Hillman, Bruce J., Catherine A. Joseph, Michael R. Mabry, Jonathan H. Sunshine, Stephen Kennedy, and Monica Noether. 1990. "Frequency and Costs of Diagnostic Imaging in Office Practice—A Comparison of Self-Referring and Radiologist-Referring Physicians." *The New England Journal of Medicine* 323(23):1604-1608.

In another study Hillman found that physicians who own imaging equipment use diagnostic imaging to evaluate their patients between 1.7 and 7.7 times more frequently than doctors who refer their patients to radiologists and they charged more per unit of service as well. Hillman, Bruce J., George T. Olson, Patricia E. Griffith, Jonathan H. Sunshine, Catherine A. Joseph, Stephen D. Kennedy, et al. 1992. "Physicians' Utilization and Changes for Outpatient Diagnostic Imaging in a Medicare Population." *Journal of the American Medical Association* 268(15):2050-2054.

[53]Fee-for-service practice can be construed as part of self-referral broadly defined. Despite its limitations, fee-for-service is still considered desirable by many individuals because of the flexibility and choice it provides patients. Rather than prohibit fee-for-service practice altogether, it is better to regulate it and encourage other forms of payment that avoid self-referral conflicts.

[54]In certain exceptional situations, volume may be a good index of quality and could be used as a quality measure. For example, tissue committees in hospitals can gauge poor practice by whether a surgeon removes an abnormally high rate of tissue. But, most likely this volume measure will be part of a more comprehensive assessment. My objection is not to the use of volume measures in general, but to volume measures for services when volume is not established as an adequate measure of quality.

For a first-rate discussion of trade-offs between incentives and rules see, Hillman, Alan L. 1991. "Managing the Physician: Rules Versus Incentives." *Health Affairs*10(4); 138–146.

For the views of some proponents of financial incentives see, Frankford, David M. 1989. "Creating and Dividing the Fruits of Collective Economic Activity." *Columbia Law Review* 89(8):1861–1938.

Havighurst, Clark C. 1988. *Health Care Law and Policy: Readings, Notes and Questions*. Westbury: Foundation Press.

[55]It is probably not possible to devise a completely neutral payment system that neither encourages nor discourages providing services. But the ideal is worth striving for, and many payment systems have less distorting effects than fee-for-service or the seven practices we have discussed.

[56]Physicians paid on a per capita basis are at risk for their own time, and time, for many physicians, is money. Under capitation payment, doctors do not increase their income by spending more time with a patient, so this might lead them to shorten visits, especially if no limits were placed on the number of patients allowable in their practice. Physicians could then increase their income by building a larger practice, spending less time on each patient, and requiring long waits for patients to obtain appointments.

If physicians serve a population with more severe medical problems than average, it may also be appropriate to limit the amount of risk that primary care physicians bear. For example, if a primary care doctor served a particularly unhealthy patient pool that required the doctor to spend significantly more time with them than usual, then provisions should compensate physicians for this extra effort by paying a higher capitation fee and limiting the size of the practice. The same approach could be used for patients with chronic, catastrophic, or unusually costly illness.

[57]The average physician salary in 1990 was $155,000. Suppose this were the base line for a physician in an HMO with a risk-sharing plan that could increase or decrease his pay by 2%. Then the physician could increase or decrease his income by $3100.00 Thus his income would be between $151,900 and $158,100. By sharing risk and making financially driven choices, he could affect his income by $6,200.

[58]Harvard Medical Practice Study Group. 1990. *Patients, Doctors, and Lawyers: Medical Injury, Malpractice Litigation, and Patient Compensation in New York.*

[59]*Moore v. Regents of University of California*, 51 Cal. 3rd 120, 793 P. 2d 479, 271 Cal. Reptr. 147 (1990).

[60]Morreim, E. Haavi. 1990. "Physician Investment and Self-Referral: A Philosophical Analysis of a Contentious Debate." *Journal of Medicine and Philosophy* 15(4):425-448.

[61]A variation on this theme is for courts to shift the burden of proof under the legal doctrine of *res ipsa loquitur*. In civil cases plaintiffs typically have the burden of proving their case. But courts sometimes shift the burden. If such a rule were used, the defendant, i.e., the doctor, would have to prove that they were not responsible for a bad outcome. Shifting the burden of proof would be an

approach midway between the traditional negligence standard and strict liability.

[62]Brinkley, Joel. 1986. "State Medical Boards Discipline Record Number of Doctors in 1985." *The New York Times* (November 9):1,26.

Reaves, Randolph P. 1984. *The Law of Professional Licensing and Certification.* Charlotte: Publications For Professionals.

Morris, William O. 1984. *Revocation of Professional Licenses by Governmental Agencies.* Charlottesville: The Michie Company.

Schware v. Board of Bar Examiners, 353 U.S. 232. (1957).

[63]Fox, Daniel M. and Daniel C. Schaffer. 1991. "Tax Administration as Health Policy: Hospitals, the Internal Revenue Service, and the Courts." *Journal of Health Politics, Policy and Law* 16(2):251-279.

Fox, Daniel M. and Daniel C. Schaffer. 1987. "Tax Policy as Social Policy: Cafeteria Plans: 1978-1985." *Journal of Health Politics, Policy and Law* 12(4):609-64.

[64]In the summer of 1992 two proposals for health care financing reform proposed by Democratic party presidential candidate Bill Clinton and Senate Majority Leader George Mitchell included provisions that would have a federal agency or quasi-governmental board establish pay rates for hospitals and doctors. Although not proposed, such an agency could also be given authority to address physicians' conflicts of interests. For a discussion of the proposals see McIllrath, Sharon. 1992. "Dems' Reform Bills Bump into Each Other." *American Medical News* (July 20):1,32-33.

[65]H.R. 4464, Introduced May 1990. The bill would have required that the Secretary of the Department of Health and Human Services develop a mechanism to certify physicians unless the medical profession developed its own recertification programs for each specialty. Although many medical specialties already have some sort of recertification program, the bill was opposed by many medical groups and not enacted. But Representative Stark , reportedly, plans to link the issue to any proposals for malpractice reform legislation.

[66]This approach might also be used for nursing homes and other institutional providers.

[67]The results of the Columbus Surgical Society auditing program are discussed in Chapter 2.

[68]The federal government has used this approach for assessing the impact of policies and projects on the environment. First proposed in 1966, environmental impact assessment became written into law in the National Environmental Policy Act passed in 1969. It has been a standard feature of government since then and emulated by legislation in many countries.

See Caldwell, Lynton K. 1966. "Problems of Applied Ecology: Perceptions, Institutions, Methods, and Operational Tools." *BioScience* 16(8):524-527.

Hearings Before the Committee on Interior and Insular Affairs, United States Senate, 91st Congress, 1st Session, on S. 1075, S. 237 and S. 1752, April 16, 1969. Testimony of Lynton Caldwell, p. 116.

National Environmental Policy Act, 42 U.S.C. Section 4332.

[69]Stone, Deborah. A. 1988. *Policy Paradox and Political Reason*. Glenview: Scott, Foresman/Little Brown College Division. "Inducements." pp. 212-230.

[70]Cousins, Norman. 1979. *Anatomy of An Illness: As Perceived by a Patient*. New York: W. W. Norton.

Benson, Herbert and Mark D. Epstein. 1975. "The Placebo Effect: A Neglected Asset in the Care of Patients." *Journal of the American Medical Association* 232(12):1225-7.

Shapiro, A.K. 1961. "Factors Contributing to the Placebo Effect." *American Journal of Psychotherapy* 18(1):73-88.

Beecher, H.K. 1956. "Evidence for Increased Effectiveness of Placebos with Increased Stress." *American Journal of Physiology* 187(1):163-9.

Lasagna, L. 1956. "Placebos." *Scientific American* 193(2):68-71.

Beecher, H.K. 1955. "The Powerful Placebo." *Journal of the American Medical Association*. 159(17):1602-1606.

Wolf, S. 1954. "Effects of Placebo Administration and Occurrence of Toxic Reactions." *Journal of the American Medical Association* 155(4):339-341.

[71]For a discussion of how a public spirited motivation can affect policy-making see, Kelman, Steven. 1987. *Making Public Policy: A Hopeful View of American Government*. New York: Basic Books.

[72]The economist Kenneth Arrow has argued that professional codes can promote efficiency and proper conduct in cases of market failure. See Arrow, Kenneth J. 1973. "Social Responsibility and Economic Efficiency." *Public Policy* 16(2):303-17.

[73]*Canterbury v. Spense* 464 F. 2d 772 (D.C. Cir.1972). *Cobbs v. Grant*, 502 P. 2d 1 (Cal. 1972).

[74]Courts have developed disclosure requirements over many years. However, a major transformation occurred in the 1970s in a series of cases. These cases marked a major legalization of the patient-physician relationship.

[75]There would still be room for the medical profession and individual physicians to develop their own ethical perspectives within the context of conflict-of-interest law, just as they have for informed consent.

[76]Lawrence M. Friedman also uses the term "legalizing" to describe the process by which law brings increasing numbers of issues into court and spreads its influence to places it has not penetrated before. Friedman, Lawrence M. 1984. *American Law: An Introduction*. New York: W. W. Norton. p. 78.

[77]Todd, James S. 1992. "Must the Law Assure Ethical Behavior?" *Journal of the American Medical Association* 268(1):98.

[78]de Tocqueville, Alexis. 1969. *Democracy in America*, J.P. Mayer, ed. (George Lawrence, trans.) New York: Doubleday. p. 270. (Originally published 1835.)

The actual quote uses the word *political*. But de Tocqueville uses the word "political" in an expanded sense to refer to the whole range of social and political matters.

[79]347 U.S. 483 (1954).

[80]The Boston Women's Health Book Collective. *The New Our Bodies Ourselves*. 1984.

Scotch, Richard K. 1984. *From Good Will to Civil Rights: Transforming Federal Disability Policy*. Philadelphia: Temple University Press.

DeJong, Gerban. 1979. "Independent Living: From Social Movement to Analytic Paradigm." *Archives of Physical Medicine and Rehabilitation* 60(10): 435-436.

[81]Malone, Thomas W. and Barbara Paul. 1991. "The Consumer Movement."

Appendix A

[1]For thoughtful discussions of the concept of conflict of interest, see, Knight, Frank H. 1961. "Some Comments on the Assumption Underlying the Conflict-of-Interest Concept." *University of Chicago Law School Conference on Conflict of Interest*. Conference Series No. 17. pp. 92-98.

Schotland, Roy A. 1980. "Introduction," in *Abuse on Wall Street: Conflicts of Interest in the Securities Markets*. Report to Twentieth Century Fund Steering Committee on Conflicts of Interest in the Securities Markets. Westport: Quorum Books.

[2]Hohfeld, Wesley Newcomb. 1978. *Fundamental Legal Conceptions*. Westport: Greenwood Press.

[3]One exception is Michael Davis who has advocated using the lawyers' Code of Professional Responsibility as a model for conflicts of interest of other professionals. Davis, Michael. 1982. "Conflict of Interest." *Business & Professional Ethics Journal* 1(4):17-27.

[4]Margolis, Joseph. 1979. "Conflict of Interest and Conflicting Interests," in *Ethical Theory and Business*, Tom L. Beauchamp and Norman E. Bowie, eds. Englewood Cliffs: Prentice-Hall. pp. 361-372.

[5]Macklin, Ruth. 1983. "Conflicts of Interest," in *Ethical Theory and Business*, Tom L. Beauchamp and Norman E. Bowie, eds. Englewood Cliffs: Prentice-Hall. pp. 240-246. In an unpublished paper from which this article was excerpted, Macklin includes another interest: "interests deriving from professional roles or group membership."

The first of Macklin's interests (the actor's personal interests) is equivalent to personal interests. Macklin's second interest (interests of the actor's organization) is an example of divided loyalties, as are interests deriving from professional roles or group membership, which she identifies in her unpublished paper. Macklin's third interest (society's or the public's interests) is an examples of general moral conflict and therefore much broader than what I define as conflict of interest.

[6]McGuire says a conflict of interest exists "when a subsystem attempts deliberately to enhance its own interests or those of an alien system to the detriment of a larger system of which it is part." McGuire, Joseph M. 1978. "Conflicts of Interest: Whose Interest? and What Conflict?" in *Ethics, Free Enterprise, and Public Policy: Original Essays on Moral Issues in Business*, Richard T. DeGeorge and Joseph A. Pichler, eds. New York: Oxford University Press. pp. 215-231 at 216.

[7]There is a literature that has developed around hospital institutional review boards which monitor research. The classical work in this field is Levine, Robert J. 1986. *Ethics and the Regulation of Clinical Research* (Second Edition). Urban & Schwarzenberg: Baltimore-Munich.

There is also the journal *IRB: A Review of Human Subjects Research*. Although the ethics of human experimentation is premised on concern that physicians may act in ways that are contrary to the interests of their patients, the particular issues discussed are rarely conceptualized in terms of conflicts of interest.

[8]Francis Miller focuses on the potential for secondary income from recommended treatments. Miller, Frances H. 1983. "Secondary Income from Recommended Treatment: Should Fiduciary Principles Constrain Physician Behavior?" In *The New Health Care for Profit: Doctors and Hospitals in a Competitive Environment*, B. Gray, ed. Washington, D.C.: National Academy Press. pp. 153-170.

[9]Relman, Arnold S. 1987. "Doctors and the Dispensing of Drugs." *The New England Journal of Medicine* 317(5):311-12.

[10]Arnold Relman is an exponent of this view. See Relman, Arnold S. 1983. "The Future of Medical Practice." *Health Affairs* 5-19.

Relman, Arnold S. 1985. "Cost Control, Doctor's Ethics, and Patient Care." *Issues in Science and Technology* (Winter):103-111; Relman, Arnold S. 1987. "Doctors and the Dispensing of Drugs." *The New England Journal of Medicine* 317(5):311-12.

Relman, Arnold S. 1980. "The New Medical-Industrial Complex." *The New England Journal of Medicine* 303(17):963-970; Relman, Arnold S., and Uwe Reinhardt. 1986. "An Exchange on For-Profit Health Care" in *For-Profit Enterprise in Health Care*, B.H. Gray, ed. Washington, D.C.: National Academy Press. pp. 209-23.

Relman, Arnold S. 1985. "Economic Considerations in Emergency Care: What Are Hospitals For?" *The New England Journal of Medicine* 312(6):372-3.

Relman, Arnold S. 1981. "Faculty-Practice Plans." *The New England Journal of Medicine* 304(5):292-3.

Relman, Arnold S. 1985. "Editorial: Dealing With Conflicts of Interest." *The New England Journal Of Medicine* 313(12):749-751.

Relman, Arnold S. 1988. "Salaried Physicians and Economic Incentives." *The New England Journal of Medicine* 319(12):784.

Relman, Arnold S. 1987. "Practicing Medicine in The New Business Climate." *The New England Journal of Medicine* 316(18):1150-51.

See, also, Veatch, Robert M. 1983. "Ethical Dilemmas of For-Profit Enterprise in Health Care" in *The New Health Care for Profit: Doctors and Hospitals in a Competitive Environment*,   B. Gray, ed., Washington, D.C.: National Academy Press. pp. 140-141.

[11]See, Berenson, Robert A. 1986. "Capitation and Conflict of Interest." *Health Affairs* 5(1):141-146.

Berenson, Robert A. 1987. "Hidden Compromises in Paying Physicians." *Business and Health* (July): 18-19, 22.

Stone, Alan A. 1985. "Sounding Board, Law's Influence on Medicine and Medical Ethics." *The New England Journal of Medicine* 312(5):309-12.

For a contrary view, see Begley, Charles E. 1987. "Prospective Payment and Medical Ethics." *Journal of Medicine and Philosophy* 12(2):107-22.

[12]Capron, Alexander M. 1986. "Containing Health Care Costs: Ethical and Legal Implications of Changes in the Methods of Paying Physicians."*Case Western Reserve Law Review* 36(4):708-59. See especially p. 748.

[13]Morreim, E. Haavi. 1985. "The MD and the DRG." *Hastings Center Report*, (June): 30-38.

Morreim, E. Haavi. 1985. "Cost Containment: Issues of Moral Conflict and Justice for Physicians." *Theoretical Medicine* 6(3):257-79.

[14]See for example, Boyle, J.F. 1984. "Should We Learn to Say No?" *Journal of the American Medical Association* 252(6):782-784.

Angell, Marcia. 1987. "Medicine: The Endangered Patient-Centered Ethic." *Hastings Center Report* 17(1):S12-S13.

Furrow, Barry R. 1988. "The Ethics of Cost Containment: Bureaucratic Medicine and the Doctor as Patient-Advocate." *Notre Dame Journal of Law, Ethics and Public Policy* 3(2):187-225.

[15]McGuire, Joseph M. 1978.

[16]Margolis, Joseph. 1979.

[17]Macklin distinguishes between: (1) personal interests of the agent; (2) interests belonging to one's organization or institution; and (3) interests pertaining to society as a whole: the public interest. Macklin, Ruth. 1983.

[18]Davis suggests that the professional's role defines his or her obligations to clients. His formulation of conflict of interest is similar to mine: namely a conflict of interest exists whenever there is a reasonable probability that the professional's independent judgment will be adversely affected. Davis, Michael. 1982.

[19]Bowie, Norman E. 1986. "Accountants, Full Disclosure, and Conflicts of Interest." *Business & Professional Ethics Journal.* 5(3 & 4): 60-73.

[20]Bowie, Norman E. 1982. "'Role' As A Moral Concept In Health Care." *Journal of Medicine and Philosophy.* 7(1): 56-63.

[21]Margolis states that "the concept of conflict of interest in business and professional ethics is singularly ignored and analysis of the concept breaks new ground." Margolis, Joseph. 1979. p. 361. Davis agrees that the concept is not discussed much in the philosophic literature although it is well-developed in lawyer's professional codes. Davis, Michael. 1982. p. 17. Macklin also notes that "there is not very much in the way of systematic writing on moral problems of conflicts of interest." Macklin, Ruth. 1983. p. 241.

Appendix B

[1]For a discussion of conflicting roles, see Field, Mark. 1953. "Structured Strain in the Role of the Soviet Physician."*American Journal of Sociology* 58(5):493-502.

Levinsky, Norman G. 1984. "The Doctor's Master." *The New England Journal of Medicine* 311(24):1573-1575.

Toulmin, Stephen. 1986. "Divided Loyalties and Ambiguous Relationships." *Social Science and Medicine* 23(8):783-787.

[2]It is also possible that as a result of pursuing these other roles, physicians can, and often do, have either direct or indirect financial interests that prompt them to act in ways that are inconsistent with the interests of a particular patient.

[3]Levine, Robert J. 1985. "The Physician-Researcher: Role Conflicts," in *Alzheimer's Dementia: Dilemmas in Clinical Research.* V. L. Melnick and N. N. Dubler, eds. Clifton, N.J.: Humana Press. pp. 41-50.

[4]Szasz, Thomas Stephen. 1963. *Law, Liberty and Psychiatry: An Inquiry into the Social Uses of Mental Health Practices.* New York: Macmillan.

[5]*Tarasoff v. Regents of the University of California,* 17 Cal.3d, 425 (1976). In order to preserve his patient's confidences, a psychiatrist did not reveal the patient's intent to kill a named individual. The patient did murder the individual, and the deceased person's family brought suit. The California Supreme Court held that a psychiatrist has a duty to warn an individual known to be at risk of imminent harm and stated that this duty overrides the patient's right to confidentiality.

[6]Many states have statutes requiring that physicians report certain sexually transmitted diseases.

[7] AMA, Council on Ethical and Judicial Affairs. 1988. "Ethical Issues Involved in the Growing AIDS Crisis." *Journal of the American Medical Association* 259(9): 1360-1361.

But see *Doe v. Health/Kansas City, Inc.* C.A. No. 88C-5149 (Judge Marion W. Chipman), October 17, 1988, District Court, Johnson City, Kansas. In this case, the court enjoined physicians in an HMO from notifying a man's former wife of his HIV status.

[8] Daniels, Norman. 1986. "Why Saying No to Patients in the United States Is so Hard: (Cost Containment, Justice, and Provider Autonomy)." *The New England Journal of Medicine* 314(21):1381-1383.

Leaf, Alexander. 1984. "The Doctor's Dilemma—and Society's Too." *The New England Journal of Medicine* 310(11):718-721.

[9] Reagan, Michael D. 1987. "Physicians as Gatekeepers." *The New England Journal of Medicine* 317(27):1731-1734.

Somers, Anne R. 1983. "And Who Shall Be the Gate Keeper? The Role of the Primary Physician in the Health Care Delivery System." *Inquiry* 20:301.

Stone, Deborah A. 1979. "Physicians as Gatekeepers: Illness Certification as a Rationing Device." *Public Policy* 27(2):227-254.

[10] Winslow, G. R. 1982. *Triage and Justice.* Berkeley: University of California Press.

[11] Zawacki, Bruce E. 1985. "ICU Physician's Ethical Role in Distributing Scarce Resources." *Critical Care Medicine* 13(1):57-60.

[12] Walsh, Diana Chapman. 1988. *Corporate Physicians.* New Haven: Yale Uni-versity Press.

Walsh, Diana Chapman. 1986. "Divided Loyalties in Medicine: The Ambi-valence of Occupational Medical Practice." *Social Science and Medicine* 23(8): 789-796.

[13] Howe, Edmund G. 1986. "Ethical Issues Regarding Mixed Agency of Military Physicians." *Social Science and Medicine* 23(8):803-815.

Daniels, Arlene K. 1972. "Military Psychiatry: The Emergence of a Sub-specialty," in *Medical Men and Their Work,* Eliot Friedson and Judith Lorber, eds. Chicago: Aldine.

[14] Murray, Thomas H. 1984. "Divided Loyalties in Sports Medicine." *The Physician and Sports Medicine* 12(8):134-140.

[15] The Uniform Anatomical Gift Act, 8 U.L.A. 15 (1968), adopted by 50 states and the District of Columbia, establishes procedures for organ donation.

Martyn, Susan, Richard Wright, Leo Clark, and Arthur Caplan. 1988. "Required Request for Organ Donation: Moral, Clinical, and Legal Problems." *The Hastings Center Report* 18(2):27-34.

Appendix C

[1]There is a dearth of literature on the history of bioethics. The most comprehensive account is by Rothman. See Rothman, David J. 1991. *Strangers at the Bedside: A History of How Law and Bioethics Transformed Medical Decision-making*. New York: Basic Books;

Rothman, David J. 1990. "Human Experimentation and the Origins of Bioethics in the United States," in *Social Science Perspectives on Medical Ethics*, George Weisz, ed. Dordrecht: Kluwer Academic Publishers. pp. 185-200.

In recounting the history, I have drawn on his work, as well as a review of the bioethics literature. A few articles were particularly helpful.

Callahan, Daniel. 1980. "Shattuck Lecture—Contemporary Biomedical Ethics." *The New England Journal of Medicine* 302(22):1228-1233.

Callahan, Daniel. 1988. "The Waning of Old Ethical Models," in *Bioethics Today: A New Ethical Vision*, James E. Walters, ed. Loma Linda: Loma Linda University Press. pp. 1-12.

Childress, James F. 1989. "Introduction to the Legal System and Bioethics." *Biolaw* R1-R15.

Clouser, K. Danner. 1978. "Bioethics," in *Encyclopedia of Bioethics*, Warren T. Reich, ed. London: Macmillan & Free Press. pp. 115-127.

Clouser, K. Danner. 1980. *Teaching Biothics: Strategies, Problems and Resources*. Hastings on Hudson: Hastings Center.

Fox, Renee C. 1990. "The Evolution of American Bioethics: A Sociological Perspective," in *Social Science Perspectives on Medical Ethics*, George Weisz, ed. Dordrecht: Kluwer Academic Publishers. pp. 201-217.

Fox, Renee C., and Judith P. Swazey. 1984. "Medical Morality Is not Bioethics—Medical Ethics in China and the United States." *Perspectives in Biology and Medicine* 27(3):336-360.

Gorovitz, Samuel. 1986. "Baiting Bioethics." *Ethics* 96(2):356-374.

Toulmin, Stephen. 1988. "Medical Ethics in Its American Context: An Historical Survey," *Annals of the New York Academy of Sciences* (Biomedical Ethics: An Anglo American Dialogue) 530:7-15.

[2]Fox, Daniel M. 1979. "The Segregation of Medical Ethics: A Problem in Modern Intellectual History." *The Journal of Medicine and Philosophy* 4(1):81-97.

[3]Karl Menninger quoted by Joseph Fletcher in the forward to his book. Fletcher, Joseph F. 1954. *Morals and Medicine: The Moral Problems of the Patient's Right to Know the Truth, Contraception, Artificial Insemination, Sterilization, Euthanasia*. Princeton: Princeton University Press. pp. viii-ix.

[4]45 C.F.R. 46.

[5]See, e.g., Engelhardt, H. Tristram, Jr. 1986. *The Foundations of Biomedical Ethics*. New York: Oxford University Press. p. 7.

⁶Engelhardt, H. Tristram, Jr. 1986.

Veatch, Robert M. 1981. *A Theory of Medical Ethics*. New York: Basic Books.

Beauchamp, Tom L., and James P. Childress. 1979. *Principles of Biomedical Ethics*. New York: Oxford University Press.

⁷Toulmin, Stephen. 1988. "Medical Ethics."

⁸Walker, Robert M., Laura Weiss Lane, and Mark Siegler. 1989. "Development of a Teaching Program in Clinical Medical Ethics at the University of Chicago." *Academic Medicine: Journal of the Association of American Medical Colleges* 64(12):1.

⁹Toulmin, Stephen. "How Medicine Saved the Life of Ethics." *Perspectives in Biology and Medicine* 25(4):736-750.

¹⁰Callahan, Daniel. 1988. "Waning of Old Ethical Models."

¹¹Brennan, Troyen A. 1991. *Just Doctoring: Medical Ethics in the Liberal State*. Berkeley: University of California Press.

Emanuel, Ezekiel J. 1991. *The Ends of Human Life: Medical Ethics in a Liberal Polity*. Cambridge: Harvard University Press.

¹²Lilla, Mark. 1981. "Ethos, 'Ethics' and Public Service."*The Public Interest* 63:3-18.

¹³A recent edition of *Academic Medicine* is devoted to teaching medical ethics. The journal includes a survey of the literature and articles on different programs. *Academic Medicine: Journal of the Association of American Medical Colleges*. 1989. "Special Issue: Teaching Medical Ethics." 64(12).

Some other relevant articles include the following:

Frader, Joel, Robert Arnold, John Coulehan, et al. 1989. "Evolution of Clinical Ethics Teaching at the University of Pittsburgh."*Academic Medicine* 64(12):747-750.

Perkins, Henry S. 1989. "Teaching Medical Ethics During Residency." *Academic Medicine* 64(12):263-266.

Puckett, Andrew C., Dole G. Graham, Lois A. Pounds, et al. 1989. "The Duke University Program for Integrating Ethics and Human Values into Medical Education." *Academic Medicine* 64(12):231-235.

Bickel, Janet. 1987. "Human Values Teaching Programs in the Clinical Education of Medical Students." *Academic Medicine* 62:369-378.

Veatch, Robert M. 1987. "Medical Ethics Education," in *Encyclopedia of Bio-Ethics*, Warren T. Reich, ed. London: Free Press.

Culver, Charles M., K. Danner Clouser, Bernard Gert, et al. 1985. "Basic Curricular Goals in Medical Ethics."*The New England Journal of Medicine* 312(4):253-256.

¹⁴The Association of American Medical Colleges in consultation with the Society for Health and Human values has suggested guidelines for medical ethics programs. Thomasma, David C. 1982. "Report of Group II on the Future of Medical Humanities Programs," in *The Humanities and Human Values in Medical Schools: A Ten-year Overview*, E. D. Pellegrino and T. K. McElhinney, eds. Washington, D.C.: Institute on Human Values in Medicine of the Society for

Health and Human Values. pp. 66-79. But a recent survey of medical ethics teaching in medical schools shows variations in the approach and content of programs. See *Academic Medicine*. 1989. "Special Issue: Teaching Medical Ethics."

[15]I list topics that appear most frequently and are more central. A comprehensive list of the content of the medical education included in a survey article in *Academic Medicine* follows. While the list indicates that "economic incentives" is a topic, the articles cited either focus on cost containment or do not indicate that the ethics of incentives get more than a passing reference in the program. See Miles, Steven H., Laura Weiss Lane, Janet Bickel, et al. 1989. *Academic Medicine: Journal of the Association of American Medical Colleges* 64(12):705-714.

Ethical Theory and Humanities
    Basic bioethical concepts
    Religious theory and medicine
    Humanities
    Professional Ethos
    Codes of ethics in medicine
    Physician bias about patient's quality of life
    Duty to treat HIV-infected persons
    Compassion
    Rights and duties of doctors
    Determination of death
    Pain control
    Organ donation, requests, selecting recipients
    Innovative technology
    Physicians and cost constraints or economic incentives
Multidisciplinary Issues
    Impaired colleagues
    Consultation and team ethics
    Differences with colleagues
    Relations with lawyers, nurses, and reporting agencies
    Use of ethics consultants and committees
Patient Autonomy and Clinical Dilemmas
    Autonomy and personhood
    How patients relate to risk values
    Obtaining consent
    Patients' refusal of recommended treatments
    Truth telling and withholding information from patients
    Patient privacy and confidentiality
    Evaluation of decision-making capacity
    Proxy consent, informed consent, coerced consent
    Roles of families in treatment decisions

Sexual responsibility
Abortion
Defective newborns
Maternal-fetal conflicts
Rights of children, psychiatric patients, and handicapped persons
Artificial insemination, in vitro fertilization
Care of the dying, comatose, or hopelessly ill
Foregoing life support
Euthanasia
Student Physicians
Academic integrity
Revealing student's health status to patients
Student's feelings of excess entitlement
Disclosure of new information to patients
Role of student physicians
Academic Medicine
Authorship
Research ethics
Social Issues
Preventive medicine; health and disease concepts
Justice and health care
Legal medicine, forensic medicine, malpractice
Nuclear war
Genetics
Community service

[16]For example, the University of California, San Francisco.

[17]Self, Donnie, J., Frederic D. Wolinsky, and DeWitt C. Baldwin. 1989. "The Effects of Teaching Medical Ethics on Medical Students' Moral Reasoning." *Academic Medicine* 64(12):755-759.

[18]For example, a recent issue of *Academic Medicine* that reviewed nine medical school teaching programs on medical ethics does not even mention conflicts of interest in passing. However, an article reviewing the literature on medical ethics education does indicate four articles that discuss physicians and cost constraints or economic incentives. See Miles, Steven H., Laura Weiss Lane, Janet Bickel, et al. 1989. "Medical Ethics Education; Coming of Age." *Academic Medicine* 64(12):705-714. But a reading of these articles reveals that they do not discuss conflicts of interest except in passing.

Appendix D

[1]In one case, a medical facility was structured as a limited partnership owned by 200 separate corporations, each of which had one physician shareholder. See State of Florida Health Care Cost Containment Board and Department of Economics and Department of Finance, Florida State University. 1991. *Joint Ventures Among Health Care Providers in Florida: Volume II.* State of Florida Health Care Cost Containment Board. Tallahassee, FL.

[2]State of Florida Health Care Cost Containment Board and Department of Economics and Department of Finance, Florida State University. 1991. *Joint Ventures Among Health Care Providers in Florida: Volume II.* State of Florida Health Care Cost Containment Board. Tallahassee, FL.

Acknowledgments

My principal indebtedness is to my fine colleagues at Brandeis University and Boston University who guided the study: Deborah A. Stone and Saul Touster, as well as Tamar Frankel, Leonard Glantz, and Irving K. Zola. They encouraged me to tackle an unconventional topic using an unusual approach. Each offered special insights and criticism, carefully read what I wrote, made very helpful suggestions, and spent considerable time discussing these issues with me.

Several colleagues in health policy at Brandeis University and Boston University in the Pew Health Policy program also provided valuable help. These include Stuart H. Altman, Margarete Arndt, Helen Batten, Egon Bittner, Stephen C. Crane, Richard Egdhal, Sol Levine, Jeffrey M. Prottas, Joseph D. Restuccia, Bruce Spitz, Stanley S. Wallack, and Diana C. Walsh

I also wish to thank my colleagues at Indiana University for their support: Deborah Freund, Eleanor D. Kinney, and David Smith, in particular, provided helpful comments on drafts. Dean A. James Barnes, Dean Charles Wise, and James Buher arranged for summer research support from the School of Public and Environmental Affairs. They also made sure I had the resources I needed to revise the study and produce camera-ready copy. A Research and University Graduate School grant from Indiana University provided funds for preparation of the index and help with proofreading.

Several people read the whole manuscript and provided helpful comments. These include George Annas, Troyen Brennan, Dan W. Brock, Allan E. Buchanan, Baruch Brody, Eliot Friedson, Daniel Fox, Mark Hall, Peter Hiam, Al Jonson, Martin Kessler, John D. Lantos, Frances Miller, Arnold S. Relman, Walter Wadlington, and several anonymous reviewers. Thanks also are due to my editor at Oxford University Press, Jeffrey W. House.

In addition, many other people commented on one or more chapters, educated me about issues in various fields, met with me to discuss issues bearing on conflict of interests, and helped me find documents and other information.

On the history of the conflicts of interest and the organized American medical professions' response I am grateful for help from Allan M. Brandt, Chester R. Burns, Paul Cleary, Jackson C. Coker, Daniel M. Fox, Albert R. Jonsen, Ted Marmor, David Rosner, David J. Rothman, and Rosemary Stevens. At the AMA, Betty Jane Anderson, Marguritte Fallucco, and David Orentlicher were helpful in illuminating current and past policy and providing access to documents. Maureen Conklin and Peter Van Schoonhoven at the Joint Commission on Accreditation of Health Care Institutions provided information on their policies.

On issues of biomedical ethics and other ethical issues, I learned much from Sissela Bok, Norman E. Bowie, Dan W. Brock, Allen E. Buchanan, Courtney S. Campbell, Daniel Callahan, James F. Childress, K. Danner Clouser, Norman Fost, Renee C. Fox, Albert R. Jonsen, Craig M. Lawson, John D. Lantos, Tom H. Murray, Ruth Purtilo, Stephen Toulmin, and Dennis F. Thompson.

Numerous physicians provided insights and help. Arnold S. Relman deserves thanks for his leadership in making physicians' conflicts of interest a respectable subject in medicine and health policy and encouraging others to pursue this as an area of scholarly research. Other physicians I consulted include William Andereck, Felix M. Balasco, Robert A. Berenson, David Blumenthal, Ron Bronow, Mary Margaret Chren, Kenneth V. Iseron, Richard Egdahl, Tom Hoban, David Hyman, Henry E. Jones, John D. Lantos, Nicole Lurie, Philip R. Lee, Joanne Lynn, Barry M. Manuel, Gordon McCloud, William F. McNary, Eugene C. Rich, David Schiedermayer, Benjamin Siegel, Lynn Soffer, John D. Stoeckle, Alan Stone, Susan W. Tolle, and Peyton E. Weary.

A number of knowledgeable practitioners working in health and public policy and other fields also provided insights. These include Tom Antoine at the National Association of Medical Equipment Suppliers; Jill Bernstein, Janet M. Corrigan, and Lauren B. LeRoy at the Physician Payment Review Commission; Joyce Bullock at the Council on Governmental Ethics Laws; Mark Briant, Randall W. Gott, and Charles Woeple at Jackson and Coker; Mark N. Cooper, Consumer Federation of America; Gary Edwards at the Ethics Resource Center; James L. Flore at Physicians Clinical Services, Ltd.; Marsha Gold at the Group Health Association of America; Brian Gordon and John Roberts at the MR

Cooperative; Lynn R. Gruber at Interstudy; Paul A. Gurney and Joan Stieber at the Public Citizen Health Research Group; Charles Harker at the American Physical Therapy Association; Ron Kovak at Technicore; Kathryn M. Langwell at the Congressional Budget Office; Linda B. Miller at the Volunteer Trustees of Non-Profit Hospitals; Janet G. Newport at FHP Health Care, Inc.; John M. Rector at the National Association of Retail Druggists; Neil Schlackman at U.S. HealthCare; John Steiner at the American Hospital Association; and Doug Wilson at the Controlled Risk Insurance Company and Joel Wittenberg, Wittenberg Investment Management.

In the Office of Representative Pete Stark, I received help from Stephen H. Bandeian, Dan McCormick, and Bill Vaughan. David S. Abernethy, professional staff member on the Committee on Ways and Means, Subcommittee on Health also provided continuing help. At the Department of Health and Human Services Inspector General's Office, I met attorneys and staff including Tom Crane, David Hsia, Barry Steely, Penny Thompson and Harvey Yampolski. At the Government Accounting Office, I spoke with Tom Dodwell.

A number of attorneys in practice provided insights. These include Richard Beckler, Richard S. Boskey, Robert S. Bromberg, Harold Corlew, Max Dean, Hope S. Foster, Marcy Kass, Marek L. Laas, Jane Ley, Howard Marderosian, Ronald J. Nessim, Randall E. Robbins, Alan M. Sandals, T.J. Sullivan, Ann Treimer, Helen R. Trilling, and Daniel Waugh. At the Office of Governmental Ethics, I spoke to Jack Covaleski and others.

Other legal scholars I consulted include Judith Areen, Charles H. Baron, Thomas F. Bergin, Troyen Brennan, Robert J. Condlin, Richard Daynard, Barry R. Furrow, Dwight Golan, Jeffrey Gordon, Peter D. Jacobson, Sylvia A. Law, John Leubsdorf, Maxwell J. Mehlman, Frances H. Miller, Edward P. Richards, Rand E. Rosenblatt, Joanne B. Stern, Walter J. Wadlington, Calvin Woodard, and Adam Yarmolinski.

Other scholars who were helpful include Gordon C.F. Bearn, Edward N. Beiser, Robert J. Blendon, Robert Cohen, Rashi Fein, Stan N. Finkelstein, Regina A. Herzlinger, Sheldon Krimsky, Jean Mitchell, E. Haavi Morreim, James E. Post, Harvey M. Sapolsky, Eve Spangler, Andrew Stark, Steven Thomas, and several anonymous reviewers.

Some journalists wrote stories that provided important leads. These include Joe Rosenblum of "Frontline" (WGBH TV); Dan Haney and Fred Bayles of the, Associated Press; and Walt Bogdanich and Mike Waldholtz of *The Wall Street Journal*.

Mark Hulbert provided a home and an office for me in Washington, D.C., during my several trips there, offered insightful comments on the project along the way, and reviewed a draft. Hilbert Fefferman, Vesta Kimble, Milly McLean, and Brian Thomas made editing suggestions on the research proposal. Molly McQuade provided exceptional editorial help. Margaret Willard copy-edited Chapter 2 for *The Milbank Quarterly*. Helen Greenberg copy-edited the manuscript for Oxford Press. Susan Baker also provided help with copy editing. Barbara Nagy and Nancy Feldman helped out with numerous issues at Brandeis.

Camera-ready copy was produced at the School of Public and Environmental Affairs, Indiana University. Rita Fortner organized support for typing the manuscript even before I arrived. Many people chipped in, but my secretary, Bobby Brooking, took the brunt of the burden and did a superb job with typing revisions of the manuscript cheerfully and quickly. Pam Solie also provided valuable typing assistance, and help with the Index. Frank Novak helped track down articles and prepare the index. Al Sohlstrom arranged for converting computer files and solved many other difficult computer problems. Cynthia Mahigian Moorhead did a superb job of turning the manuscript into camera-ready copy, quicker, better, and with more flexibility than any publisher could. Erin Cornish helped with proof-reading.

A fellowship from the Pew Charitable Trust lured me from private practice of law into health policy research at Brandeis University's Heller School. During the fellowship, I started the project. The federal government waived fees for several Freedom of Information requests at the Department of Health and Human Services, the Department of Justice, and the Department of Veterans Affairs. My family chipped in with income subsidies to complement income from my part-time employment, none of which was from groups that would remotely have a financial interest in the issues discussed. I received no other funding from any organization or individual and thus avoided even the appearance of conflicts of interest.

My family heard more about the project than makes for good dinner conversation. Lloyd, Victor, and Julie all commented on drafts. Wendy read it all several times and combined wisdom with proofreading and editorial advice. Nadine encouraged me and had faith in the project from the start.

Librarians at Brandeis and Boston universities, the Brandeis Institute for Health Policy, and the Kennedy Institute for Bioethics and Indiana University helped me with bibliographic work. I particularly wish to thank Judith Humphreys, Sylvia Pendleton, Patricia M. McCarrick, and Rhonda Thomas.

Some special teachers played more of a role than they suspect. Thanks are due to Charles Chatfield, Robin Cohen, Ernest Gelhorn, Dwight and Anna Heath, Robert Kaplan, Charles Merrill, Edward Ryerson, Arnold Weinstein, and Philip Quinn.

Thanks are no doubt also due to others whom I may have inadvertently failed to mention.

Permissions: Chapter two appeared in a slightly shortened and altered form in *The Milbank Quarterly* which holds the copyright. Rodwin, Marc A. 1992. "The Organized American Medical profession's Response to Financial Conflicts of Interest: 1890-1992."*Milbank Quarterly* 70(4):703-741. The discussion of disclosure in Chapter 8 is adapted from Rodwin, Marc A. 1992. "Conflicts of Interest: The Limitations of Disclosure," *The New England Journal of Medicine* 321:1406-1408.

Permission to reprint the Norman Rockwell illustrations "Doctor and Doll" and "Before the Shot" was granted by the Norman Rockwell Family Trust. Photographs of the print courtesy of the Norman Rockwell Museum at Stockbridge. The Daumier engraving is printed courtesy of Bibliothèque Nationale, Paris France. *Health Care Financial Management* granted permission to reprint its August 1990 cover. The cover design is by Jim Lienhart and the photograph by Michael Slaughter. The illustration on the January 15, 1990 cover of *Modern Health Care* is by Roger Schillestrom, reprinted with permission from Modern Health Care, copyright Crain Communications, Inc., 740 N. Rush Street, Chicago, Il 60611.

About the Author

Marc A. Rodwin has practiced law and worked as a consultant on health and environmental policy. He has taught in the Legal Studies Program at Brandeis University and the Community Health Program at Tufts University. Now Associate Professor of Public and Environmental Affairs, specializing in law and public policy at Indiana University's School of Public and Environmental Affairs, he lives in Bloomington, Indiana with his wife, Wendy Schoener, and their daughter, Nina Sophia.

His current research focuses on the relation between law, ethics, markets, and regulation. His degrees include a B.A. in analytical method and policy from Brown University; a B.A. and M.A. in philosophy, politics, and economics from Oxford University; a J.D. from the University of Virginia Law School; and a Ph.D. in social policy from the Brandeis University Heller School.

Index

Abbott Laboratories, 221
Adversary system, 180, 200, 208
Agent, 180, 183
Alexander, M., 179
Alexian Brothers Hospital, 72
Allied health professionals, 66
American Bar Association (ABA), 200, 202
American Clinical Laboratory Association, 127
American College of Nuclear Medicine, 127
American College of Physicians, 134
American College of Radiology, 127
American College of Surgeons (ACS), 20, 28-29, 32-35, 38, 40, 45, 51, 241, 266-267
American Health Care Management, 59
American Home Products Corporation, 60-61
American Hospital Association, 151
American Medical Association (AMA), 20, 257
  conflict-of-interest guidelines, 20, 41-45, 120, 213, 266-267
  fee-splitting, 20, 22-28, 30-37, 40, 51, 92
  gifts, 91-92, 108, 131-133
  House of Delegates, 21, 23, 27, 36, 45

Judicial Council/Council on Ethical and Judicial Affairs, 21-22, 25, 30-31, 33, 35, 39-41, 45
  organizational structure, 21
  physician ownership, 39
  principles and codes of ethics, 21-22, 26, 30, 33, 35-36, 40, 269-270
  risk-sharing, 43, 149
  self-referral, 13, 21, 39, 44-45, 51, 126
  survey on conflicts of interest, 42
  survey on fee-splitting, 24-25
  survey on state medical society discipline, 43
American Medical News, 133
American Pain and Stress, Inc., 71
American Psychiatric Association, 257
American Surgical Association, 134
Ancillary Medical Services, 16, 102
Annals of Internal Medicine, 108
Antitrust law, 33, 46, 78, 129-130
Aristotle, 212
Assistant surgeons, *See* 7, 16, 23, 7, 24, 37-38
Associated Press, 145
Austell Physical Therapy Center, 66
Av-Med, 157
Avorn, Jerry, 109

Bad-faith, breach of obligations, 234
Balasco, Felix, 62-63